Diseases of the Biliary Tract

Editor

J. BART ROSE

SURGICAL CLINICS
OF NORTH AMERICA

www.surgical.theclinics.com

Consulting Editor
RONALD F. MARTIN

April 2019 • Volume 99 • Number 2

ELSEVIER

1600 John F. Kennedy Boulevard • Suite 1800 • Philadelphia, Pennsylvania, 19103-2899

http://www.surgical.theclinics.com

SURGICAL CLINICS OF NORTH AMERICA Volume 99, Number 2

April 2019 ISSN 0039–6109, ISBN-13: 978-0-323-68249-7

Editor: John Vassallo, j.vassallo@elsevier.com

Developmental Editor: Meredith Madeira

Photocopying

Single photocopies of single articles may be made for personal use as allowed by national copyright laws. Permission of the Publisher and payment of a fee is required for all other photocopying, including multiple or systematic copying, copying for advertising or promotional purposes, resale, and all forms of document delivery. Special rates are available for educational institutions that wish to make photocopies for non-profit educational classroom use. For information on how to seek permission visit www.elsevier.com/permissions or call: (+44) 1865 843830 (UK)/(+1) 215 239 3804 (USA).

Derivative Works

Subscribers may reproduce tables of contents or prepare lists of articles including abstracts for internal circulation within their institutions. Permission of the Publisher is required for resale or distribution outside the institution. Permission of the Publisher is required for all other derivative works, including compilations and translations (please consult www.elsevier.com/permissions).

Electronic Storage or Usage

Permission of the Publisher is required to store or use electronically any material contained in this periodical, including any article or part of an article (please consult www.elsevier.com/permissions). Except as outlined above, no part of this publication may be reproduced, stored in a retrieval system or transmitted in any form or by any means, electronic, mechanical, photocopying, recording or otherwise, without prior written permission of the Publisher.

Notice

No responsibility is assumed by the Publisher for any injury and/or damage to persons or property as a matter of products liability, negligence or otherwise, or from any use or operation of any methods, products, instructions or ideas contained in the material herein. Because of rapid advances in the medical sciences, in particular, independent verification of diagnoses and drug dosages should be made.

Although all advertising material is expected to conform to ethical (medical) standards, inclusion in this publication does not constitute a guarantee or endorsement of the quality or value of such product or of the claims made of it by its manufacturer.

Surgical Clinics of North America (ISSN 0039–6109) is published bimonthly by Elsevier Inc., 360 Park Avenue South, New York, NY 10010-1710. Months of publication are February, April, June, August, October, and December. Business and Editorial Offices: 1600 John F. Kennedy Blvd., Suite 1800, Philadelphia, PA 19103-2899. Periodicals postage paid at New York, NY and additional mailing offices. Subscription prices are $417.00 per year for US individuals, $845.00 per year for US institutions, $100.00 per year for US students and residents, $507.00 per year for Canadian individuals, $1071.00 per year for Canadian institutions, $536.00 for international individuals, $1071.00 per year for international institutions and $250.00 per year for Canadian and foreign students/residents. To receive student/resident rate, orders must be accompanied by name of affiliated institution, date of term, and the *signature* of program/residency coordinator on institution letterhead. Orders will be billed at individual rate until proof of status is received. Foreign air speed delivery is included in all *Clinics* subscription prices. All prices are subject to change without notice. POSTMASTER: Send address changes to *Surgical Clinics*, Elsevier Health Sciences Division, Subscription Customer Service, 3251 Riverport Lane, Maryland Heights, MO 63043. **Customer Service (orders, claims, online, change of address): Telephone: 1-800-654-2452 (U.S. and Canada); 314-447-8871 (outside U.S. and Canada). Fax: 314-447-8029. E-mail: journalscustomerservice-usa@elsevier.com (for print support); journalsonline support-usa@elsevier.com (for online support).**

Reprints. For copies of 100 or more, of articles in this publication, please contact the Commercial Reprints Department, Elsevier Inc., 360 Park Avenue South, New York, New York 10010-1710. Tel. 212-633-3874, Fax: 212-633-3820, E-mail: reprints@elsevier.com.

The Surgical Clinics of North America is also published in Spanish by McGraw-Hill Interamericana Editores S.A., P.O. Box 5-237 06500 Mexico D.F. Mexico; and in Portuguese by Interlivros Edicoes Ltda., Rua Comandante Coelho 1085, CEP 21250, Rio de Janeiro, Brazil; and in Greek by Paschalidis Medical Publications, Athens Greece.

The Surgical Clinics of North America is covered in *MEDLINE/PubMed (Index Medicus), EMBASE/Excerpta Medica, Current Contents/Clinical Medicine, Current Contents/Life Sciences, Science Citation Index*, and *ISI/BIOMED.*

Contributors

CONSULTING EDITOR

RONALD F. MARTIN, MD, FACS
Colonel (ret.), United States Army Reserve, Department of Surgery, York Hospital, York, Maine, USA

EDITOR

J. BART ROSE, MD, MAS
Assistant Professor, Division of Surgical Oncology, Director of the Pancreatobiliary Disease Center at UAB, The University of Alabama, Birmingham, Alabama, USA

AUTHORS

JAD E. ABOU-KHALIL, MD, MSc, FRCSC
Assistant Professor of Surgery, Hepatobiliary and Pancreatic Surgery Unit, University of Ottawa, The Ottawa Hospital, Ottawa, Ontario, Canada

FARZAD ALEMI, MD, FACS
St. Vincent Medical Center, Transplant and Hepatopancreatobiliary Institute, Los Angeles, California, USA

SUBHASHINI AYLOO, MD, MPH, FACS
Rutgers, New Jersey Medical School, Newark, New Jersey, USA

RACHEL E. BEARD, MD
Department of Surgery, Rhode Island Hospital, Providence, Rhode Island, USA

KIMBERLY A. BERTENS, MD, MSc, FRCSC
Assistant Professor of Surgery, Hepatobiliary and Pancreatic Surgery Unit, University of Ottawa, The Ottawa Hospital, Ottawa, Ontario, Canada

KEVIN P. CHARPENTIER, MD
Department of Surgery, Rhode Island Hospital, Providence, Rhode Island, USA

CLANCY J. CLARK, MD
Assistant Professor of Surgery, Associate Program Director, General Surgery Residency, Assistant Professor of Anatomy, Surgical Director, Center for Applied and Experiential Learning, Wake Forest Baptist Health, Winston-Salem, North Carolina, USA

JOSHUA T. COHEN, MD
Department of Surgery, Rhode Island Hospital, Providence, Rhode Island, USA

CARLO CONTRERAS, MD, FACS
Associate Professor, Division of Surgical Oncology, Department of Surgery, The University of Alabama at Birmingham, Birmingham, Alabama, USA

LEIGH ANNE DAGEFORDE, MD, MPH
Assistant Professor, Department of Surgery, Harvard Medical School, Assistant Surgeon,
Division of Transplant Surgery, Massachusetts General Hospital, Boston, Massachusetts,
USA

AUSTIN R. DOSCH, MD
Department of Surgery, University of California, Irvine, Irvine, California, USA

WILLIAM SCOTT HELTON, MD
Virginia Mason Medical Center, Seattle, Washington, USA

LAURA HICKMAN, MD
Division of Surgical Oncology, Department of Surgery, The University of Alabama at
Birmingham, Birmingham, Alabama, USA

DAVID K. IMAGAWA, MD, PhD
Department of Surgery, University of California, Irvine, Irvine, California, USA

ZELJKA JUTRIC, MD
Department of Surgery, University of California Irvine, Irvine, California, USA; Assistant
Professor, Hepatobiliary and Pancreas Surgery, University of California, Irvine, Orange,
California, USA

ZAHEER S. KANJI, MD, MSc, FRCSC
Section of General, Thoracic and Vascular Surgery, Virginia Mason Medical Center,
Seattle, Washington, USA; Division of General Surgery, Department of Surgery,
Royal Inland Hospital, University of British Columbia, Kamloops, British Columbia,
Canada

ADEEL S. KHAN, MD, MPH, FACS
Assistant Professor, Department of Surgery, Section of Abdominal Transplant Surgery,
Washington University in St. Louis, St. Louis, Missouri, USA

RAJESH KRISHNAMOORTHI, MD
Digestive Diseases Institute, Virginia Mason Medical Center, Seattle, Washington, USA

CHRISTINA W. LEE, MD
Division of Surgical Oncology, General Surgery Resident, Department of Surgery,
University of Wisconsin School of Medicine and Public Health, University of Wisconsin,
Madison, Wisconsin, USA

LEE M. OCUIN, MD
Assistant Professor of Surgery, Division of Hepatopancreatobiliary Surgery, Atrium
Health/Carolinas Medical Center – Northeast, Concord, North Carolina, USA

SUSHANTH REDDY, MD, FACS
Assistant Professor, Surgery, The University of Alabama at Birmingham, Birmingham,
Alabama, USA

FLAVIO G. ROCHA, MD, FACS
Section of General, Thoracic and Vascular Surgery, Virginia Mason Medical Center,
Seattle, Washington, USA

MARGARET M. ROMINE, MD, MS
Resident PGY 5, General Surgery, Division of Transplantation, The University of Alabama
at Birmingham, Birmingham, Alabama, USA

SEAN RONNEKLEIV-KELLY, MD
Assistant Professor, Division of Surgical Oncology, Department of Surgery, University of Wisconsin School of Medicine and Public Health, University of Wisconsin, Madison, Wisconsin, USA

ANDREW ROSS, MD
Digestive Diseases Institute, Virginia Mason Medical Center, Seattle, Washington, USA

DOMINIC E. SANFORD, MD, MPHS
Assistant Professor of Surgery, Division of Hepatobiliary, Pancreatic, and Gastrointestinal Surgery, Washington University School of Medicine, St Louis, Missouri, USA

NATALIE SEISER, MD, PhD
St. Vincent Medical Center, Transplant and Hepatopancreatobiliary Institute, Los Angeles, California, USA

JESSE K. SULZER, MD, PhD
Division of Hepatopancreatobiliary Surgery, HPB Surgery Fellow, Department of Surgery, Atrium Health/Carolinas Medical Center, Charlotte, North Carolina, USA

JARED WHITE, MD, FACS
Associate Professor, General Surgery, Division of Transplantation, The University of Alabama at Birmingham, Birmingham, Alabama, USA

RUI ZHENG-PYWELL, MD
Surgery, The University of Alabama at Birmingham, Birmingham, Alabama, USA

Contents

Video content accompanies this article at http://www.surgical.
theclinics.com.

Consensus guidelines recommend patients with symptomatic cholelithiasis and suspected choledocholithiasis have common bile duct exploration (CBDE) at the time of cholecystectomy to prevent downstream
problems. Despite superiority of single-stage cholecystectomy with
CBDE, 2-stage precholecystectomy/postcholecystectomy with endoscopic clearance of the duct is commonly practiced. This is related to
inadequate training in minimally invasive techniques, lack of technical support for efficient and safe CBDE, and surgeons' inexperience with complex
biliary pathologic condition. This article provides a framework for evaluating and treating patients with CBD pathologic condition with an
emphasis on technical aspects of CBDE and preoperative planning and
preparation.

Common bile duct injury is a feared complication of cholecystectomy, with
an incidence of 0.1% to 0.6%. A majority of injuries go unnoticed at index
operation, and postoperative diagnosis can be difficult. Patient presentation can vary from vague abdominal pain to uncontrolled sepsis and peritonitis. Diagnostic evaluation typically begins with ultrasound or CT scan in
the acute setting, and source control is paramount at time of presentation.
In a stable patient, hepatobiliary iminodiacetic acid scan can be useful in
identifying an ongoing bile leak, which requires intervention. A variety of
diagnostic techniques define biliary anatomy. Treatment often requires a
multidisciplinary approach.

Although the most common presentation of biliary disorder in North America is secondary to gallstone disease, an awareness of benign biliary cystic
neoplasms is important because of the risk of malignant transformation.
The incidence of premalignant cystic neoplasms of the bile duct is not
well characterized and they often are detected incidentally for suspicion
of other abdominal disorders. This article describes the 4 most common
premalignant biliary cystic neoplasms: biliary mucinous cystic neoplasms,
intraductal papillary mucinous neoplasms of the bile duct, intraductal
tubular papillary neoplasms of the bile duct, and choledochal cysts.

Cholangiocarcinoma is a rare malignancy and accounts for 2% of all malignancies. Incidence is on the increase in the Western world. Cholangiocarcinoma arises from the malignant growth of the epithelial lining of the

bile ducts and can be found all along the biliary tree. It can be classified into subtypes based on location: intrahepatic (arising from the intrahepatic biliary tract in the hepatic parenchyma), perihilar (at the hilum of the liver involving the biliary confluence) and distal (extrahepatic, often in the head of the pancreas). Margin status and locoregional lymph node metastases are the most important determinants of postsurgical outcomes.

Gallbladder cancer (GBC) is an often lethal disease, but surgical resection is potentially curative. Symptoms may be misdiagnosed as biliary colic; over half of new diagnoses are made after laparoscopic cholecystectomy for presumed benign disease. Gallbladder polyps >1 cm should prompt additional imaging and cholecystectomy. For GBC diagnosed after cholecystectomy, tumors T1b and greater necessitate radical cholecystectomy. Radical cholecystectomy includes staging laparoscopy, hepatic resection, and locoregional lymph node clearance to achieve R0 resection. Patients with locally advanced disease (T3 or T4), hepatic-sided T2 tumors, node positivity, or R1 resection may benefit from adjuvant chemotherapy. Chemotherapy increases survival in unresectable disease.

Compared with other periampullary tumors, cancers of the ampulla of Vater are rare. These tumors tend to present earlier than their pancreatic and distal bile duct brethren. In addition to the hypothesis that they are also less biologically aggressive, ampullary cancers tend to have better survival than other types of periampullary cancers. The mortality from this disease remains high, and much can still be learned about ampullary cancers.

Endoscopic retrograde cholangiopancreatography (ERCP) has evolved from a diagnostic and therapeutic tool to a predominantly therapeutic tool. There is a limited role for diagnostic ERCP with widespread availability of magnetic resonance cholangiopancreatography and endoscopic ultrasound (EUS). Since its introduction, EUS evolved from a diagnostic imaging modality to one with combined diagnostic and therapeutic capabilities. Currently, ERCP remains the standard of care for biliary decompression. In future, it is possible that EUS guided transmural biliary drainage may replace ERCP for certain indications. Given the risk of adverse events related with these more invasive endoscopic procedures, a multidisciplinary team-based approach is recommended.

Orthotopic liver transplantation (OLT) has many roles in biliary disease. OLT provides excellent results for patients with unresectable hilar cholangiocarcinoma. OLT prolongs survival in primary biliary cirrhosis not responsive to therapy and improves quality of life. OLT remains the durable option for patients with primary sclerosing cholangitis and complications of end-stage liver disease or recurrent cholangitis secondary to biliary obstruction. Indications for OLT after bile duct injury are chronic liver disease secondary to biliary cirrhosis and acute liver failure from associated vascular injury. OLT is treatment of choice for Caroli disease and syndrome when fibrosis leads to portal hypertension and esophageal varices.

SURGICAL CLINICS
OF NORTH AMERICA

SERIES OF RELATED INTEREST

Advances in Surgery
Available at: www.advancessurgery.com
Surgical Oncology Clinics
Available at: www.surgonc.theclinics.com
Thoracic Surgery Clinics
Available at: www.thoracic.theclinics.com

THE CLINICS ARE AVAILABLE ONLINE!
Access your subscription at:
www.theclinics.com

Foreword
Biliary Issue

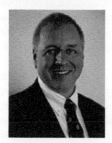

Ronald F. Martin, MD, FACS
Consulting Editor

For those of you who have read this series for some time, you will be aware that we are always trying to explore the boundary between what belongs in the realm of the generalist and what belongs on the realm of the specialist. Mostly, this line is more of a poorly defined "area" rather than an easily identified sharp demarcation. In some areas, the areas have narrowed sharply: cardiac surgery, transplantation, perhaps even vascular, while other areas remain difficult to be so clear about: gastric surgery, colorectal surgery, breast surgery, and perhaps even most of all, biliary surgery.

There are many reasons to explain why we might have difficulty deciding where the line between specialist care and generalist care should be drawn for operative biliary care. Wide differences in "local" availability of other specialty support (biliary endoscopy, interventional radiology, advanced imaging capacity, and so forth) may influence one's willingness to approach certain operations. Institutional commitment and financial resources to maintain a broad-based program may be a factor. The ability to care for, and to have the coverage to care for, sometimes complex patients may play a role in decision making.

While all of the above are good reasons to favor or shy away from taking on complex biliary patients, they probably pale in comparison to one other major determinant: the advent of laparoscopy, and to a lesser extent, biliary endoscopy, created a generation of surgeons who have not had much exposure to what were once common, though challenging, biliary procedures. Operations of varying difficulty for cholecystectomy, intraoperative cholangiography, and common bile duct exploration were once so common that residents in training learned them early in their training cycle. In fact, those operations were frequently the procedures where residents learned their more complex operative skills that prepared them for even more challenging operations of all types. One would probably be hard pressed to find anybody who feels that the development of either laparoscopy or endoscopy was anything other than an overwhelming boon to humankind; still, even the best advances have unintended consequences.

Surg Clin N Am 99 (2019) xiii–xv
https://doi.org/10.1016/j.suc.2019.02.001
0039-6109/19/© 2019 Published by Elsevier Inc.

surgical.theclinics.com

Since the advent of laparoscopic cholecystectomy in the mid-late 1980s, depending upon whose criteria one wishes to use, to its nearly complete adoption by the very early 1990s, there has been a precipitous decline in open biliary operations performed for garden variety gallstone-related maladies. The somewhat more gradual development of endoscopic retrograde cholangiopancreatography and magnetic resonance cholangiopancreatography has provided both diagnostic and therapeutic alternatives to operative procedures. These advances collectively have nearly eliminated the need for open cholecystectomy, open common duct exploration, and intraoperative cholangiography (perhaps more controversial), thereby effectively removing what was once a fundamental foundation piece of operative training.

The flip side of that process was a change in the risk-benefit equation that favored increased use of laparoscopic cholecystectomy. With this surge in demand for procedures, the surgical and engineering communities rapidly developed better videoscopic equipment and tools that further expanded our ability to avoid open procedures. Again though, this further distilled the remaining procedures that were not amenable to videoscopic approach to be the most challenging forms of their types. The unintended consequence being that for many surgeons on their developmental arc, the first open biliary procedures they would be involved with would be the most difficult to perform and the most difficult from which to learn.

This is where the concept of "transferrable skills" enters our conversation. The skills associated with open cholecystectomy and common bile duct exploration are generally quite transferrable to biliary reconstruction and resection for less common benign issues and malignant disorders. In selected cases, the videoscopic counterparts are also transferrable but on a much more constricted scale at the present time. As a result, a full range of technical capacity for biliary operations that used to be widely disseminated has now coalesced into a diminishing number of locations and centers.

If most biliary operations were similar to those for transplantation, for instance, this probably would not be a big deal. However, despite the advances in preoperative evaluation mentioned above, it is not always clear when one is getting into a challenging biliary situation. Depending on availability and quality of preoperative evaluation, one can easily find oneself in over his/her head in a hurry. Also, even when we think we know what we are going to find, it can be a lot worse than predicted even in the best of preoperative circumstances. Situations such as xanthogranulomatous cholecystitis and unexpected Mirizzi syndrome leap to mind when I think of how people have been caught off guard, not to mention the unexpected neoplasm.

To say that it is *unlikely* we will ever go back to a day in which surgeons will develop their skills performing routine open biliary procedures is an understatement of epic proportions. Despite that, we all need to find a way to develop our understanding of biliary disorders and conditions that will keep us alert to situations we could find ourselves in. We also need to have a clear-eyed sense of our own personal and institutional capabilities as well as those skill sets of our colleagues. To that end, we are deeply appreciative of this issue that Dr Rose and his colleagues have prepared for us. I hope you will find it equally interesting as a refresher in some things we may take for granted as well as deeply insightful into newer concepts and classifications of problems that have been refined in recent years.

How we distribute health care resources and why will remain a multifaceted discussion for some time. No doubt, politics (both within and outside of medicine), finances, shifting generational expectations, and other societal factors will all play their roles. We surgeons must maintain our own level of expertise and understanding of these sometimes complicated matters if we have any hope of contributing to the larger conversation in a meaningful way. We at the *Surgical Clinics of North America* remain committed to providing our readership with content placed into context to allow us all to help our communities on multiple levels.

Ronald F. Martin, MD, FACS
Colonel (ret.), United States Army Reserve
Chief of Surgery
Department of Surgery
York Hospital
16 Hospital Drive, Suite A
York, ME 03909, USA

E-mail address:
rmartin@yorkhospital.com

Preface

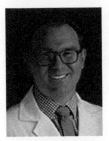

J. Bart Rose, MD, MAS
Editor

Diseases of the biliary tract includes some of the most common and rarest pathology in mankind. Management of these conditions can be extremely rewarding or devastating for both patients and providers alike. Cholecystectomies are the most often performed surgical procedure in the United States and can provide significant relief to suffering patients. However, iatrogenic injury to the bile duct resulting from this operation is one of the most litigious complications facing general surgeons.

Many of the first successful intra-abdominal operations performed were for surgical management of biliary diseases. In the modern era, new minimally invasive techniques have improved outcomes, reduced morbidity, and improved quality of life for patients. Percutaneous, endoscopic, and laparoscopic modalities have drastically changed management of these diseases in the last two decades. Open cholecystectomy is now rarely performed, endoscopic management of choledocholithiasis has become standard of care in most instances, and biliary bypasses are usually deferred in lieu of endobiliary stenting.

While we have made significant strides in the treatment of these complex diseases in the past century, more work needs to be done. Cancers of the bile duct and gall-bladder, while thankfully rare, are usually advanced at presentation and have a generally poor prognosis. We are in dire need of better systemic treatment and screening modalities for these malignancies.

These topics and others are discussed in this issue of Surgical Clinics of North America. I would like to thank the authors that contributed their time and expertise to this project. We hope that this is not only a review of current knowledge, but also highlights areas were data is lacking, thereby encouraging others to answer the unknown. I would

Surg Clin N Am 99 (2019) xvii–xviii
https://doi.org/10.1016/j.suc.2018.12.010
0039-6109/19/© 2018 Published by Elsevier Inc.

surgical.theclinics.com

also like to thank the editorial staff and Elsevier for their guidance, as well as my family for their patience. I hope everyone who reads this finds it is fascinating and useful as I did.

J. Bart Rose, MD, MAS
Division of Surgical Oncology
UAB The University of Alabama
1808 7th Avenue South
BDB 605
Birmingham, AL 35233-3411, USA

E-mail address:
jbrose@uabmc.edu

Embryology, Anatomy, and Imaging of the Biliary Tree

Jad E. Abou-Khalil, MD, MSc, FRCSC*, Kimberly A. Bertens, MD, MSc, FRCSC

KEYWORDS

- Biliary tree • Extrahepatic • Hepatic diverticulum • Intrahepatic

KEY POINTS

- The anatomy of the biliary tree is notoriously variable. This variation is the bane of the hepatobiliary surgeon, to whom an understanding of biliary anatomic variation is key to the planning and safe conduct of liver surgery, from oncological resections to split-liver transplantation.
- The hepatic diverticulum, also termed "the liver bud," is the first semblance of the biliary system in the human embryo.
- As development ensues, the hepatic diverticulum acquires a distinct distal bud. It is commonplace to label the cranial part of the hepatic diverticulum as the pars hepatica and the caudal bud as the pars cystica.
- A variety of techniques used in the mid twentieth century for imaging the biliary tree have since been abandoned in favor of more practical, safer, less invasive, and more sensitive and specific contemporary methods.

EMBRYOLOGY OF THE BILIARY TREE
Overview

During the fourth week of human embryonic development, the hepatic diverticulum, which is the first anlage of the liver and bile ducts, appears from the ventral foregut. The hepatic diverticulum can be further divided into the cranial pars hepatica and the caudal pars cystica. The former becomes the liver and intrahepatic ducts, whereas the latter forms the extrahepatic biliary tree and gallbladder. The distal-most right and left hepatic ducts develop as part of the extrahepatic bile duct around the 12th week of gestation, whereas the intrahepatic ducts form from the ductal plate along the path of the developing portal veins. The central intrahepatic ducts are the first to form with progressive expansion toward the periphery of the liver as gestation progresses. The most peripheral of the intrahepatic biliary tree are not yet fully matured at the time of birth.

The authors have nothing to disclose.
Hepatobiliary and Pancreatic Surgery Unit, The University of Ottawa, The Ottawa Hospital, 501 Smyth Road, Box 202, Ottawa, Ontario K1H8L6, Canada
* Corresponding author.
E-mail address: jaboukhalil@toh.ca

The hepatic diverticulum

The hepatic diverticulum, also termed "the liver bud," is the first semblance of the biliary system in the human embryo. It begins as a thickening of the ventral wall of the caudal end of the primitive foregut, in an area designated the intestinal portal. Between the third and fourth week of gestation, the hepatic diverticulum is a well-developed structure composed of endoderm, which lengthens and branches into the surrounding mesenchyme of the septum transversum.[1] The septum transversum is an embryonic structure composed of a thick mass of mesenchymal tissue that separates the pericardial and peritoneal cavities.

As development ensues, the hepatic diverticulum acquires a distinct distal bud. It is commonplace to label the cranial part of the hepatic diverticulum as the pars hepatica and the caudal bud as the pars cystica. The former is the primordium to the liver and intrahepatic ducts and the latter to the gallbladder, cystic duct, and common bile duct. Sprouting endodermal cells from the pars hepatica extend to the septum transversum and serve to become the earliest anlage of the liver.[2]

Development of the extrahepatic bile ducts and gallbladder

The pars cystica continues to grow in length for up to 8 weeks of gestation.[3] Contrary to previously held beliefs, the common bile duct and gallbladder remain patent throughout development, and there is not a "solid stage" of endodermal occlusion. The conclusion of earlier studies that the lumen of common bile duct (CBD) is obliterated and later recannulates is likely the result of suboptimal tissue preservation techniques available in that time period. The biliary epithelium is fragile, and tissue loss occurs quickly after death, which likely resulted in plugging of the CBD with denuded epithelium.[3]

By 29 days gestation the primordial gallbladder is discernible as an anterolateral dilatation to the right of the hepatic diverticulum, and by 34 days the cystic duct is also present. Out pockets form on the outside of the gallbladder wall, resulting in the development of folds on the inside wall. Mesenchymal cells condense around the epithelium of the gallbladder anlage, culminating in the 3-layer wall of the mature gallbladder. As the extrahepatic biliary tree lengthens, an outgrowth from the dorsal wall of the choledochus gives rise to the ventral pancreatic bud, explaining the close approximation of the 2 structures. At approximately the fifth week of development, the duodenum rotates in a counter-clockwise manner, and the CBD comes to rest on the dorsal side of the duodenum.

By the fifth gestational week, the common hepatic duct undergoes active remodeling and becomes a broad, funnel-shaped structure at the hepatic hilum in contact with the primordial liver. At this point of gestation there is not a discernible left and right hepatic duct. Rapid endodermal proliferation ensues in the dilated funnellike structure above the level of the CBD and cystic duct. This leads to folding of the tissue, and the formation of multiple channels at the level of the porta hepatis. This process of remodeling at the hilum has been postulated to give rise to the vast anatomic variation in how the left and right hepatic ducts join together, with the "normal" Y-shaped configuration only present in 56% of people. The distal portion of the left and right hepatic ducts form as an extension of the extrahepatic biliary tree and are clearly defined tubular structures by 12 weeks of gestation. Tan and Moscoso also refuted the earlier belief from mouse studies, suggesting that the extra- and intrahepatic ducts developed in a discontinuous fashion and joined late in development. They showed that from the beginning of organogenesis, the extra- and intrahepatic biliary tree maintains luminal continuity, although the process is still not well understood.[3]

Development of the intrahepatic bile ducts

The intrahepatic ducts do not start to form until sometime between the fifth and ninth gestational weeks. Over time, many theories regarding the evolution of the intrahepatic ducts and their relationship with the extrahepatic biliary tree have been postulated. The theory most commonly accepted at present time is that the intrahepatic biliary tree develops from hepatoblasts, which are the precursor cells to both the hepatocyte and biliary epithelium. The location of the branching portal veins determines the anatomic pattern of the intrahepatic biliary tree. There is a thin double layer of cells surrounding the portal vein branches termed "the ductal plate." The ductal plate is the precursor from which the biliary radicles form.[4] This phenomenon explains why biliary anatomy typically follows that of the aberrant portal venous anatomy.

From the 12th gestational week onwards, there is ongoing remodeling of the ductal plate; proliferation of the surrounding mesenchyme leads the ductal plates to separate from the surrounding liver parenchyma.[5] Eventually the cells of the ductal plate that do not form the biliary tubules regress. The development of the intrahepatic ducts starts at the large portal vein branches near the hepatic hilum and continues throughout gestation toward the periphery of the liver.[1] In fact, the most peripheral ducts continue to develop from immature ductal plates up until 4 weeks following birth.[6]

Ductal plate malformations Ductal plate malformation (DPM) is a broad term encompassing a range of human diseases including biliary atresia, Caroli disease, Meckel syndrome, and Alagille syndrome. Normal development of the intrahepatic biliary tree results from a carefully timed sequence of events where ducts develop from the primitive ductal plate along the portal vein branches from the hilum outwards. If remodeling of the ductal plate fails to occur properly, this results in the embryonic ductal plate configuration failing to regress. These abnormalities are associated with abnormalities in the branching pattern of the portal blood vessels.

Biliary atresia Biliary atresia (BA) is a well-known case of DPM. The exact inciting cause remains contested. Previously, it was a commonly held belief that BA was a congenital anomaly that resulted from a failure in recanalization of the biliary tree at the hepatic hilum. However, because the "solid stage" of biliary development has now been proved to be nonexistent, this theory no longer holds. Many other models have been proposed, including exposure to an unknown virus after birth. Recently, Tan and Moscoso[5] suggested a new theory to explain the inciting event leading to BA. The investigators postulated that between the 11th and 13th week of gestation, there is a failure of the normal biliary duct development at the hepatic hilum, which leads to small primitive ducts that lack surrounding mesenchyme. When these fragile ducts are subjected to biliary flow nearing the end of gestation, they rupture, which results in bile leakage and inflammatory scaring.

ANATOMY OF THE BILIARY TREE
Overview

The anatomy of the biliary tree is notoriously variable. This variation is the bane of the hepatobiliary surgeon, to whom an understanding of biliary anatomic variation is key to the planning and safe conduct of liver surgery, from oncological resections to split-liver transplantation. An understanding of the common variants of biliary anatomy is also important to the general surgeon, who will inevitably encounter the wide breadth of variation in biliary configurations at cholecystectomy during their career. This article illustrates the common anatomic types and configurations of the left and right biliary tree, the biliary confluence, and point out common and relevant anatomic variants.

An exploration of conventional and variant gallbladder and extrahepatic biliary anatomy will then follow.

The intrahepatic biliary tree

Anatomy of the left biliary system Segments 2, 3, and 4 drain into the left bile duct. Corrosion casting of the left biliary tree demonstrates 4 common variants of its anatomy.[7] The most common configuration, observed in 55% of livers, sees segment 2 and 3 bile ducts join to form a left lateral section[8] duct close to the umbilical fissure (**Fig. 1**A). In this variant, the confluence of the segment 2 and 3 ducts occurs at the umbilical fissure 5% of the time, medial to the umbilical fissure 50% of the time, and laterally to the fissure 45% of the time, with the left lateral segment bile duct (LLS) then joining a single segment 4 duct to form the left hepatic duct. In the second most common configuration, occurring 30% of the time, the LLS forms close to the umbilical fissure and is then joined by 2 separate segment 4 ducts, one closer to the umbilical fissure and one closer to the confluence with the right hepatic duct (**Fig. 1**B). In a third configuration, observed in 10% of patients, there is no LLS, and a segment 3 duct is joined by a segment 4 duct lateral to the umbilical fissure, with the segment 2 duct joining the left hepatic duct closer to the hilum (**Fig. 1**C). A fourth configuration sees a short LLS at the umbilical fissure rapidly joined by a segment 4 duct, almost as a trifurcation (**Fig. 1**D). In approximately 30% of patients, a segment 4 biliary radical crosses the umbilical fissure to meet the LLS. This is most commonly seen in the second configuration of the left biliary system described earlier.

The relationship of the biliary tree to the portal veins has been initially described by Rex, as well as studies by Healey and Shroy (1952) and by Couinaud in his corrosion casts and comparative anatomic studies. The proximal left hepatic ducts are universally superior to the portal vein (epiportal or supraportal), a relationship that allows for the Hepp-Couinaud lowering of the hilar plate to access the left hepatic duct. This relationship is mostly maintained through the rest of the left biliary system, with the biliary ducts being superior to the portal vein. However, between 3% and 8% of patients have a hypoportal, or caudal, location of the segment 3 duct. This variant is documented by Couinaud in 9/108 (8.3%) of his corrosion casts, by Kitamura in studies of 166 computed tomography (CT) scan (3.6%)[9] and more recently by Ozden and his colleagues (6%).[10] They document an association between the presence of a parenchymal bridge or fibrous band over Rex's recess and the presence of an infraportal or hypoportal segment 3 bile duct—of the 6 patients with an infraportal segment 3 duct, 5 had a liver parenchymal bridge or fibrous band (83%) compared with 9/75 (12%) in patients with a supraportal duct. Of note, the segment 3 duct does not run through the parenchymal bridge, and the absence of a bridge does not guarantee a conventional position of the segment 3 duct. The fact that the segment 2 duct is never found in an infraportal position is thought to be related to the embryologic development of the liver, with segment 3 and 4 originating together as a left anterior (paramedian) sector while segment 2 arising separately as a posterior (lateral) sector, leading segment 3 to lie anteriorly and caudally to the umbilical portion of the left portal vein, explaining why the segment 3 duct is more likely to be found in an infraportal position than the segment 2 duct.

Particular attention should be paid to these variations in resections of segments 2 and 3, extended right hepatectomies, as well as in split-liver and reduced-liver transplantation where an understanding of these anatomic variants is critical to the safe conduct of these procedures.

Anatomy of the biliary confluence and the right biliary system The right hepatic duct drains segments 5, 6, 7, and 8. Segments 5 and 8 drain into a right anterior bile duct

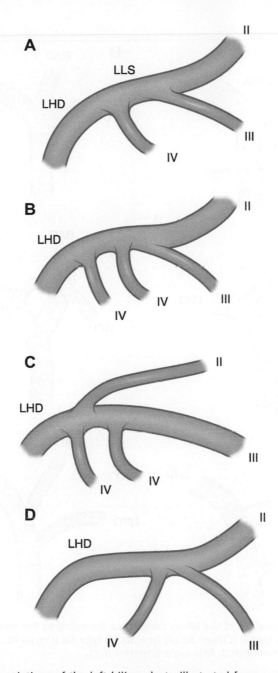

Fig. 1. Anatomic variations of the left biliary ducts, illustrated from a caudal perspective. LHD, left hepatic duct; LLS, left lateral segment bile duct.

and segments 6 and 7 into a right posterior bile duct. There are 4 drainage patterns of the right liver described by Varotti and colleagues[11] and, in another classification system, by Nakamura and colleagues.[12] In the conventional pattern, seen in 56% of livers, the right anterior and right posterior section ducts meet to form the right hepatic duct,

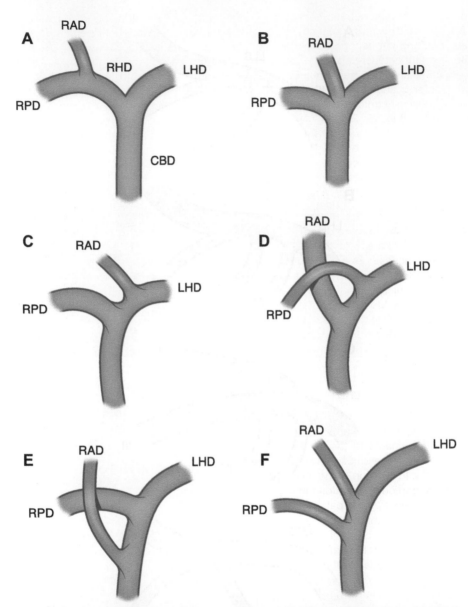

Fig. 2. Anatomic variation of the biliary confluence according to the Nakamura classification. (*A*) Type 1; (*B*) type 2; (*C*) type 3a; (*D*) type 3b; (*E*) type 4a; (*F*) type 4b. LHD, left hepatic duct; RAD, right anterior duct; RPD, right posterior duct.

which in turn joins the left hepatic duct to form the common hepatic duct (**Fig. 2**A). This configuration is known as type 1, and whereas the right anterior bile duct lies anteriorly to the right anterior portal vein, the right posterior duct hooks around the right anterior portal vein, a configuration described by Hjortsö and named eponymously after him. Awareness of this configuration is key to the safe conduct of extended left hepatectomies, as is the realization that the right posterior duct can variably lie in a hypoportal position. The right hepatic duct is usually epiportal but can be hypoportal in 20% of livers. Type 2, with a frequency of 14%, is a trifurcation of the right posterior, right anterior, and left hepatic ducts, with no right hepatic duct (**Fig. 2**B). In type 3a and 3b, the right anterior and posterior section ducts join the left hepatic duct respectively with a 5% and 15% frequency (**Fig. 2**C, D. respectively), and in types 4a and 4b the right anterior and right posterior hepatic ducts respectively join the common hepatic duct below the confluence—a configuration known as *convergence etagée* or shelved confluence (**Fig. 2**E, F). The existence of biliary radicals draining directly into the gallbladder from the liver parenchyma has been disproved, and the term "duct of Luschka" should be avoided. The term "subhepatic duct" is now used to describe a variety of anatomic conditions where bile ducts lie in close proximity to the cystic plate. These ducts can be injured during a cholecystectomy if the dissection plane violates the cystic plate, accounting for a significant portion of bile leaks after cholecystectomy.

Anatomy of the caudate ducts The caudate lobe is divided into the spiegel lobe, the paracaval caudate, and the caudate process, with a visible notch separating the caudate process from the Spigelian lobe in 50% of livers. The paracaval and caudate process, considered one unit and equated with Couinaud's segment 9, and the Spigelian lobe, Couinaud's segment 1, each drain via 1 to 3 ducts, with up to 5 ducts for the entire caudate. Most of the time, Spiegel's lobe drains into the left hepatic duct and the paracaval caudate drains into the right posterior section duct or the right hepatic duct. However, there are frequent right-left dissociations of the drainage patterns of the caudate ducts, with more than one-third of Spigelian lobe ducts draining into the right hepatic duct or the right posterior section duct. This is usually observed when the right posterior section duct inserts into the left hepatic duct. Similarly, a third of paracaval caudate ducts drain into the left hepatic duct or its tributaries.[13]

Biliary configuration with right-sided round ligaments In the presence of a right-sided round ligament, a rare variation occurring in 0.2% to 1.2% of adults, the round ligament connects to the right paramedian portal vein instead of its conventional attachment to the umbilical portion of the left portal vein, causing a right dominance of the liver. In addition to the known variations of the portovenous and hepatic arterial systems, particular attention must be paid to the configuration of the biliary tree when planning liver surgery in patients with a right-sided round ligament. Four configurations are described in this setting by Nishitai and colleagues[14]: in the symmetric configuration, observed in 56% of patients, the right anterior and posterior bile ducts join together into a right hepatic duct before joining with the left hepatic duct. In 26% of patients, the independent right lateral configuration is observed, with the right posterior section ducts draining independently into the common hepatic duct, below the confluence of the left and right anterior ducts. A total left configuration, where a single thick biliary duct drains the left liver and then passes along the umbilical fissure to drain the right through smaller biliary radicals, is seen 13% of the time, with a total right configuration seen more rarely.

The gallbladder and extrahepatic biliary tree
Gallbladder anatomy and variant anatomy The gallbladder lies on the inferior aspect of the liver, its longitudinal axis aligned with the Rex-Cantlie's line bisecting the right and left hemiliver, straddling the border between segments 4b and 5. Its fundus and body, mostly extrahepatic and lying on a fibrous area known as the cystic plate, stretch toward the liver hilum into an infundibulum that empties into the cystic duct, the lumen of which is lined by spiral valves of Heister. The cystic duct meets with

the common hepatic duct in a variety of configurations, running parallel to the hepatic duct for a variable distance and sometimes spiraling posteriorly before inserting. The cystic duct can also insert into the right hepatic duct or the posterior section duct in 4% of livers. The surgeon must be mindful of this variant, because inadvertent encircling and amputation of a right posterior section duct on which the gallbladder is inserting is a known pattern of biliary injury and complications at cholecystectomy. Because of variations of cystic duct insertions, it is unnecessary to visualize the cystic duct-CBD junctions at the time of cholecystectomy, and attempting to do so may cause unnecessary trauma. The cystic artery most commonly arises from the right hepatic artery but can also originate from the hepatic artery proper or a replaced or aberrant right hepatic artery when present. Care must be taken at the time of cholecystectomy not to inadvertently ligate the right hepatic artery—hence the importance of lifting the gallbladder off the cystic plate over 30% of its length and to clear the hepatocystic triangle of all fibrofatty tissues to ensure that any structure to be amputated is truly going only into the gallbladder, and not entering the liver. This method of identifying the cystic duct and artery is known as the Critical View of Safety and has gained wide acceptance within the community of surgeons as the method of choice for identification of the cystic duct and artery.[15]

Gallbladder agenesis is a very rare anatomic variant, thought to occur in 1/6000 live births. Gallbladder duplication is a more common variant, estimated to occur in 1/4000 humans. The preoperative identification of a duplicate gallbladder is difficult, with most cases identified intraoperatively. Ultrasonography and magnetic resonance cholangiopancreatography (MRCP) are the most sensitive modalities for preoperative detection, with a sensitivity of 66% and 99%, respectively.[16] Gallbladder duplications occur on a spectrum and are classified into types by Harlaftis and colleagues,[17] likely mirroring the embryologic stage at which gallbladder development was disrupted. These variants do not seem to be associated with any other congenital anomalies or known syndromes. There are 2 patterns of type 1 duplications: the "Y" type, where 2 distinct gallbladders have 2 cystic ducts that join before entering the CBD and likely resulting from early division of the pars cystica. A later division of the pars cystica results in the second pattern of type 1 duplications, a bilobed gallbladder, also known as *vesica divisa*, wherein a septum divides a gallbladder that otherwise has a single cystic duct. Type 1 accounts for 43% of duplicated gallbladders. Type 2, accounting for 50% of gallbladder duplications, occurs when the cystic duct enters the CBD (ductular type) or the intrahepatic ducts (trabecular type) separately. This type can be difficult to differentiate from a Todani type 2 choledochal cyst, and although the presence of an anomalous pancreaticobiliary junction suggests the diagnosis of a choledochal cyst, the definitive distinction between a type 2 Todani choledochal cyst and a type 2 gallbladder duplication is made at histopathologic analysis of the specimen by identification of the presence or absence of a muscularis layer. Type 3 are variants where more than 2 gallbladders are present and type 4 are duplicate gallbladders without communication to the remaining biliary tree.

The gallbladder can adopt a variety of positions *vis a vis* the liver bed, from completely intrahepatic gallbladders, to gallbladders with little to no attachment to the liver, suspended by a mesentery and at a risk of torsion in addition to rare case reports of retroduodenal gallbladders. These variations of gallbladder position could be caused by disordered migration of the pars cystica, but they are often associated with other anatomic variations of liver anatomy. A left-sided gallbladder (sinistroposition), most commonly, is in fact associated with the presence of a right-sided round ligament; it is therefore not a "true" left-sided gallbladder because the gallbladder in fact maintains the relationship of its long axis to the Rex-Cantlie's line between the

2 hemilivers and represents an anomaly of the round ligament and not of the gall-bladder. In the case of a right-sided round ligament, the gallbladder is to the left of the round ligament, its long axis at a 30° angle.[18] A true left-sided gallbladder in the absence of a right-sided round ligament is very rare and in one case report is associated with other anomalies of the portal vein and biliary tree such as an infraportal segment 2 bile duct.[19]

Extrahepatic bile ducts The confluence of left and right biliary systems is usually extra-hepatic in the hilum of the liver, with the right and left ducts exiting the liver in their Glissonian sheath along with corresponding portal vein and hepatic arterial branches, and meeting to become the common hepatic duct, joins the cystic duct, and which courses anterolaterally within the hepatoduodenal ligament as the CBD. The CBD will typically join with the pancreatic duct at the ampulla of Vater and drain into the second portion of the duodenum. The left hepatic duct, measuring 2 to 5 cm, has a longer, more horizontal extrahepatic course than the right hepatic duct, which, if present at all, has but a short extrahepatic course of 1 cm. The CBD usually crosses anteriorly to the right hepatic artery as it traverses the upper porta hepatis obliquely to enter the liver, but 25% of the time it crosses behind the artery. Along its course toward the ampulla, the CBD receives paired arterial tributaries from the gastroduodenal artery inferiorly and the right hepatic artery superiorly, in a plexus that runs parallel to the CBD. It courses posteriorly to the head of the pancreas, which surrounds or encases it over a variable length.

IMAGING OF THE BILIARY TREE
Overview

A variety of techniques used in the mid twentieth century have since been abandoned in favor of more practical, safer, less invasive, and more sensitive and specific contemporary methods. Oral cholecystography was a popular method of ruling out the presence of gallstone but has largely fallen out of use in favor of ultrasonography. Some more modern techniques of mapping the biliary tree have fallen out of usage due to inavailability of the contrast agents: CT of the abdomen following the administration of meglumine biotrexate, known commercially as Biliscopin, can yield accurate images of the biliary tree,[20] assisting in the identification of biliary anatomy, but is no longer in common use because of the unavailability of the intravenous contrast agent.

Although ultrasonography is the initial modality through which biliary pathologies are investigated, more detailed anatomic assessment of the biliary tree usually requires other forms of cholangiography techniques.

Hepatobiliary scintigraphy
The accidental discovery that ^{99m}Tc hepatobiliary iminodiacetic acid (HIDA) radiopharmaceuticals cleared through the hepatobiliary system led to the development in the 1960s of imaging methods that still find clinical use today. A ^{99m}Tc HIDA scan consists of the intravenous injection of the radiopharmaceutical followed by timed scintigraphic imaging of the liver and proximal gastrointestinal tract. The primary utility of a ^{99m}Tc HIDA scan is in the workup of gallbladder disease, specifically in documenting filling and emptying of the gallbladder. Lack of filling of the gallbladder demonstrates the primary pathologic process of acute cholecystitis, namely cystic duct obstruction. The diagnostic accuracy of ^{99m}Tc HIDA scan for the diagnosis of acute cholecystitis is high, with a higher sensitivity and specificity than ultrasonography.[21] Dynamic studies of gallbladder emptying and measurement of gallbladder ejection fraction (GBEF) in response to cholecystokinin are performed to rule out functional gallbladder disorders;

however, the evidence base supporting a GBEF of less than 38% as a traditional benchmark for normal function is not strong, GBEF measurement is poorly reproducible,[22] and the interpretation of the GBEF can be difficult.[23] Moreover, ultrasonography has supplanted ^{99m}Tc HIDA scan as the modality of choice for the diagnosis of acute cholecystitis and other gallbladder disorders in the emergency department.

Ultrasonography of the gallbladder and biliary tree
Ultrasonography uses the differential echogenicity of organs and tissues to obtain 2 dimensional imaging of tissues. Traditionally these images are obtained by a transabdominal probe, but the biliary system can also be imaged by endoscopic ultrasound as well as intraoperatively, using either open or laparoscopic ultrasound probes. The gallbladder should be anechoic, with thin walls of 3 mm or less. In a nonfasted state, the gallbladder can be collapsed and therefore the walls may seem thicker. A normal CBD measures less than 6 mm at the level where it crosses the right hepatic artery, but in elderly individuals it can be as dilated as 8 mm even without any associated pathologies. It lies in the porta hepatis where, in its lower aspect, it forms the ear of a "mickey mouse sign," with the right ear being the hepatic artery and the face being the portal vein. In the absence of biliary dilatation, the intrahepatic bile ducts are difficult to visualize by ultrasonography. Ultrasonography is the best initial diagnostic modality for the diagnosis of gallbladder and biliary tract disease. However, it is unable to provide detailed anatomic information on biliary configuration to assist in surgical planning, and in such cases MRCP is the modality of choice. Three-dimensional ultrasonography is promising but has yet to be adopted widely and validated against MRCP.

Magnetic resonance cholangiopancreatography and liver MRI
MRCP is a rapid, noninvasive means of imaging the biliary tree that does not use ionizing radiation. Using T2-weighted imaging, MRCP provides a visualization of fluid-filled structures of the abdomen and when coupled with T1-weighted imaging of the soft tissues, yields both a luminal evaluation allowing a reconstruction for the biliary anatomy as well as valuable soft tissue assessment. MRCP equals or exceeds the diagnostic sensitivity and specificity of endoscopic retrograde cholangiopancreatography (ERCP) in the detection of choleodcholithiasis, with sensitivities of 90% to 100% and specificities of 92% to 100% and negative predictive values of 96% to 100%.[24] MRCP and MRI of the liver are now the modality of choice to clarify biliary anatomy, with T2-weighted MRCP being the modality of choice for this purpose. T1-weighted imaging of the liver with hepatobiliary agents such as gadolinium ethoxybenzyl diethylenetriamine pentaacetic acid (known commercially as Primovist and Eovist) has also been used to generate images of the biliary tree and to clarify biliary anatomy. Although not in common use for this purpose, it may improve second-order bile duct visualization and the prediction of the number of bile duct orifices in live donor liver transplantation.[25] Gadolinium-enhanced T1-weighted imaging of the abdomen is a sensitive means of diagnosing benign and malignant conditions of the gallbladder and biliary systems.[26]

Endoscopic retrograde cholangiopancreatography and percutaneous transhepatic cholangiography
Introduced in 1968, ERCP is an invasive technique of imaging the biliary tree that is at the core of diagnosis and treatment of both benign and malignant conditions of the biliary tree. ERCP is associated with procedural risks such as pancreatitis, which occurs in 3% to 10% of patients, perforation, and hemhorrage.[27] With the rising popularity of noninvasive imaging modalities of the biliary tree such as MRCP, it is therefore no surprise that ERCP has taken on a more prominent role as a therapeutic

and interventional modality rather than the first-line imaging modality. ERCP provides a luminal view of the biliary tree, with no anatomic detail of surrounding vascular structures. For example, although the branching pattern of the biliary tree can be clarified, it cannot yield any information regarding variant relationship of the bile ducts to the portal vein branches. Cholangiographic images can also be obtained by percutaneous transhepatic cholangiography, another invasive technique wherein the bile ducts are accessed percutaneously under ultrasound and x-ray guidance, and similarly to ERCP offer a luminal view of the biliary tree. These invasive techniques give access to the biliary tree for interventions such as the relief of malignant obstruction, the dilatation of biliary strictures, and biliary drainage.

In the intraoperative context, a direct cholangiogram can be a valuable tool to clarify the anatomy and integrity of the biliary tree before, for example, amputating a structure identified as the cystic duct. This is performed using a cholangiogram catheter inserted through a small ductotomy, with radiopaque contrast injection and x-ray imaging of the liver and extrahepatic biliary tree. An adequate cholangiogram demonstrates the contrast entering the duodenum inferiorly and filling the second-order biliary radicals into the liver, with no overlying obscuring radiopaque objects. In some instances, filling of the intrahepatic biliary tree is facilitated by placing the patient in a Trendelenburg position. Intraoperative cholangiograms are a popular, if not divisive, adjunctive method used by some surgeons to mitigate the risk of a bile duct injury.[28]

REFERENCES

1. Roskams T, Desmet V. Embryology of extra- and intrahepatic bile ducts, the ductal plate. Anat Rec (Hoboken) 2008;291(6):628–35.
2. Severn CB. A morphological study of the development of the human liver. II. Establishment of liver parenchyma, extrahepatic ducts and associated venous channels. Am J Anat 1972;133(1):85–107.
3. Tan CE, Moscoso GJ. The developing human biliary system at the porta hepatis level between 29 days and 8 weeks of gestation: a way to understanding biliary atresia. Part 1. Pathol Int 1994;44(8):587–99.
4. Van Eyken P, Sciot R, Callea F, et al. The development of the intrahepatic bile ducts in man: a keratin-immunohistochemical study. Hepatology 1988;8(6):1586–95.
5. Tan CE, Moscoso GJ. The developing human biliary system at the porta hepatis level between 11 and 25 weeks of gestation: a way to understanding biliary atresia. Part 2. Pathol Int 1994;44(8):600–10.
6. Blankenberg TA, Lund JK, Ruebner BH. Normal and abnormal development of human intrahepatic bile ducts. An immunohistochemical perspective. Perspect Pediatr Pathol 1991;14:143–67.
7. Reichert PR, Renz JF, D'Albuquerque LAC, et al. Surgical anatomy of the left lateral segment as applied to living-donor and split-liver transplantation: a clinicopathologic study. Ann Surg 2000;232(5):658–64.
8. Abu Hilal M, Aldrighetti L, Dagher I, et al. The Southampton consensus guidelines for laparoscopic liver surgery: from indication to implementation. Ann Surg 2018;268(1):11–8.
9. Kitamura H, Mori T, Arai M, et al. Caudal left hepatic duct in relation to the umbilical portion of the portal vein. Hepatogastroenterology 1999;46(28):2511–4.
10. Ozden I, Kamiya J, Nagino M, et al. Clinicoanatomical study on the infraportal bile ducts of segment 3. World J Surg 2002;26(12):1441–5.

11. Varotti G, Gondolesi GE, Goldman J, et al. Anatomic variations in right liver living donors11No competing interests declared. J Am Coll Surg 2004;198(4):577–82.
12. Nakamura T, Tanaka K, Kiuchi T, et al. Anatomical variations and surgical strategies in right lobe living donor liver transplantation: lessons from 120 cases. Transplantation 2002;73(12):1896–903.
13. Kitami M, Murakami G, Ko S, et al. Spiegel's lobe bile ducts often drain into the right hepatic duct or its branches: study using drip-infusion cholangiography-computed tomography in 179 consecutive patients. World J Surg 2004;28(10): 1001–6.
14. Nishitai R, Shindoh J, Yamaoka T, et al. Biliary architecture of livers exhibiting right-sided ligamentum teres: an indication for preoperative cholangiography prior to major hepatectomy. HPB (Oxford) 2016;18(11):929–35.
15. Strasberg SM, Brunt LM. Rationale and use of the critical view of safety in laparoscopic cholecystectomy. J Am Coll Surg 2010;211(1):132–8.
16. Darnis B, Mohkam K, Cauchy F, et al. A systematic review of the anatomical findings of multiple gallbladders. HPB (Oxford) 2018;20(11):985–91.
17. Harlaftis N, Gray SW, Skandalakis JE. Multiple gallbladders. Surg Gynecol Obstet 1977;145(6):928–34.
18. Shindoh J, Akahane M, Satou S, et al. Vascular architecture in anomalous right-sided ligamentum teres: three-dimensional analyses in 35 patients. HPB (Oxford) 2012;14(1):32–41.
19. Ishii H, Noguchi A, Onishi M, et al. True left-sided gallbladder with variations of bile duct and cholecystic vein. World J Gastroenterol 2015;21(21):6754–8.
20. Alibrahim E, Gibson RN, Vincent J, et al. Spiral computed tomography-intravenous cholangiography with three-dimensional reconstructions for imaging the biliary tree. Australas Radiol 2006;50(2):136–42.
21. Ziessman HA. Hepatobiliary scintigraphy in 2014. J Nucl Med 2014;55(6): 967–75.
22. Rose JB, Fields RC, Strasberg SM. Poor reproducibility of gallbladder ejection fraction by biliary scintigraphy for diagnosis of biliary dyskinesia. J Am Coll Surg 2018;226(2):155–9.
23. Ziessman HA. Sincalide cholescintigraphy–32 years later: evidence-based data on its clinical utility and infusion methodology. Semin Nucl Med 2012;42(2):79–83.
24. Fulcher AS, Turner MA. MR cholangiopancreatography. Radiol Clin North Am 2002;40(6):1363–76.
25. Cai L, Yeh BM, Westphalen AC, et al. 3D T2-weighted and Gd-EOB-DTPA-enhanced 3D T1-weighted MR cholangiography for evaluation of biliary anatomy in living liver donors. Abdom Radiol (NY) 2017;42(3):842–50.
26. Gore RM, Yaghmai V, Newmark GM, et al. Imaging benign and malignant disease of the gallbladder. Radiol Clin North Am 2002;40(6):1307–23.
27. Anderson MA, Fisher L, Jain R, et al. Complications of ERCP. Gastrointest Endosc 2012;75(3):467–73.
28. Flum DR, Dellinger E, Cheadle A, et al. Intraoperative cholangiography and risk of common bile duct injury during cholecystectomy. JAMA 2003;289(13):1639–44.

Cholangitis
Causes, Diagnosis, and Management

Jesse K. Sulzer, MD, PhD[a], Lee M. Ocuin, MD[a,b],*

KEYWORDS

- Acute cholangitis • Biliary obstruction • Choledocholithiasis • Biliary infection

KEY POINTS

- Improvements in endoscopic management and critical care have decreased mortality from acute cholangitis but the disease remains lethal.
- Knowledge of advancements in drainage techniques being used in biliary drainage during acute cholangitis can improve care.
- Modern diagnostic schemes and treatment algorithms can reduce mortality from acute cholangitis.

INTRODUCTION

Acute cholangitis has long been recognized as a potentially lethal medical emergency characterized by obstruction and subsequent infection of the biliary tree.[1] Before recent advancements in critical care, diagnostic modalities and strategies, and expansion of less invasive means by which to decompress the bile duct system, mortality was reported to be more than 50% for acute cholangitis.[2,3] Utilization of these new tools in the diagnosis and care of patients with acute cholangitis have contributed to a significant decrease in mortality from this disease. The significant decrease in mortality emphasizes the importance of early and accurate diagnosis and proper selection and timing of interventions when needed. A working knowledge of common etiologies and updated diagnostic criteria can enable the practitioner to not only make this critical diagnosis early but appropriately assess the severity of the disease process and thus the urgency and scope of interventions.

Disclosures: The authors have nothing to disclose.
[a] Division of Hepatopancreatobiliary Surgery, Department of Surgery, Atrium Health/Carolinas Medical Center, Charlotte, NC, USA; [b] Division of Hepatopancreatobiliary Surgery, Atrium Health/Carolinas Medical Center – Northeast, 200 Medical Park Drive, Suite 430, Concord, NC 28025, USA
* Corresponding author. Division of Hepatopancreatobiliary Surgery, Atrium Health/Carolinas Medical Center – Northeast, 200 Medical Park Drive, Suite 430, Concord, NC 28025.
E-mail address: lee.ocuin@atriumhealth.org

Surg Clin N Am 99 (2019) 175–184
https://doi.org/10.1016/j.suc.2018.11.002
0039-6109/19/© 2018 Elsevier Inc. All rights reserved.

CAUSES
Pathophysiology

Partial or complete obstruction of the bile duct and subsequent infection is the key factor in the development of acute cholangitis.[4] Under normal circumstances, the continuous flow of bile and immunologic defenses of the biliary epithelial cells keep the biliary tree sterile. Obstruction and the resulting increase in bile duct pressure to greater than 25 cm H_2O can lead to a breakdown of these defenses and subsequent infection and septicemia from bacterial translocation into the bloodstream.[5,6] Seeding of the biliary tree can occur via retrograde entry of bacteria from the gastrointestinal track or the portal vein.[7] The impact of retrograde infection of the biliary tree is evidenced by the fact that higher positive bile duct culture rates are observed in cases of partial obstruction when compared with complete obstruction.[8] Gram-negative bacteria, including *Escherichia coli* and *Klebsiella pneumoniae,* are the most commonly identified bacteria in acute cholangitis.[9] In patients with indwelling stents, *Enterococcus* species are the most commonly detected bacteria, and high rates of *Candida* species are also reported.[10]

Etiology of Obstruction

There are multiple disease processes that can result in biliary obstruction with resultant cholangitis (**Box 1**). Benign etiologies include stone-related disease and resultant complications, and strictures related to chronic pancreatitis, prior biliary surgery, and primary sclerosing cholangitis. Biliary obstruction most commonly occurs from choledocholithiasis, representing roughly half of cases.[11] Mirizzi syndrome, defined by obstruction of the extrahepatic bile ducts by a gallstone in the neck of the gallbladder or cystic duct, has also been reported as a cause of acute cholangitis.[12] Malignant etiologies include biliary strictures related to periampullary cancers, hilar cholangiocarcinoma, or gallbladder cancers. Acute cholangitis resulting from malignant obstruction accounts for 10% to 30% of cases.[8] Endoluminal or percutaneous instrumentation of the biliary tree is another known risk factor for development of acute cholangitis. Complications have decreased significantly following endoscopic biliary procedures, and acute cholangitis following these procedures represents 0.5% to

---

Box 1
Causes of acute cholangitis

- Benign
  - Choledocholithiasis
  - Benign biliary stricture
  - Congenital abnormalities
  - Postoperative stricture
  - Pancreatitis

- Malignant
  - Bile duct cancer
  - Gallbladder cancer
  - Pancreatic cancer
  - Ampullary cancer
  - Duodenal cancer

- Other
  - Autoimmune/inflammatory disease
  - External compression (Mirizzi/Lemel syndromes)
  - Sump syndrome

2.4% of cases.[13] Infrequent causes of obstruction and cholangitis include duodenal diverticula, which can cause mechanical obstruction of the common bile duct (Lemmel syndrome),[14,15] parasitic infections, acquired immunodeficiency syndrome cholangiopathy, and autoimmune/immunoglobulin G4–associated cholangitis.[16]

DIAGNOSIS
Diagnostic Criteria

Numerous definitions and diagnostic criteria exist to establish a diagnosis of acute cholangitis. These range from purely clinical approaches encompassing the Charcot triad (fever, right upper quadrant pain, and jaundice), to greater focus on documentation of biliary obstruction.[17] The Tokyo Guidelines have attempted to establish a common definition and diagnostic criteria consisting of a mix of clinical, laboratory, and imaging findings (**Box 2**).[18]

Clinical Presentation

Fever and right upper quadrant pain are the most common presenting symptoms and occur in patients 80% of the time.[19] Jaundice, the third component of the traditionally taught Charcot triad, is observed in 60% to 70% of cases.[17,19] The Charcot triad has been reported to have high specificity (95.9%) but lacks sensitivity (26.4%) for acute cholangitis.[17,20] A 2017 study by Kiriyama and colleagues[21] that included more than 6000 patients with acute cholangitis found the Charcot triad to be positive only 21.2% of the time. Likewise, the Reynold pentad (Charcot triad plus septic shock and mental status changes) has been reported to be found in only 4% to 8% of patients with severe cholangitis.[17] The Tokyo Guidelines (see **Box 2**), originally published in 2007 and revised in 2013 and 2018, have attempted to provide an additional data-driven diagnostic framework for the clinical diagnosis of acute cholangitis.[21,22] The Tokyo Guidelines retain the presence of the Charcot triad as a definitive diagnostic criterion. However, given the variable presentation of this clinical constellation, the guidelines incorporate the addition of laboratory and imaging findings consistent with biliary obstruction in the diagnostic criteria.[8,22] The Tokyo Guidelines have been shown to provide accurate diagnosis on 90% of cases.[21]

Box 2
Diagnostic criteria

A. Systemic inflammation
  - A-1. Fever higher than 38°
  - A-2. Laboratory evidence of inflammation (white blood cell count <4 or >10, C-reactive protein >1)

B. Cholestasis
  - B-1. Jaundice (Total bilirubin >2 mg/dL)
  - B-2. Abnormal liver function tests (elevation > 1.5 × Standard deviation of alkaline phosphatase, glutamate pyruvate transaminase, aspartate aminotransferase, or alanine aminotransferase)

C. Imaging
  - C-1. Biliary dilation
  - C-2. Evidence of etiology of obstruction

Suspected diagnosis: One item in A + 1 item in either B or C.
Definite diagnosis: One item in A, 1 item in B, and 1 item in C.
From Kiriyama S, Takada T, Strasberg SM, et al. TG13 guidelines for diagnosis and severity grading of acute cholangitis (with videos). J Hepatobiliary Pancreat Sci 2013;20:28; with permission.

Laboratory Findings

Laboratory tests consistently associated with acute cholangitis include white blood cell count greater than 10×10^9/L and elevated blood levels of bilirubin, alkaline phosphatase, aspartate aminotransferase and alanine aminotransferase, and these tests should be routinely sent in all suspected cases.[11,17,19] Alkaline phosphatase is the most consistently elevated marker, with elevations found in 74% to 93% of cases of acute cholangitis. Alkaline phosphatase also exhibits a quicker recovery pattern following successful drainage than other markers of obstruction, such as bilirubin, and may provide a more accurate early indicator of adequate drainage.[23] Other laboratory findings, such as elevated amylase and prothrombin time, have been more variable.[19] The tumor marker carbohydrate antigen 19-9 (CA19-9) has been reported with a broad range of both frequency and values,[24–26] and high levels (>9000 IU/mL) have been observed in confirmed cases of cholangitis with rapid resolution following successful treatment.[26] We do not recommend routine analysis of amylase, prothrombin time, or CA19-9 in context of workup and management of acute cholangitis. Elevation of additional markers of inflammation/infection, including C-reactive protein and procalcitonin, are regularly observed and values can provide additional guidance on choice of therapeutic interventions and for prognosis. Procalcitonin has recently received much attention in the diagnosis of and management of sepsis. In cases of acute cholangitis, procalcitonin has been shown to be a more accurate predictor of severe disease than conventional biomarkers.[27] Furthermore, high procalcitonin levels have the potential to expose the need to perform emergency decompression in cases that may otherwise not be classified as severe based on other clinical data.[28–30]

Blood cultures are often collected as part of the initial investigation in patients with suspected infection. Positive blood cultures in acute cholangitis have been reported over a range from 21% to 71% of cases.[22] However, these positive cultures most often do not provide additional clinically relevant information in routine cases of community-acquired intra-abdominal infection.[31] A study of the impact of blood cultures taken in the emergency department for patients with suspected infection found that positive cultures resulted in changes to clinical management in a small minority of cases.[32] Thus, both the Tokyo Guidelines and the Guidelines by the Surgical Infection Society/Infectious Diseases Society of America do not routinely recommend blood cultures.[31,33] An exception to this is the toxic or immunocompromised patient or in high-severity infections when culture results may change therapy or guide duration.

Imaging

Initial radiographic studies rely on indirect findings of bile duct obstruction in support of the diagnosis of acute cholangitis. Transabdominal ultrasound is often a first-line diagnostic study, given its ready availability and low cost. Findings of biliary ductal dilation can support the diagnosis, but sensitivity for detection of common bile duct stones is less than 30%.[20] Contrast-enhanced computed tomography (CT) scan also can provide indirect support for the diagnosis of cholangitis in suspected cases, including findings of biliary stones, ductal dilation, hepatic abscess, or pneumobilia.[18] The ability of CT to detect stones in the biliary tree has been reported at 42%.[5] Hepatic parenchymal changes have been noted as a more specific finding of acute cholangitis. Inhomogeneous hepatic parenchymal enhancement caused by a decrease in portal blood flow is observed in acute cholangitis.[34] In addition, CT allows for evaluation of the entire liver, enabling diagnosis of complications of cholangitis, such as liver abscesses. MRI/magnetic resonance cholangiopancreatography (MRCP) provides another noninvasive diagnostic method. MRCP has been demonstrated to reveal ductal pathology in acute cholangitis in more than 80% of cases but is limited in its sensitivity to detect stones smaller than 6 mm.[5]

Endoscopic ultrasound (EUS) and endoscopic retrograde cholangiopancreatography (ERCP) are invasive tests that can provide additional diagnostic information. ERCP has the additional advantage of allowing for therapeutic intervention. EUS has a sensitivity approaching 100% and a specificity of more than 90%, with an overall accuracy of 96.9% for the detection of bile duct stones.[35,36] EUS has the advantage of portability and the possibility of performing ERCP during the same session.[37] Purulence emanating from the major papilla encountered on ERCP remains the gold standard for diagnosis of acute cholangitis.[20] Furthermore, ERCP may elucidate additional information regarding the etiology of the episode and allows for therapeutic intervention.[5]

Grading

The Tokyo Guidelines divide acute cholangitis into 3 grades (**Box 3**): mild (grade I), moderate (grade II), and severe (grade III). The grades are defined by initial response to medical treatment and associated organ dysfunction. Grade I acute cholangitis is defined by response to initial medical treatment. Grade II acute cholangitis does not respond to initial medical treatment but is not associated with additional organ dysfunction. Grade III acute cholangitis is associated with organ dysfunction. Accurate diagnosis and grading can assist with prognosis and help guide management. Mortality has been demonstrated to increase significantly with rising severity staging ranging from 1% in grade I to 5% or more in grade III.[17,18]

MANAGEMENT
Antibiotics

Aggressive resuscitation and early antibiotic administration remain the initial therapeutic steps in cases of suspected or confirmed acute cholangitis.[38,39] Antibiotics are administered to limit systemic sepsis and local inflammation as well as complications associated with acute cholangitis, such as intrahepatic abscess formation.[33] Current guidelines recommend initial treatment with a penicillin/beta-lactamase inhibitor, third-generation cephalosporin, or carbapenem.[33,38] Regional variations in the microbiology profile and drug-resistance patterns can further guide antibiotic selection. In patients with indwelling biliary stents or with other potential for hospital-acquired infection, it is reasonable to add antifungal coverage, and bile culture with Gram stain should be obtained when possible to guide the antimicrobial regimen.[9,33]

Box 3
Severity grading

- Grade I
  - Responds to initial medical management

- Grade II
  - Does not respond to initial medical treatment but without evidence of organ dysfunction

- Grade III
  - Acute cholangitis associated with evidence of organ dysfunction defined as follows:
    - Hypotension requiring pressor use
    - Altered mental status
    - Pao_2/Fio_2 ratio less than 300
    - Acute kidney injury
    - Prothrombin time–international normalized ratio greater than 1.5
    - Thrombocytopenia

Drainage Procedures

Biliary drainage is recommended for all but the mildest cases of acute cholangitis that respond effectively to antibiotics and supportive care. Drainage can be accomplished endoscopically, percutaneously, or surgically. In addition to improvements in care of the septic patient, advances in endoscopic biliary drainage have been credited with the decrease in mortality from acute cholangitis.[40]

Endoscopic Retrograde Cholangiopancreatography

Endoscopic transpapillary biliary drainage should be first-line therapy for decompression in acute cholangitis. This can be accomplished by endoscopic biliary stenting or placement of a nasobiliary tube. Several studies have demonstrated clinical equivalence between these 2 techniques but increased patient discomfort and greater electrolyte abnormalities in patients who underwent nasobiliary drainage.[41,42] Advantages of the nasobiliary approach include continued monitoring of bile output and ability for flushing of purulent bile. Endoscopic biliary stenting involves placement of a 7-Fr to 10-Fr plastic stent after selective biliary cannulation to provide internal drainage. This can be performed alone as a drainage procedure or with other interventions to clear the bile duct of stones in cases of choledocholithiasis.[40]

Endoscopic sphincterotomy, commonly performed for stone extraction, can be used as an adjunct to stent placement. When performed before large-bore stent placement, sphincterotomy can possibly prevent occlusion of the pancreatic duct and had been suggested to help prevent post-ERCP pancreatitis. Studies have failed to demonstrate any difference unless multiple stents are required; however, with post-ERCP pancreatitis rates of 3% to 4% following ERCP whether sphincterotomy was performed or not.[43] Sphincterotomy when performed at the time of biliary drainage can decrease the duration of symptoms and hospital stay.[44] A major concern with performing endoscopic sphincterotomy is bleeding. The combination of severe sepsis, biliary obstruction, and hepatic dysfunction in acute cholangitis can lead to increased rates of hemorrhage following sphincterotomy.[45] This increased risk has been demonstrated in the absence of any associated coagulopathy.[46] The Tokyo Guidelines recommend against sphincterotomy in severe acute cholangitis, reserving sphincterotomy and stone extraction combined with biliary drainage for patients with mild or moderate disease.[40]

Percutaneous transhepatic cholangiography

Percutaneous transhepatic cholangiography (PTC) is an additional safe and effective technique for biliary drainage. It is currently considered second-line therapy after failed ERCP, in the setting of surgically altered anatomy, or when a therapeutic endoscopist is not available.[47] Procedural success has been reported at 95% with dilated hepatic ducts and at 70% with nondilated ducts. Internal drainage and stone removal have technical success rates of 90% following successful cannulation.[48] Complications of PTC, including sepsis, hemorrhage, peritonitis, and pancreatitis, have been reported in 1.2% to 2.5% of patients.[49]

Endoscopic Ultrasound–Guided Biliary Drainage

In cases when endoscopic access to the ampulla is not possible, either from altered surgical anatomy or failed cannulation, an alternative to ERCP is endoscopic ultrasound–guided biliary drainage (EUS-BD). This approach has been used to attempt to limit the potential complications associated with PTC. EUS-BD can be accomplished in several ways, including transgastric or transjejunal intrahepatic biliary drainage, transduodenal or transgastric extrahepatic biliary drainage, or EUS-guided antegrade stenting. The multiple approaches can be tailored to the patient's pathology. Meta-analysis of EUS-BD studies demonstrates a high technical and functional success rate. Importantly, a success rate of more than 90% was achieved in high-volume centers following failed ERCP.[50] The procedure is associated with an adverse event rate of 25%, with hemorrhage and bile leak being the most common morbidities. Other serious complications have been reported, including perforation and sepsis. It is therefore recommended to reserve EUS-BD for cases in which ERCP has failed, and it should be performed only by a therapeutic endoscopist trained in the technique.[20,40]

Surgical Drainage

Open surgical drainage was once the mainstay of treatment of biliary obstruction and cholangitis, but currently has no role in the treatment of severe acute cholangitis. A randomized trial by Lai and colleagues[51] that compared ERCP with surgical decompression demonstrated a significantly higher rate of complications (66% vs 34%) and mortality (32% vs 10%) in the surgical drainage group. Endoscopic and percutaneous biliary drainage have since remained first-line and second-line therapeutic choices, with open surgical drainage as a last resort. Recently there has been an increased interest in early laparoscopic common duct exploration with cholecystectomy.[52] Studies have demonstrated feasibility of this approach, although current recommendations reserve this approach only for nonsevere acute cholangitis.[53]

Drainage in the Setting of Surgically Altered Anatomy

Patients with surgically altered anatomy, such as after a Roux-en-Y gastric bypass, present a unique challenge for nonsurgical drainage of the biliary tree. Several approaches have been devised to circumvent the altered anatomy, including balloon enteroscopy–assisted ERCP, EUS-BD, and transgastric ERCP. Balloon enteroscopy–assisted ERCP is the first-line recommendation in the Tokyo Guidelines.[40] PTC, EUS-BD, and laparoscopic common bile duct exploration can provide additional techniques when there is no available therapeutic endoscopist or when balloon enteroscopy–assisted ERCP fails.

SUMMARY

A thorough understanding of the etiology and pathophysiology of acute cholangitis coupled with utilization of modern diagnostic schema can assist the practitioner in making this urgent diagnosis in an accurate and timely fashion. Furthermore, evolving methods of biliary drainage add to the armamentarium available to prevent mortality in this potentially lethal disease. Further ongoing refinements of these diagnostic and prognostic criteria will continue to aid in targeted intervention and reduction in patient morbidity and mortality.

REFERENCES

1. Lipsett PA, Pitt HA. Acute cholangitis. Front Biosci 2003;8:s1229–39.
2. Andrew DJ, Johnson SE. Acute suppurative cholangitis, a medical and surgical emergency. A review of ten years experience emphasizing early recognition. Am J Gastroenterol 1970;54(2):141–54.
3. Shimada H, Nakagawara G, Kobayashi M, et al. Pathogenesis and clinical features of acute cholangitis accompanied by shock. Jpn J Surg 1984;14(4):269–77.
4. Reynolds BM, Dargan EL. Acute obstructive cholangitis; a distinct clinical syndrome. Ann Surg 1959;150(2):299–303.

5. Buyukasik K, Toros AB, Bektas H, et al. Diagnostic and therapeutic value of ERCP in acute cholangitis. ISRN Gastroenterol 2013;2013:191729.
6. Leung JW, Ling TK, Chan RC, et al. Antibiotics, biliary sepsis, and bile duct stones. Gastrointest Endosc 1994;40(6):716–21.
7. Ahmed M. Acute cholangitis - an update. World J Gastrointest Pathophysiol 2018; 9(1):1–7.
8. Kimura Y, Takada T, Kawarada Y, et al. Definitions, pathophysiology, and epidemiology of acute cholangitis and cholecystitis: Tokyo Guidelines. J Hepatobiliary Pancreat Surg 2007;14(1):15–26.
9. Reuken PA, Torres D, Baier M, et al. Risk factors for multi-drug resistant pathogens and failure of empiric first-line therapy in acute cholangitis. PLoS One 2017;12(1):e0169900.
10. Lübbert C, Wendt K, Feisthammel J, et al. Epidemiology and resistance patterns of bacterial and fungal colonization of biliary plastic stents: a prospective cohort study. PLoS One 2016;11(5):e0155479.
11. Gigot JF, Leese T, Dereme T, et al. Acute cholangitis. Multivariate analysis of risk factors. Ann Surg 1989;209(4):435–8.
12. Beltrán MA. Mirizzi syndrome: history, current knowledge and proposal of a simplified classification. World J Gastroenterol 2012;18(34):4639–50.
13. Kimura Y, Takada T, Strasberg SM, et al. TG13 current terminology, etiology, and epidemiology of acute cholangitis and cholecystitis. J Hepatobiliary Pancreat Sci 2013;20(1):8–23.
14. Desai K, Wermers JD, Beteselassie N. Lemmel syndrome secondary to duodenal diverticulitis: a case report. Cureus 2017;9(3):e1066.
15. Kang HS, Hyun JJ, Kim SY, et al. Lemmel's syndrome, an unusual cause of abdominal pain and jaundice by impacted intradiverticular enterolith: case report. J Korean Med Sci 2014;29(6):874–8.
16. Lim JH. Liver flukes: the malady neglected. Korean J Radiol 2011;12(3):269–79.
17. Wada K, Takada T, Kawarada Y, et al. Diagnostic criteria and severity assessment of acute cholangitis: Tokyo guidelines. J Hepatobiliary Pancreat Surg 2007;14(1): 52–8.
18. Kiriyama S, Kozaka K, Takada T, et al. Tokyo guidelines 2018: diagnostic criteria and severity grading of acute cholangitis (with videos). J Hepatobiliary Pancreat Sci 2018;25(1):17–30.
19. Boey JH, Way LW. Acute cholangitis. Ann Surg 1980;191(3):264–70.
20. Ramchandani M, Pal P, Reddy DN. Endoscopic management of acute cholangitis as a result of common bile duct stones. Dig Endosc 2017;29(Suppl 2):78–87.
21. Kiriyama S, Takada T, Hwang TL, et al. Clinical application and verification of the TG13 diagnostic and severity grading criteria for acute cholangitis: an international multicenter observational study. J Hepatobiliary Pancreat Sci 2017;24(6): 329–37.
22. Takada T, Strasberg SM, Solomkin JS, et al. TG13: updated Tokyo guidelines for the management of acute cholangitis and cholecystitis. J Hepatobiliary Pancreat Sci 2013;20(1):1–7.
23. Watanapa P. Recovery patterns of liver function after complete and partial surgical biliary decompression. Am J Surg 1996;171(2):230–4.
24. Ker CG, Chen JS, Lee KT, et al. Assessment of serum and bile levels of CA19-9 and CA125 in cholangitis and bile duct carcinoma. J Gastroenterol Hepatol 1991; 6(5):505–8.
25. Albert MB, Steinberg WM, Henry JP. Elevated serum levels of tumor marker CA19-9 in acute cholangitis. Dig Dis Sci 1988;33(10):1223–5.

26. Korkmaz M, Ünal H, Selçuk H, et al. Extraordinarily elevated serum levels of CA 19-9 and rapid decrease after successful therapy: a case report and review of literature. Turk J Gastroenterol 2010;21(4):461–3.
27. Umefune G, Kogure H, Hamada T, et al. Procalcitonin is a useful biomarker to predict severe acute cholangitis: a single-center prospective study. J Gastroenterol 2017;52(6):734–45.
28. Shinya S, Sasaki T, Yamashita Y, et al. Procalcitonin as a useful biomarker for determining the need to perform emergency biliary drainage in cases of acute cholangitis. J Hepatobiliary Pancreat Sci 2014;21(10):777–85.
29. Shah T, Zfass A. Predicting cholangitis with procalcitonin: procrastinate or procedure? Dig Dis Sci 2018. https://doi.org/10.1007/s10620-018-5098-0.
30. Lee YS, Cho KB, Park KS, et al. Procalcitonin as a decision-supporting marker of urgent biliary decompression in acute cholangitis. Dig Dis Sci 2018;63(9): 2474–9.
31. Solomkin JS, Mazuski JE, Bradley JS, et al. Diagnosis and management of complicated intra-abdominal infection in adults and children: guidelines by the Surgical Infection Society and the Infectious Diseases Society of America. Clin Infect Dis 2010;50(2):133–64.
32. Kelly AM. Clinical impact of blood cultures taken in the emergency department. J Accid Emerg Med 1998;15(4):254–6.
33. Gomi H, Solomkin JS, Schlossberg D, et al. Tokyo guidelines 2018: antimicrobial therapy for acute cholangitis and cholecystitis. J Hepatobiliary Pancreat Sci 2018;25(1):3–16.
34. Arai K, Kawai K, Kohda W, et al. Dynamic CT of acute cholangitis: early inhomogeneous enhancement of the liver. AJR Am J Roentgenol 2003;181(1):115–8.
35. Meeralam Y, Al-Shammari K, Yaghoobi M. Diagnostic accuracy of EUS compared with MRCP in detecting choledocholithiasis: a meta-analysis of diagnostic test accuracy in head-to-head studies. Gastrointest Endosc 2017;86(6):986–93.
36. de Lédinghen V, Lecesne R, Raymond JM, et al. Diagnosis of choledocholithiasis: EUS or magnetic resonance cholangiography? A prospective controlled study. Gastrointest Endosc 1999;49(1):26–31.
37. Chen YI, Martel M, Barkun AN. Choledocholithiasis: should EUS replace MRCP in patients at intermediate risk? Gastrointest Endosc 2017;86(6):994–6.
38. Okamoto K, Takada T, Strasberg SM, et al. TG13 management bundles for acute cholangitis and cholecystitis. J Hepatobiliary Pancreat Sci 2013;20(1):55–9.
39. Mayumi T, Okamoto K, Takada T, et al. Tokyo guidelines 2018: management bundles for acute cholangitis and cholecystitis. J Hepatobiliary Pancreat Sci 2018; 25(1):96–100.
40. Mukai S, Itoi T, Baron TH, et al. Indications and techniques of biliary drainage for acute cholangitis in updated Tokyo guidelines 2018. J Hepatobiliary Pancreat Sci 2017;24(10):537–49.
41. Lee DW, Chan AC, Lam YH, et al. Biliary decompression by nasobiliary catheter or biliary stent in acute suppurative cholangitis: a prospective randomized trial. Gastrointest Endosc 2002;56(3):361–5.
42. Park SY, Park CH, Cho SB, et al. The safety and effectiveness of endoscopic biliary decompression by plastic stent placement in acute suppurative cholangitis compared with nasobiliary drainage. Gastrointest Endosc 2008;68(6): 1076–80.
43. Tarnasky PR, Cunningham JT, Hawes RH, et al. Transpapillary stenting of proximal biliary strictures: does biliary sphincterotomy reduce the risk of postprocedure pancreatitis? Gastrointest Endosc 1997;45(1):46–51.

44. Hui CK, Lai KC, Wong WM, et al. A randomised controlled trial of endoscopic sphincterotomy in acute cholangitis without common bile duct stones. Gut 2002;51(2):245–7.
45. Lee MH, Tsou YK, Lin CH, et al. Predictors of re-bleeding after endoscopic hemostasis for delayed post-endoscopic sphincterotomy bleeding. World J Gastroenterol 2016;22(11):3196–201.
46. Freeman ML. Complications of endoscopic retrograde cholangiopancreatography: avoidance and management. Gastrointest Endosc Clin N Am 2012;22(3): 567–86.
47. Itoi T, Tsuyuguchi T, Takada T, et al. TG13 indications and techniques for biliary drainage in acute cholangitis (with videos). J Hepatobiliary Pancreat Sci 2013; 20(1):71–80.
48. Saad WE, Wallace MJ, Wojak JC, et al. Quality improvement guidelines for percutaneous transhepatic cholangiography, biliary drainage, and percutaneous cholecystostomy. J Vasc Interv Radiol 2010;21(6):789–95.
49. Burke DR, Lewis CA, Cardella JF, et al. Quality improvement guidelines for percutaneous transhepatic cholangiography and biliary drainage. J Vasc Interv Radiol 2003;14(9 Pt 2):S243–6.
50. Wang K, Zhu J, Xing L, et al. Assessment of efficacy and safety of EUS-guided biliary drainage: a systematic review. Gastrointest Endosc 2016;83(6):1218–27.
51. Lai EC, Mok FP, Tan ES, et al. Endoscopic biliary drainage for severe acute cholangitis. N Engl J Med 1992;326(24):1582–6.
52. Sun Z, Zhu Y, Zhu B, et al. Controversy and progress for treatment of acute cholangitis after Tokyo Guidelines (TG13). Biosci Trends 2016;10(1):22–6.
53. Atstupens K, Plaudis H, Fokins V, et al. Safe laparoscopic clearance of the common bile duct in emergently admitted patients with choledocholithiasis and cholangitis. Korean J Hepatobiliary Pancreat Surg 2016;20(2):53–60.

Autoimmune Diseases of the Biliary Tract: A Review

Christina W. Lee, MD, Sean Ronnekleiv-Kelly, MD*

KEYWORDS

- Primary biliary cirrhosis • Primary sclerosing cholangitis
- IgG4-related sclerosing cholangitis • Biliary tract

KEY POINTS

- Autoimmune cholestatic liver diseases represent a small portion of hepatobiliary disorders characterized by a progressive, inflammatory destruction of bile ducts.
- Continued investigation is required for improved diagnosis and treatment of these cholestatic diseases.
- The medical management of autoimmune diseases of the biliary tract is limited to ursodeoxycholic acid for primary biliary cirrhosis (PBC) and primary sclerosing cholangitis (PSC), and corticosteroids for IgG4-related hepatobiliary disease.
- Liver transplantation remains the most definitive source of treatment of PBC and PSC with varying survival outcomes, influenced by the nature of disease and risk of recurrence post-transplantation.

INTRODUCTION

Autoimmune diseases of the biliary tract are broadly defined as progressive, immune reactive, and inflammatory diseases of the bile ducts. The three main forms of autoimmune biliary diseases include primary biliary cirrhosis (PBC), primary sclerosing cholangitis (PSC), and IgG4-related hepatobiliary diseases (IgG4-HBD). These represent a small proportion of hepatobiliary disorders among which, the molecular interactions with and subsequent dysregulation of hepatic immune homeostatic processes remain poorly understood. The clinical sequelae of disease include progressive obliteration of bile ducts, which is ultimately followed by cholestasis.[1]

The initial stages of disease are often asymptomatic. Laboratory abnormalities often prompt suspicion for cholestasis, characterized by elevated alkaline phosphatase (ALP) (>1.5 times the upper limit of normal) and/or elevated γ-glutamyltranspeptidase

The authors have nothing to disclose.
Division of Surgical Oncology, Department of Surgery, University of Wisconsin School of Medicine and Public Health, University of Wisconsin, 600 Highland Avenue, Madison, WI 53792, USA
* Corresponding author. Division of Surgical Oncology, University of Wisconsin, 600 Highland Avenue, BX 7375, K4/748 CSC, Madison, WI 53792.
E-mail address: ronnekleiv-kelly@surgery.wisc.edu

Surg Clin N Am 99 (2019) 185–201
https://doi.org/10.1016/j.suc.2018.11.003
0039-6109/19/Published by Elsevier Inc.

(>3 times the upper limit of normal).[1,2] Elevated hyperbilirubinemia often presents later in the course of disease. As with any disease, a complete and careful history and physical examination are essential, followed by imaging to further delineate extrahepatic and/or intrahepatic ductal anatomy. If imaging studies fail to demonstrate a cause of obstruction, serum testing for autoimmune antibodies and liver biopsy may be considered.

Autoimmune and immune-mediated hepatobiliary diseases have undoubtedly attracted increasing attention because of the significant effort in understanding the basic biologic mechanisms responsible for disease pathogenesis. In part, identification and recognition of diagnostic markers has led to an improved understanding of the clinical significance of disease.

CLINICAL PRESENTATION AND EPIDEMIOLOGY

There are various overlapping characteristics among PBC, PSC, and IgG4-related HBD, yet each disease presents within a distinct demographic group and distribution, requiring a disease-specific approach to diagnosis and work-up. **Table 1** provides a summary of disease-specific definitions, epidemiologic, and clinical findings reviewed in this article.

Primary Biliary Cirrhosis

PBC is the most common autoimmune disorder of the liver, characterized by a progressive, inflammatory destruction of small intrahepatic bile ducts resulting in cholestasis and fibrosis.[3] Hepatic cirrhosis and liver failure present as late-stage, untreated or refractory disease. PBC most commonly presents in patients between the ages of 40 and 50, with a significant female predominance (female to male ratio of 10:1).[3] The overall reported prevalence of PBC ranges from 19.1 to 40.2 cases per 100,000 people with higher rates in Europe and North America, in comparison with Asia.[4]

Clinical presentation

Up to 20% to 60% of cases are diagnosed in the absence of symptoms.[5] The most common symptoms accompanying PBC are fatigue and pruritis, which may also include hyperpigmentation, hepatosplenomegaly, and xanthelasmas.[6] Up to 70% of patients with PBC have been reported to present with other autoimmune-related syndromes, including Hashimoto disease, celiac disease, keratoconjunctivitis sicca, Raynaud phenomenon, and systemic sclerosis.[6] The most commonly associated syndromes are keratoconjunctivitis sicca and Raynaud phenomena, which has been detected in up to 75% and 32% of patients, respectively.[7,8]

Primary Sclerosing Cholangitis

PSC is a chronic, progressive cholestatic disease of the liver characterized by progressive, obliterative inflammation and fibrosis of the intrahepatic and extrahepatic bile ducts leading to cirrhosis.[9] The result, ultimately, is fibrosis and eventual decompensated cirrhosis over an approximate course of 10 to 15 years. The underlying mechanism of disease remains elusive at best, but is conceptualized as an immune-mediated disease as opposed to an autoimmune disease. By definition, the latter involves gender predilection, response to immunosuppressive medications, and highly selective pathogenic autoantibodies.[10]

Patients often present between 35 and 47 years of age, with a 62% to 70% male predilection.[11-15] A recent meta-analysis of population-based studies from Europe, the United Kingdom, Canada, and the United states reported a cumulative estimated

Table 1
Overview of biliary autoimmune diseases by definition, epidemiologic, and clinical presentations

Disease Type	Definition	Gender Predilection	Incidence	Clinical Presentation
Primary biliary cirrhosis	Autoimmune liver disease of progressive, inflammatory destruction of small intrahepatic biliary ducts	Female > male 10:1	19.1–40.2 cases per 100,000 persons	Presentation: Ages 40–50 y Often asymptomatic Most develop fatigue, pruritis, hyperpigmentation, hepatosplenomegaly, xanthelasmas Associated syndromes (<70%): Hashimoto disease, Raynaud syndrome, keratoconjunctivitis, celiac disease, systemic sclerosis
Primary sclerosing cholangitis	Chronic, progressive, immune-mediated, obliterative inflammatory process of intrahepatic and extrahepatic biliary ducts	Immune-mediated disease with a male predilection	0.9–13.6 cases per 100,000 persons	Presentation: Ages 35–47 y May be asymptomatic Develop right upper quadrant abdominal pain, bacterial cholangitis, fatigue, pruritis, jaundice, weight loss Associated syndromes: Highly associated with inflammatory bowel disease Highly regarded as a premalignant lesion for hepatobiliary and colorectal malignancy
IgG4-related sclerosing cholangitis	Multiorgan, steroid-responsive, immune-mediated, inflammatory mural lymphocytic infiltration of the bile duct	None	United States: unknown Asia: 0.9 per 100,000 persons	Presentation: Ages 60–70 y Painless, obstructive jaundice May develop abdominal pain, weight loss, steatorrhea, diabetes mellitus Associated diseases: Autoimmune pancreatitis

incidence of PSC to be 1 in 100,000 persons; the highest incidence is in Norway, where 1.3 in 100,000 persons is affected.[15] In the United states, the current age- and gender-adjusted incidence of PSC is approximately 0.9 per 100,000 persons and a prevalence of 13.6 in 100,000 persons.[13] The prevalence of PSC is approximately three times lower than that of PBC.[12] Among the most feared potential manifestations of PSC is the development of cholangiocarcinoma. Recent reports estimate

Table 2 Multisystem organ involvement in immunoglobulin G4-related hepatobiliary diseases	
Hepatobiliary Organs	**Extrahepatobiliary Organs**
Pancreas (autoimmune pancreatitis)	Salivary glands
Bile ducts	Periorbital tissues
Gallbladder	Lungs
	Lymphatics
	Skin
	Thyroid
	Vasculature (aorta)
	Breast
	Prostate
	Retroperitoneum (kidneys, ureter)

that cholangiocarcinoma occurs in 9% to 20% of individuals with PSC, wherein the annual estimated risk rests at the upper range of 1.5%.[16–18]

Clinical presentation

The dominant initial symptoms afflicting patients with PSC are pruritis and fatigue, which often progress toward abdominal pain, jaundice, and weight loss. Biliary strictures present in later stages of disease and confer fevers, chills, and right upper quadrant pain consistent with bacterial cholangitis.[19] Forty percent to 56% of patients, however, are asymptomatic at the time of diagnosis.[13] Incidental identification of biliary ductal dilation (intrahepatic and extrahepatic) on cross-sectional imaging and the investigation of serum laboratory abnormalities has contributed to the increased incidence of reported cases of PSC.[3] Among asymptomatic patients, the estimated survival without decompensated cirrhosis at 7 years is 75% compared with 96% for age- and gender-matched healthy individuals.[20]

Typically, elevated serum liver abnormalities present as increased ALP, aspartate aminotransferase, and alanine aminotransferase in the range of two to three times the upper limit of normal.[9] Additionally, various nonspecific autoantibodies have been correlated with PSC, such as antinuclear antibodies, anticardiolipin antibodies, thyroperoxidase, rheumatoid factor, and smooth muscle antibodies. Although the detection of these antibodies is not liver specific, the detection of these suggests an underlying immune dysregulation. Peripheral antineutrophil cytoplasmic antibodies have been detected in 30% to 80% of patients with PSC; however, they lack disease specificity.[21] None of the aforementioned autoantibodies carries clinical or pathologic significance to reflect disease severity or progression and are therefore not routinely used for PSC.

Immunoglobulin G4-Related Hepatobiliary Diseases

Immunoglobulin G4-related sclerosing cholangitis (ISC) is recognized as a hepatic presentation of a multiorgan, steroid responsive, immune-mediated inflammatory disease, characterized by its responsiveness to steroid therapy.[9,22] These inflammatory lesions are characterized by lymphocytic infiltration of the bile duct walls along the pancreaticobiliary tract, in addition to elevated IgG4 serum levels.[23] The term IgG4-related disease encompasses a spectrum of IgG4-related histopathologic features across numerous organ systems (**Table 2**). As such, more than one organ system may be affected at any one time, either simultaneously or in sequence. The histopathologic features across the various organ systems remain largely similar, consisting primarily of richly abundant IgG4-bearing cells, which tie these disease conditions together, in addition to elevated serum IgG4 levels.[23] At present, the pathophysiologic mechanisms underpinning ISC remain largely unknown.

Patients with ISC are predominantly male in their sixth to seventh decade of life.[9,24] Most (>50%) patients with ISC also have concurrent involvement of the pancreas, namely autoimmune pancreatitis (AIP).[9,25,26] Limited data exist on the incidence and prevalence of ISC in the United States. However, national data from Japan may serve as a starting estimate of its global distribution through the study of AIP, from which the estimated prevalence of AIP is reported as 2.2 per 100,000 inhabitants, and annual incidence rate of 0.9 per 100,000 persons.[27] At present, there remains a need to clarify whether prevalence rates between Asia and North America are similar or comparable.

Clinical presentation

Classically, most patients present with painless, obstructive jaundice. Other symptoms may include mild to moderate abdominal pain and weight loss.[22,25,28] Concurrent AIP may result in new-onset diabetes mellitus or steatorrhea.[22] An association with inflammatory bowel disease (IBD) is rare, whereas association with AIP is common.[24,26] IgG4-related sclerosing cholangitis is responsive to corticosteroids, and relapse is common following withdrawal.[9]

PATHOPHYSIOLOGY
Primary Biliary Cirrhosis

The geographic variation in incidence of PBC is highly suggestive of strong environmental influences on its development and progression. The pathophysiology of PBC remains incompletely understood and likely involves a complex combination of genetic and environmental factors. Early epidemiologic studies investigating genetic relationships among monozygotic twins (concordance rate of 63%) and families (4% incidence in first-degree relatives) suggest an association between PBC and HLA, and non-HLA variant genes.[29,30] For instance, HLA-DR 7 and 8 seem to be risk factors for PBC, whereas HLA-DR 11 and 13 seem to confer protection.[31] Recent data now confirm that most gene associations are derived from strong associations with HLAs, and more interestingly, several large-scale genome-wide association studies have identified up to 27 non-HLA loci associated with PBC susceptibility.[6,32]

Primary Sclerosing Cholangitis

Genetic, autoimmune, and environmental influences have been postulated as contributing causes in the pathogenesis of PSC. PSC is well known to be associated with IBD, namely ulcerative colitis, which often precedes the development of PSC and afflicts up to two-thirds of patients with PSC. A generally accepted theory of pathogenesis involves an environmental or infectious insult as an inciting event in a genetically predisposed individual, resulting in persistent stimulation of an immune-mediated destruction of bile ducts.[33] Commonly associated insults have been linked to gastrointestinal sources of infection, culminating into increased bacterial translocation across a compromised intestinal mucosal barrier.[34] This theory, in essence, relies on the dysregulation in gut immune homeostasis, which remains poorly understood. Increased bacterial translocation subsequently encourages gut-derived memory T lymphocytes to target cholangiocytes.[17,34] This concept is supported by data demonstrating a relative protective effect on PSC progression in transplanted liver patients who have undergone prior colectomy.[35] Proctocolectomy for ulcerative colitis does not alter the course of disease among patients with PSC, as evidenced in those who develop PSC several years following proctocolectomy.[17,19] Rather, these findings suggest a shared underlying inflammatory mechanism rooted in PSC and ulcerative colitis, as opposed to a sequential order in disease pathogenesis.

Genome-wide association studies have isolated genes unique to the process of cholangiocyte and intestinal barrier function among patients with PSC.[36,37] Specifically, HLA haplotypes, HLA-DR3 and HLA-B8, have shown strong associations with PSC.[37] Various non-HLA gene polymorphisms have also been linked to increased PSC susceptibility, namely those encoding intracellular adhesions molecule 1,[13] tumor necrosis factor,[38] and matrix metalloproteinase 3.[39] Within families, there is a pattern of clustering, which supports the genetic predisposition of PSC, along with a near 100-fold increased risk of PSC among first-degree relatives.[40]

Immunoglobulin G4-Related Hepatobiliary Diseases

Optimization of therapeutic strategies against ISC requires an appreciation of the pathophysiologic mechanisms leading to the multitude of organ systems afflicted by IgG4-related diseases. However, this remains largely unknown.

IgG4 antibodies are believed to exert anti-inflammatory properties. IgG4 distinguishes itself from other classes of IgG, namely its low capacity to induce complement activation and mediate proinflammatory responses.[41] IgG4 is unique because of its bispecificity characterized by its ability to exchange a single heavy and light chain pair with another pair complex, yet function as a single monovalent antibody.[42] To further obscure the clinical relevance of IgG4 levels, serum titers have been reported to remain elevated in ISC patients in clinical remission, suggesting that IgG4 antibodies may not be directly involved in the pathogenesis of ISC.[28] At present the question similar to that of the chicken and egg remains with respect to whether IgG4-producing B cells serve as the driving force culminating in an autoimmune response versus an induced inflammatory response secondary to an unknown antigen.

Recent evidence has emerged supporting the autoimmune response of IgG4-positive B lymphocytes in the pathogenesis of ISC. Mailette de Buy Wenninger and colleagues[43] initially identified a highly expanded group of IgG4-positive B-cell clones within B-cell receptor population in patients afflicted with ISC as compared with healthy control subjects. These data were confirmed via in vivo studies that demonstrated expression of B-cell heavy and light chains from these expanded B-cell plasma blasts in IgG4-related cholangitis are in fact self-reactive, confirming that this population is largely autoreactive.[44]

Further research is needed to identify possible target antigens for autoimmune diseases of the biliary tract. It is therefore critical to continue the pursuit and investigation of the influence of environmental factors on immune response pathogenesis in IgG4-RD.

DIAGNOSIS
Primary Biliary Cirrhosis

PBC has become more frequently diagnosed at earlier stages because of greater recognition of disease; earlier detection of serum laboratory abnormalities; and more widespread use of serum markers, such as antimitochondrial antibody (AMA).[45,46] Most cases are diagnosed among asymptomatic women between the ages of 30 and 65 years, who have been found to demonstrate increased ALP levels (ALP >1.5 upper limit of normal for more than 24 weeks). On physical examination, patients may present with hepatomegaly. In contrast, fatigue and pruritis are the two most common forms of symptom presentation.

The serologic hallmark of PBC is positive detection of AMA.[1,46] More specifically, the diagnosis of PBC is qualified by a titer of greater than 1:40, although natural variation in titers between patients are not suggestive of disease severity, nor is it used as a marker in response to therapy.[1] AMA carries a 98% specificity for PBC, and AMAs target a group of autoantigens, collectively referred to as the M2 subtype of mitochondrial autoantigens.[46] These autoantigens consist of the E2 dehydrogenase complex, the ketoglutarate-dehydrogenase complex, and the hydrolipoamide dehydrogenase binding protein.[46] In addition to a positive AMA, serum IgM and hypercholesterolemia may be present.

Liver biopsy necessity is frequently debated in the diagnosis of PBC. It is not mandatory in the setting of a classic biochemical profile and positive AMA titer. A biopsy, however, may be considered to evaluate the degree of biliary destruction and cirrhosis. The histologic findings characterize PBC into four stages that occur in sequence with disease progression. These include (1) portal inflammation with or without inflammatory infiltrate/necrosis around the bile ducts, (2) presence of inflammatory infiltrate with interface hepatitis, and (3) consequent hepatic architecture distortion or (4) cirrhosis.[31]

Primary Sclerosing Cholangitis

The gold standard for the diagnosis of PSC is cholangiography. Classic radiographic findings include multifocal, short annular strictures alternating between normal and dilated intervening segments resulting in the classically reported appearance of "beads on a string" (**Fig. 1**).[3] Longer stricture segments can also present and are worrisome for cholangiocarcinoma. PSC involves intrahepatic and extrahepatic biliary ducts, wherein isolated intrahepatic ductal involvement (25%) occurs more frequently than sole extrahepatic involvement (<5%).[19] Magnetic resonance cholangiopancreatography (MRCP) is routinely recommended as the initial imaging study of choice for diagnosis. The benefits of MRCP are conferred through the lack of radiation, improved cost effectiveness, and comparable sensitivity (80%–90%) and specificity (>90%) versus endoscopic retrograde cholangiopancreatography (ERCP)[9]; however, MRCP

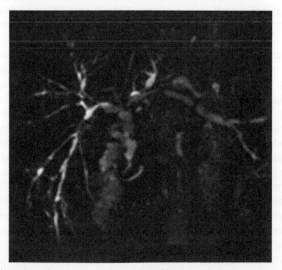

Fig. 1. Primary sclerosing cholangitis. Classic beads on a string.

does not offer the option for intervention. In contrast, ERCP is a diagnostic procedure associated with potential complications, such as pancreatitis and cholangitis, and may require hospitalization. For symptomatic patients, however, ERCP is recommended because of the likelihood of requiring intervention, such as stent placement and/or sphincterotomy.

Liver biopsy is not required to confirm the diagnosis of PSC in patients that present with classic cholangiographic findings. It is, however, useful for the purposes of staging disease where profound inflammation and fibrosis may result in fibrosis. Histologic analysis is critical, however, in the diagnosis of small-duct PSC and in those patients with overlap syndromes, such as autoimmune hepatitis.

Immunoglobulin G4-Related Hepatobiliary Diseases

Establishing ISC is challenging, because ISC shares several clinical, radiographic, and laboratory manifestations to other more common diagnoses, such as biliary malignancy and PSC. Radiographically, cholangiography provides the best representation of ductal anatomy. The classic cholangiographic finding is that of multilevel bile duct narrowing. The distribution of stenosis ranges from hilar stenosis to distal and diffuse distributions of stenoses (**Fig. 2**). Common differential diagnoses include Klatskin tumors (hilar stenosis), PSC (diffuse structuring), chronic pancreatitis, pancreatic malignancy, or cholangiocarcinoma (distal stenosis). Distinguishing characteristics leading to a diagnosis of ISC require the association of clinical symptoms, such as its lack of clear association with IBD, and common association with pancreatic inflammation.

Laboratory abnormalities may demonstrate increased cholestatic values, such as ALP, γ-glutamyltranspeptidase, total bilirubin, and IgG4 levels. Elevated serum IgG4 levels are seen in 65% to 80% of patients at the time of diagnosis; however, increased serum IgG4 levels alone are not diagnostic because pancreaticobiliary malignancies share similarly elevated serum levels.[26] When elevated, a greater than four-fold increase to the upper limit of normal is suggestive of ISC.[22,24] To add to its complexity, prior reports note that approximately 20% to 25% of patients with ISC present with normal levels of serum IgG4.[26,47] Antinuclear antibody titers are positive in nearly 50% of patients with AIP or ISC, and rheumatoid factor levels are similarly raised in up to 20% of patients, although neither factor is specific.[48]

Histopathologically, IgG4-positive B cell, CD4$^+$ T cell, and differentiated plasma cell infiltration of bile ducts is visualized on liver biopsy, in addition to obliterative phlebitis and fibrosis (**Fig. 3**).[22] A widely accepted histologic cutoff for diagnosis includes greater than 10 IgG4-positive plasma cells per high-power field.[23] In general terms, the various organ systems involved demonstrate similar elements of cellular edema, loss of function, and lymphocytic infiltration with fibroinflammatory features.[24] In circumstances in which the diagnosis remains unclear or closely approaching that of another similar disease, a short trial (<2 weeks) of corticosteroids often confirms or refutes the diagnosis of ISC.[49]

Because of the lack of sensitive and/or specific markers of ISC, various diagnostic criteria have been proposed to facilitate the diagnosis of IgG4-related cholangiopathies, including the HISORt criteria,[26] the Japanese criteria,[25,50] and the International Consensus Diagnostic Criteria.[51] Independently, these criteria combine clinical, radiographic, biochemical, and histopathologic findings across various organ systems involved along with responsiveness to immunosuppressive therapy.

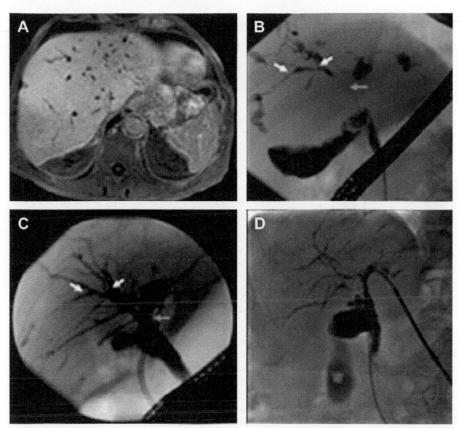

Fig. 2. IgG4-related autoimmune cholangiopathy. An 82-year-old otherwise asymptomatic man presented with elevated bilirubin and mild jaundice. (*A*) Liver MRI revealed diffusely dilated bile ducts without evidence of a mass. (*B*) ERCP demonstrates structuring at the hilum (*blue arrow*) with dilation and structuring of intrahepatic ducts (*white arrows*). (*C*) The patient had a biliary stent placed and serum IgG4 was elevated, confirming the diagnosis. He was therefore initiated on steroid therapy. Two months after his initial presentation, follow-up ERCP demonstrated resolution of the hilar stricture and smaller duct strictures. (*D*) One month later, his biliary tree appeared normal on cholangiogram, and his stents were therefore removed.

MANAGEMENT OPTIONS AND CLINICAL OUTCOMES
Primary Biliary Cirrhosis

Medical management
The sole currently approved and available therapy for PBC is ursodeoxycholic acid (UDCA). Numerous other therapeutic agents have been proposed and used with unclear benefits, such as methotrexate, colchicine, glucocorticoids, and cyclosporine and azathioprine.[1] UDCA is a naturally occurring bile acid that functions by conferring cholangiocyte protection through the reduction of bile acid cytotoxicity and stasis of bile within the hepatobiliary system. Various mechanisms of action have been proposed, including modulation of the composition of bile, and enhanced hepatobiliary secretion of bile in addition to improved hepatocyte survival via stimulation of antiapoptotic pathways.[52] Early trials comparing 13 to 15 mg/kg/d of UDCA with placebo

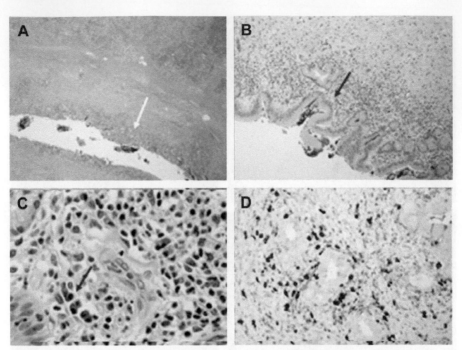

Fig. 3. Histopathologic presentation of IgG4 sclerosing cholangiopathy. (*A*) Cross-sectional view of a common bile duct in IgG4 sclerosing cholangitis, ×20 magnification (Hematoxylin and Eosin). Demonstrated is the intrapancreatic portion of the common bile duct with significant inflammatory cell infiltrate surrounding the duct (*white arrow*). (*B*) Cross-sectional view of the common bile duct at magnification of ×100 (Hematoxylin and Eosin). The inflammatory infiltrate is fairly extensive surrounding the common bile duct (*blue arrow*). (*C*) The region pertaining to the *blue arrow* from *B* is shown at ×600 magnification (Hematoxylin and Eosin). Demonstrated are the plasma cells, which are characterized by a dark round nucleus near the cell edge with significant volume of cytoplasm (*blue arrow*). (*D*) Immunohistochemistry stained for IgG4 (Immunostain); depicted in brown are the IgG4 secreting plasma cells (*blue arrow*).

revealed significant decreases in serum ALP, bilirubin, and alanine aminotransferase, and improved symptom control, such as decreased pruritis.[53–56] Overall survival and time of transplant-free survival have been evaluated in numerous randomized trials and controlled studies with conflicting results.[54,55] Studies that continued to follow patients beyond 2 years of treatment identified significant improvements in overall survival and time to transplant.[57] Delay in histologic progression has been reported in patients treated with UCDA who had early histologic stage at baseline.[53] Such improvement has not been consistently verified among patients with later stage disease.

Various agents have been tested and studied in the treatment of PBC with variable results, none of which have demonstrated significant benefit in terms of mortality or time to transplantation. Azathioprine is a purine synthesis inhibitor with immunosuppressive properties carrying proposed advantages in the treatment of PBC. Azathioprine was studied in a large multicenter, randomized, double-blind, placebo-controlled trial that failed to demonstrate a benefit of treatment in PBC.[58] These results were further supported by a Cochrane review of 10 studies and 631 patients, which did not reveal an improvement in pruritus or mortality.[56] Prednisolone and cyclosporine have also been evaluated as therapy for PBC with initial small placebo-controlled trials demonstrating a decrease in ALP in patients followed for 1 to 3 years.[59] None of these studies were able to identify a change in overall mortality rates. Colchicine has been studied in various smaller studies with variable success including improvements in biochemical parameters without histologic or survival benefits.[60] The metabolic inhibitor of folic acid, methotrexate, has known beneficial effects on the treatment of PSC (discussed later), prompting consideration of its use in PBC; however, clinical trials have demonstrated varying results.[61,62] The Primary Biliary Cirrhosis Ursodiol Plus Methotrexate or its Placebo (PUMPS) trial is the largest multicenter controlled trial revealing no benefit from the addition of methotrexate to UDCA therapy on survival without transplantation.[55]

Liver transplantation
Liver transplantation remains the most definitive source of treatment in PBC. The Mayo risk score (risk = $0.971 \log_e[\text{bilirubin mg/dL}] + 2.53 \log_e[\text{albumin g/dL}] + 0.039$ age [years] $+ 2.38 \log_e[\text{prothrombin time in seconds}] + 0.859 \log_e[\text{edema score of 0, 0.5, 1.0}]$) predicts the probability of survival in PBC, computed from the patient's age, total bilirubin, albumin, prothrombin time, and severity of edema.[63] The Model for End-Stage Liver Disease (MELD) score, however, is used more frequently in clinical practice. Liver transplantation is recommended for patients with PBC when any single criteria among the following is satisfied: total bilirubin greater than 5.0 mg/dL, albumin less than 2.8 mg/dL, signs of portal hypertension (ascites, variceal bleeding, encephalopathy), or MELD score approaching 15. Symptomatic manifestations that impact quality of life, such as uncontrolled, debilitating pruritis or osteoporosis, also warrant evaluation for liver transplantation. Of note, liver transplant patients are susceptible to recurrence, with reported rates ranging from 16% at 5 years post-transplant to up to 30% at 10 years.[64]

Primary Sclerosing Cholangitis

Medical management
As with PBC, the only drug therapy approved in the treatment of PSC is UDCA. The effect of UDCA is demonstrated through decreased bile viscosity and cholestasis, resulting in amelioration of secondary mechanisms of cell damage.[65] Early studies comparing low-dose UDCA (10–15 mg/kg/d) with placebo demonstrated only marginal outcomes in improving serum biochemical abnormalities as compared with higher doses (20–30 mg/kg/d).[38] Larger clinical trials comparing higher doses of UDCA with placebo failed to demonstrate significant clinical or survival benefits in PSC.[65]

Relief of mechanical biliary obstruction caused by stricture formation has been shown to favorably influence the prognosis and overall survival of patients with PSC.[66] Successful stenting and biliary dilation result in the relief of symptoms and normalization of serum laboratory abnormalities. The success of endoscopic decompression relies on evidence of discrete segmental stricturing within the extrahepatic or proximal intrahepatic biliary ducts seen on cholangiogram. Central and smaller distal intrahepatic biliary branches are largely inaccessible by endoscopy, hence strictures located within these peripheral ducts warrant consideration for liver transplant (or potentially resection if isolated to specific segments).[66] Endoscopy also offers the advantage to screen for cholangiocarcinoma by obtaining brushings and biopsies, which is particularly critical because malignant strictures are indistinguishable from benign strictures.

PSC has, unfortunately, been referenced as a premalignant lesion because it confers a markedly dramatic increased risk of colorectal (30-fold increased risk)[67] and hepatobiliary cancers (hepatic malignancy, 40-fold increased risk; cholangiocarcinoma, 400-fold increased risk),[68,69] with these resultant cancers reported as the leading cause of death in these patients.[40] The cumulative incidence of colorectal malignancy increases from the time of diagnosis of PSC, such that within the first 10 years, the risk of colorectal malignancy is approximately 9%, increasing to 20% to 30% at 20 years.[9] As such, surveillance colonoscopy every 1 to 2 years remains the recommended standard for colorectal malignancy screening among patients with PSC.[19] Additionally, 60% to 80% of patients with PSC have associated IBD.[11,15,70] IBD associated with PSC may have a higher incidence of backwash ileitis, rectal sparing, and more quiescent course compared with IBD alone affected individuals.[19] The challenge rests in the lack of effective medical therapy for the treatment against the progression of disease, and as a consequence, overall mortality rates among PSC have remained stable over the past two decades. Liver transplantation remains the only curative therapy at present.

Liver transplantation

Liver transplantation remains the definitive treatment of PSC, wherein the MELD score is used to assess prognosis and survival. There exist various clinical indicators for transplantation including intractable pruritis, recurrent bacterial cholangitis and sepsis with its associated septic complications, and progressive bone disease.[1]

One continued area of controversy and debate lies in the role of liver transplantation among patients with dysplastic cells identified on ERCP, or overt cholangiocarcinoma. Transplantation is controversial because of the high rate of tumor recurrence following transplant, drawing to question its utility as a true treatment option, in addition to the scarcity of resources, such as organ availability. The challenge in early diagnosis rests in the lack of methods for detection because the clinical presentation of cholangiocarcinoma in PSC is obscured by its nature to mimic benign dominant biliary strictures. However, a protocol established by the Mayo Clinic for the treatment of cholangiocarcinoma with or without PSC involves the combination of external beam radiation therapy with brachytherapy, 5-fluorouracil chemosensitization, followed by liver transplantation, and has demonstrated a significant survival benefit compared with resection for cholangiocarcinoma.[71,72] Five-year survival rates following transplantation have been noted to be 76% to 82%.[73–75]

Immunoglobulin G4-Related Hepatobiliary Diseases

Corticosteroid therapy is the first-line therapy for strictures and mass-forming lesions among patients with ISC, and responsiveness has been reported be 97%.[24,26,76] Initial treatment doses traditionally consist of prednisone at 0.6 mg/kg/d for 3 months, followed by a taper of variable duration.[27,77] No defined dosing strategy has been universally accepted because of the lack of prospective studies. However, the lowest possible dose to reach clear therapeutic response (ie, relief of symptoms, normalization of enzymes, and improvement in biliary imaging) is recommended because of the adverse effect profile of corticosteroids. As such, tapering maintenance doses and subsequent discontinuation of therapy result in up to 50% relapse rates among patients with ISC.[26,27,48,76] Various studies show a benefit with decreasing relapse rates while on maintenance therapy consisting of low-dose steroids compared with none.[76,77]

SUMMARY

The management of autoimmune cholestatic hepatic disorders is a challenging arena to navigate in the search of therapeutic advances. Although liver transplantation remains a life-saving solution for patients with end-stage disease currently, various new molecular pathways are being described to better understand the complex hepatobiliary interactions with the immune response. As clinicians become increasingly aware of the manifestations presented of autoimmune hepatic diseases, its recognition and application of therapeutics has gained greater recognition of its relevance in clinical practice. The major areas of need include the identification of reliable biomarkers to diagnose and detect disease activity in addition to the development of treatment regimens.

ACKNOWLEDGMENTS

The authors thank Kristina Matkowskyj, MD, PhD, for her contribution in providing histopathologic images in this review.

REFERENCES

1. Krok KL, Munoz SJ. Management of autoimmune and cholestatic liver disorders. Clin Liver Dis 2009;13(2):295–316.
2. Beuers U, Gershwin ME. Unmet challenges in immune-mediated hepatobiliary diseases. Clin Rev Allergy Immunol 2015;48(2–3):127–31.
3. Yeh MJ, Kim SY, Jhaveri KS, et al. Imaging of autoimmune biliary disease. Abdom Radiol (NY) 2017;42(1):3–18.
4. Boonstra K, Beuers U, Ponsioen CY. Epidemiology of primary sclerosing cholangitis and primary biliary cirrhosis: a systematic review. J Hepatol 2012;56(5): 1181–8.
5. Inoue K, Hirohara J, Nakano T, et al. Prediction of prognosis of primary biliary cirrhosis in Japan. Liver 1995;15(2):70–7.
6. Lleo A, Marzorati S, Anaya JM, et al. Primary biliary cholangitis: a comprehensive overview. Hepatol Int 2017;11(6):485–99.
7. Tsianos EV, Hoofnagle JH, Fox PC, et al. Sjögren's syndrome in patients with primary biliary cirrhosis. Hepatology 1990;11(5):730–4.
8. Marasini B, Gagetta M, Rossi V, et al. Rheumatic disorders and primary biliary cirrhosis: an appraisal of 170 Italian patients. Ann Rheum Dis 2001;60(11): 1046–9.
9. Singh S, Talwalkar JA. Primary sclerosing cholangitis: diagnosis, prognosis, and management. Clin Gastroenterol Hepatol 2013;11(8):898–907.
10. Pollheimer MJ, Halilbasic E, Fickert P, et al. Pathogenesis of primary sclerosing cholangitis. Best Pract Res Clin Gastroenterol 2011;25(6):727–39.
11. Farrant JM, Hayllar KM, Wilkinson ML, et al. Natural history and prognostic variables in primary sclerosing cholangitis. Gastroenterology 1991;100(6):1710–7.
12. Boberg KM, Aadland E, Jahnsen J, et al. Incidence and prevalence of primary biliary cirrhosis, primary sclerosing cholangitis, and autoimmune hepatitis in a Norwegian population. Scand J Gastroenterol 1998;33(1):99–103.
13. Bambha K, Kim WR, Talwalkar J, et al. Incidence, clinical spectrum, and outcomes of primary sclerosing cholangitis in a United States community. Gastroenterology 2003;125(5):1364–9.
14. Kingham JG, Kochar N, Gravenor MB. Incidence, clinical patterns, and outcomes of primary sclerosing cholangitis in South Wales, United Kingdom. Gastroenterology 2004;126(7):1929–30.
15. Molodecky NA, Kareemi H, Parab R, et al. Incidence of primary sclerosing cholangitis: a systematic review and meta-analysis. Hepatology 2011;53(5):1590–9.

16. Claessen MM, Vleggaar FP, Tytgat KM, et al. High lifetime risk of cancer in primary sclerosing cholangitis. J Hepatol 2009;50(1):158–64.
17. Cullen S, Chapman R. Primary sclerosing cholangitis. Autoimmun Rev 2003;2(6): 305–12.
18. Charatcharoenwitthaya P, Lindor KD. Primary sclerosing cholangitis: diagnosis and management. Curr Gastroenterol Rep 2006;8(1):75–82.
19. Chapman R, Fevery J, Kalloo A, et al. Diagnosis and management of primary sclerosing cholangitis. Hepatology 2010;51(2):660–78.
20. Porayko MK, Wiesner RH, LaRusso NF, et al. Patients with asymptomatic primary sclerosing cholangitis frequently have progressive disease. Gastroenterology 1990;98(6):1594–602.
21. Bansi DS, Fleming KA, Chapman RW. Importance of antineutrophil cytoplasmic antibodies in primary sclerosing cholangitis and ulcerative colitis: prevalence, titre, and IgG subclass. Gut 1996;38(3):384–9.
22. Hubers LM, Maillette de Buy Wenniger LJ, Doorenspleet ME, et al. IgG4-associated cholangitis: a comprehensive review. Clin Rev Allergy Immunol 2015; 48(2–3):198–206.
23. Deshpande V, Zen Y, Chan JK, et al. Consensus statement on the pathology of IgG4-related disease. Mod Pathol 2012;25(9):1181–92.
24. Culver EL, Chapman RW. IgG4-related hepatobiliary disease: an overview. Nat Rev Gastroenterol Hepatol 2016;13(10):601–12.
25. Ohara H, Okazaki K, Tsubouchi H, et al. Clinical diagnostic criteria of IgG4-related sclerosing cholangitis 2012. J Hepatobiliary Pancreat Sci 2012;19(5): 536–42.
26. Ghazale A, Chari ST, Zhang L, et al. Immunoglobulin G4-associated cholangitis: clinical profile and response to therapy. Gastroenterology 2008;134(3):706–15.
27. Kanno A, Masamune A, Okazaki K, et al. Nationwide epidemiological survey of autoimmune pancreatitis in Japan in 2011. Pancreas 2015;44(4):535–9.
28. Hubers LM, Beuers U. IgG4-related disease of the biliary tract and pancreas: clinical and experimental advances. Curr Opin Gastroenterol 2017;33(4):310–4.
29. Invernizzi P, Selmi C, Gershwin ME. Update on primary biliary cirrhosis. Dig Liver Dis 2010;42(6):401–8.
30. Invernizzi P, Ransom M, Raychaudhuri S, et al. Classical HLA-DRB1 and DPB1 alleles account for HLA associations with primary biliary cirrhosis. Genes Immun 2012;13(6):461–8.
31. Li M, Zheng H, Tian QB, et al. HLA-DR polymorphism and primary biliary cirrhosis: evidence from a meta-analysis. Arch Med Res 2014;45(3):270–9.
32. Liu JZ, Almarri MA, Gaffney DJ, et al. Dense fine-mapping study identifies new susceptibility loci for primary biliary cirrhosis. Nat Genet 2012;44(10):1137–41.
33. Williamson KD, Chapman RW. Primary sclerosing cholangitis: a clinical update. Br Med Bull 2015;114(1):53–64.
34. O'Mahony CA, Vierling JM. Etiopathogenesis of primary sclerosing cholangitis. Semin Liver Dis 2006;26(1):3–21.
35. Fosby B, Karlsen TH, Melum E. Recurrence and rejection in liver transplantation for primary sclerosing cholangitis. World J Gastroenterol 2012;18(1):1–15.
36. Alberts R, de Vries EMG, Goode EC, et al. Genetic association analysis identifies variants associated with disease progression in primary sclerosing cholangitis. Gut 2018;67(8):1517–24.
37. Folseraas T, Melum E, Rausch P, et al. Extended analysis of a genome-wide association study in primary sclerosing cholangitis detects multiple novel risk loci. J Hepatol 2012;57(2):366–75.

38. Mitchell SA, Bansi DS, Hunt N, et al. A preliminary trial of high-dose ursodeoxy-cholic acid in primary sclerosing cholangitis. Gastroenterology 2001;121(4): 900–7.
39. Satsangi J, Chapman RW, Haldar N, et al. A functional polymorphism of the stromelysin gene (MMP-3) influences susceptibility to primary sclerosing cholangitis. Gastroenterology 2001;121(1):124–30.
40. Bergquist A, Montgomery SM, Bahmanyar S, et al. Increased risk of primary sclerosing cholangitis and ulcerative colitis in first-degree relatives of patients with primary sclerosing cholangitis. Clin Gastroenterol Hepatol 2008;6(8):939–43.
41. Aalberse RC, Stapel SO, Schuurman J, et al. Immunoglobulin G4: an odd antibody. Clin Exp Allergy 2009;39(4):469–77.
42. van der Neut Kolfschoten M, Schuurman J, Losen M, et al. Anti-inflammatory activity of human IgG4 antibodies by dynamic Fab arm exchange. Science 2007; 317(5844):1554–7.
43. Maillette de Buy Wenniger LJ, Doorenspleet ME, Klarenbeek PL, et al. Immunoglobulin G4+ clones identified by next-generation sequencing dominate the B cell receptor repertoire in immunoglobulin G4 associated cholangitis. Hepatology 2013;57(6):2390–8.
44. Mattoo H, Mahajan VS, Della-Torre E, et al. De novo oligoclonal expansions of circulating plasmablasts in active and relapsing IgG4-related disease. J Allergy Clin Immunol 2014;134(3):679–87.
45. Kaplan GG, Laupland KB, Butzner D, et al. The burden of large and small duct primary sclerosing cholangitis in adults and children: a population-based analysis. Am J Gastroenterol 2007;102(5):1042–9.
46. Kaplan MM, Gershwin ME. Primary biliary cirrhosis. N Engl J Med 2005;353(12): 1261–73.
47. Kamisawa T, Funata N, Hayashi Y, et al. A new clinicopathological entity of IgG4-related autoimmune disease. J Gastroenterol 2003;38(10):982–4.
48. Sah RP, Chari ST. Serologic issues in IgG4-related systemic disease and autoimmune pancreatitis. Curr Opin Rheumatol 2011;23(1):108–13.
49. Moon SH, Kim MH, Park DH, et al. Is a 2-week steroid trial after initial negative investigation for malignancy useful in differentiating autoimmune pancreatitis from pancreatic cancer? A prospective outcome study. Gut 2008;57(12): 1704–12.
50. Okazaki K, Uchida K, Matsushita M, et al. How to diagnose autoimmune pancreatitis by the revised Japanese clinical criteria. J Gastroenterol 2007;42(Suppl 18): 32–8.
51. Shimosegawa T, Working Group Members of the Japan Pancreas Society, Research Committee for Intractable Pancreatic Disease by the Ministry of Labor, Health and Welfare of Japan. The amendment of the Clinical Diagnostic Criteria in Japan (JPS2011) in response to the proposal of the International Consensus of Diagnostic Criteria (ICDC) for autoimmune pancreatitis. Pancreas 2012;41(8): 1341–2.
52. Paumgartner G, Beuers U. Ursodeoxycholic acid in cholestatic liver disease: mechanisms of action and therapeutic use revisited. Hepatology 2002;36(3): 525–31.
53. Poupon R, Chrétien Y, Poupon RE, et al. Is ursodeoxycholic acid an effective treatment for primary biliary cirrhosis? Lancet 1987;1(8537):834–6.
54. Heathcote EJ, Cauch-Dudek K, Walker V, et al. The Canadian Multicenter Double-blind Randomized Controlled Trial of ursodeoxycholic acid in primary biliary cirrhosis. Hepatology 1994;19(5):1149–56.

55. Combes B, Luketic VA, Peters MG, et al. Prolonged follow-up of patients in the U.S. multicenter trial of ursodeoxycholic acid for primary biliary cirrhosis. Am J Gastroenterol 2004;99(2):264–8.

56. Gong Y, Christensen E, Gluud C. Azathioprine for primary biliary cirrhosis. Cochrane Database Syst Rev 2007;(3):CD006000.

57. Shi J, Wu C, Lin Y, et al. Long-term effects of mid-dose ursodeoxycholic acid in primary biliary cirrhosis: a meta-analysis of randomized controlled trials. Am J Gastroenterol 2006;101(7):1529–38.

58. Christensen E, Neuberger J, Crowe J, et al. Beneficial effect of azathioprine and prediction of prognosis in primary biliary cirrhosis. Final results of an international trial. Gastroenterology 1985;89(5):1084–91.

59. Wiesner RH, Ludwig J, Lindor KD, et al. A controlled trial of cyclosporine in the treatment of primary biliary cirrhosis. N Engl J Med 1990;322(20):1419–24.

60. Gong Y, Gluud C. Colchicine for primary biliary cirrhosis: a Cochrane Hepato-Biliary Group systematic review of randomized clinical trials. Am J Gastroenterol 2005;100(8):1876–85.

61. Bach N, Thung SN, Schaffner F. The histologic effects of low-dose methotrexate therapy for primary biliary cirrhosis. Arch Pathol Lab Med 1998;122(4):342–5.

62. Hendrickse MT, Rigney E, Giaffer MH, et al. Low-dose methotrexate is ineffective in primary biliary cirrhosis: long-term results of a placebo-controlled trial. Gastroenterology 1999;117(2):400–7.

63. Dickson ER, Grambsch PM, Fleming TR, et al. Prognosis in primary biliary cirrhosis: model for decision making. Hepatology 1989;10(1):1–7.

64. Liermann Garcia RF, Evangelista Garcia C, McMaster P, et al. Transplantation for primary biliary cirrhosis: retrospective analysis of 400 patients in a single center. Hepatology 2001;33(1):22–7.

65. Lindor KD, Kowdley KV, Luketic VA, et al. High-dose ursodeoxycholic acid for the treatment of primary sclerosing cholangitis. Hepatology 2009;50(3):808–14.

66. Baluyut AR, Sherman S, Lehman GA, et al. Impact of endoscopic therapy on the survival of patients with primary sclerosing cholangitis. Gastrointest Endosc 2001;53(3):308–12.

67. Broomé U, Löfberg R, Veress B, et al. Primary sclerosing cholangitis and ulcerative colitis: evidence for increased neoplastic potential. Hepatology 1995;22(5):1404–8.

68. Card TR, Solaymani-Dodaran M, West J. Incidence and mortality of primary sclerosing cholangitis in the UK: a population-based cohort study. J Hepatol 2008;48(6):939–44.

69. Boonstra K, Weersma RK, van Erpecum KJ, et al. Population-based epidemiology, malignancy risk, and outcome of primary sclerosing cholangitis. Hepatology 2013;58(6):2045–55.

70. Knight C, Murray KF. Hepatobiliary associations with inflammatory bowel disease. Expert Rev Gastroenterol Hepatol 2009;3(6):681–91.

71. Heimbach JK, Gores GJ, Haddock MG, et al. Liver transplantation for unresectable perihilar cholangiocarcinoma. Semin Liver Dis 2004;24(2):201–7.

72. Jeyarajah DR, Klintmalm GB. Is liver transplantation indicated for cholangiocarcinoma? J Hepatobiliary Pancreat Surg 1998;5(1):48–51.

73. Rea DJ, Heimbach JK, Rosen CB, et al. Liver transplantation with neoadjuvant chemoradiation is more effective than resection for hilar cholangiocarcinoma. Ann Surg 2005;242(3):451–8 [discussion: 458–61].

74. Heimbach JK, Gores GJ, Haddock MG, et al. Predictors of disease recurrence following neoadjuvant chemoradiotherapy and liver transplantation for unresectable perihilar cholangiocarcinoma. Transplantation 2006;82(12):1703–7.
75. Heimbach JK. Successful liver transplantation for hilar cholangiocarcinoma. Curr Opin Gastroenterol 2008;24(3):384–8.
76. Kamisawa T, Takuma K, Tabata T, et al. Serum IgG4-negative autoimmune pancreatitis. J Gastroenterol 2011;46(1):108–16.
77. Hart PA, Kamisawa T, Brugge WR, et al. Long-term outcomes of autoimmune pancreatitis: a multicentre, international analysis. Gut 2013;62(12):1771–6.

An Update on Biliary Dyskinesia

Clancy J. Clark, MD

KEYWORDS

- Functional gallbladder disorder • Functional sphincter of Oddi disorder
- Biliary dyskinesia • Biliary hyperkinesia • Rome IV criteria
- Post-cholecystectomy syndrome • Cholecystokinin • Cholescintigraphy

KEY POINTS

- Diagnosis of biliary dyskinesia (functional gallbladder and biliary sphincter disorders), is based on the Rome IV definition.
- Biliary dyskinesia is associated with concomitant gastrointestinal disorders.
- Cholecystokinin-stimulated cholescintigraphy is the optimal imaging study to help establish a diagnosis of biliary dyskinesia.
- Cholecystectomy can provide relief of symptoms secondary to functional gallbladder disorder in the majority of adult patients (>90%).
- In the absence of a gallbladder, functional biliary sphincter disorder requires a specialized center for treatment with less promising outcomes with invasive procedures.

INTRODUCTION

Biliary dyskinesia is a functional gastrointestinal disorder that can result in significant abdominal pain. In addition to gallbladder dyskinesia, functional biliary disorders include acalculus biliary pain, biliary dysmotility, sphincter of Oddi dysfunction, ampullary stenosis, and postcholecystectomy syndrome. Invasive procedures for biliary dyskinesia, such as cholecystectomy, are not always satisfactory resulting in controversy among gastroenterologists and surgeons. Diagnosis of this nonmalignant disorder requires the absence of stones, sludge, microlithiasis, or microcrystals within the gallbladder or biliary tree. Dysfunction of the gallbladder can be due to malignancy of the gallbladder and biliary tree, as well as distal bile duct obstruction; however, these secondary causes of biliary dyskinesia are not addressed in this article. Gallbladder dyskinesia is best described using the term functional gallbladder disorder and describes a patient with biliary pain with the gallbladder in place and without structural

Disclosure Statement: The author has nothing to disclose.
General Surgery Residency, Center for Applied and Experiential Learning, Wake Forest Baptist Health, Medical Center Boulevard, Winston Salem, NC 27157, USA
E-mail address: cjclark@wakehealth.edu

or mechanical cause for the pain. Sphincter of Oddi dyskinesia is best described using the term functional biliary sphincter of Oddi disorder and is associated with biliary pain after cholecystectomy in patients with no other underlying pathology.

DEFINITION

The symptom complex of biliary-type pain in the absence of other etiology is the hallmark of biliary dyskinesia. Given significant controversy among gastroenterologists and surgeons regarding this diagnosis, we recommend following the Rome IV consensus criteria.[1] As a diagnosis of exclusion, rigorous investigation of more common etiologies (eg, cholelithiasis, pancreatitis, malignancy) is recommended. Following Rome IV criteria (https://theromefoundation.org/rome-iv/), biliary pain is required to diagnose a functional gallbladder or sphincter of Oddi disorder.[1] Biliary pain is described as pain located in the epigastrium and/or right upper quadrant with the following characteristics: (1) builds up to a steady level and lasting 30 minutes or more, (2) occurs at different intervals (not daily), (3) severe enough to interrupt daily activity or lead to an emergency room visit, (4) not significantly related with bowel movements, and (5) not significantly relieved with postural changes or acid suppression. Supporting criteria include nausea, vomiting, pain radiating to the back, and pain resulting in waking from sleep.

The diagnostic criteria for biliary dyskinesia have evolved over the last 2 decades to help refine the diagnosis and minimize the number of patients undergoing invasive procedures. For functional gallbladder disorder, the Rome II criteria specified episodes of pain should last 30 minutes or more and required demonstration of abnormal gallbladder emptying.[2] The Rome III criteria helped to clarify the baseline diagnostic criteria for functional gallbladder disorders and sphincter of Oddi disorders.[3] Abnormal gallbladder function was no longer required for diagnosis, but a comprehensive evaluation with a thorough history and objective measure of gallbladder function were emphasized. A low gallbladder ejection fraction is now considered a supportive criterion. In the current Rome IV criteria, subtypes of sphincter of Oddi dysfunction (types I, II, and III) are no longer used. Previous type I sphincter of Oddi dysfunction (papillary stenosis) is a mechanical obstruction and should not be considered a functional disorder. In the EPISOD trial, patients with diagnosed with type III sphincter of Oddi dysfunction (normal laboratory studies, normal bile duct) did not benefit from endoscopic retrograde pancreaticocholangiography (ERCP) and sphincterotomy.[4] Rome IV diagnostic criteria for functional gallbladder disorder is outlined in **Box 1**. Rome IV diagnostic criteria for functional biliary sphincter of Oddi disorder is outlined in **Box 2**.

Box 1
Rome IV criteria for functional gallbladder disorder

Rome IV

Must include the following
1. Biliary pain
2. Absence of gallstones or other structural pathology

Supportive criteria
1. Low ejection fraction on gallbladder scintigraphy
2. Normal liver enzymes, conjugated bilirubin, and amylase/lipase

Data from Cotton PB, Elta GH, Carter CR, et al. Gallbladder and sphincter of Oddi disorders. Gastroenterology 2016;150(6):1420–9.e2.

Box 2
Diagnostic criteria for functional biliary sphincter of Oddi disorder

Rome IV

Must include the following
1. Biliary pain
2. Elevated liver enzymes or dilated bile duct, but not both
3. Absence of bile duct stones or other structural abnormalities

Supportive criteria
1. Normal amylase/lipase
2. Abnormal sphincter of Oddi manometry
3. Abnormal hepatobiliary scintigraphy

Data from Cotton PB, Elta GH, Carter CR, et al. Gallbladder and sphincter of Oddi disorders. Gastroenterology 2016;150(6):1420–9.e2.

PATHOPHYSIOLOGY

The hallmark of biliary dyskinesia is demonstrated by low gallbladder ejection fraction during cholecystokinin-stimulated cholescintigraphy (CCK-CS).[5] Although the exact etiology of biliary dyskinesia is not known, 3 hypotheses have been proposed. First, bile composition results in gallbladder inflammation leading to abnormal gallbladder motility and chronic cholecystitis associated pain. Second, functional problems of the gallbladder and sphincter of Oddi represent symptoms of a larger gastrointestinal tract disorder, such as visceral hypersensitivity seen in patients with irritable bowel syndrome. Last, biliary dyskinesia is a result of receptor or neurologic abnormality, such as altered CCK release, decreased CCK receptor sensitivity or density, or impaired smooth muscle contractility in response to CCK.[6] Altered gallbladder or sphincter of Oddi contraction then leads to inflammation and biliary pain.

Anatomy

The biliary system is composed of the intrahepatic bile ducts, extrahepatic bile duct, and gallbladder. The gallbladder temporarily stores bile (30–60 mL). The gallbladder connects with the biliary system via the cystic duct. The length and insertion point of the cystic duct is highly variable, but typically inserted into the cystic duct in a supraduodenal position in 70% of people. The common bile duct is the continuation of the hepatic duct after insertion of the cystic duct. It is approximately 8 cm in length and 4 to 9 mm in diameter. The common bile duct is divided into thirds, with the most interior third within the pancreas. The common bile duct typically joins with the pancreatic duct to exit at the sphincter of Oddi. Approximately 5% of patients have pancreatic divisum, where the common bile duct exits at the sphincter of Oddi along with the ventral pancreatic duct and the dorsal pancreatic duct exits independently at an accessory sphincter. The sphincter of Oddi has both circular and longitudinal fibers. Histologically, the sphincter of Oddi can have 4 separate sphincters depending on the junction of the bile duct and pancreatic duct. Parasympathetic innervation of the bile duct is off of the hepatic branch of the vagus nerve and the celiac plexus. Sympathetic innervation follows the fifth to ninth thoracic segments (T5–T9) through the greater splanchnic nerves to the celiac ganglion. The gallbladder can also have sensory fibers from the right phrenic nerve. Importantly, visceral organs share the same sensory innervation resulting in an inability to distinguish between gallbladder, duodenal, and pancreas-related pain.

Biliary neurohormonal regulation

Bile production is increased by gastrointestinal hormone secretin, CCK, and gastrin. The flow of bile is controlled by contraction of the sphincter of Oddi. During fasting, contractions occur 4 times per minute.[7] Normal pressure in the common bile duct is 10 to 15 mm Hg. The gallbladder fills and empties cyclically after duodenal migrating myoelectric complexes. Animal studies indicate that gallbladder distension is linked with sphincter tone via the cholecystosphincteric reflex.[8] Early studies of gallbladder function using a Guinea pig model taught us that vagal stimulation results in both gallbladder and sphincter of Oddi contraction but splachnic stimulation relaxes the gallbladder and contracts the sphincter of Oddi.[9,10]

In addition to neuronal regulation, gallbladder and sphincter of Oddi function are regulated by hormones produced within the gastrointestinal tract (**Fig. 1**). Secretin increases the production of bile and pancreatic juice. The release of secretin from the proximal small bowel S cells is stimulated by ingestion of protein and exposure of the duodenum to acid. CCK–pancreozymin, or more commonly CCK, produces gallbladder contraction and pancreatic enzyme production. CCK is secreted by I cells within the proximal small bowel. CCK is not only found in the duodenum and jejunum, but also found in neurons in the distal ileum, colon, and brain. It can increase gut motility, but also results in pyloric contraction and decreased gastric emptying. Secretion of CCK is stimulated by protein and fat ingestion. The action of CCK is outlined in **Box 3**.

Gallbladder and sphincter of Oddi motility depend on the hormones motilin and CCK, as well as neural reflexes with eating. Clearly, gallbladder and sphincter of

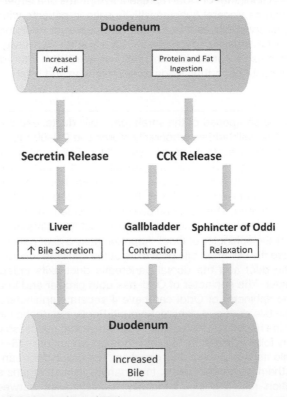

Fig. 1. Function of cholecystokinin (CCK).

Box 3
Action of cholecystokinin.

Contraction and emptying of the gallbladder

Relaxation of the sphincter of Oddi

Increase in pancreatic enzyme secretion

Increase in secretion of insulin, glucagon, and somatostatin by Islet cells

Inhibition of gastric emptying by contraction of the pyloric sphincter

Increase in hepatic bile secretion

Increase in intestinal peristalsis

Increase in intestinal blood flow

Suppression of appetite

Decrease in systolic blood pressure

Data from Krishnamurthy S, Krishnamurthy GT. Biliary dyskinesia: role of the sphincter of Oddi, gallbladder and cholecystokinin. J Nucl Med 1997;38(11):1825.

Oddi motility is influenced by multiple factors. Dysregulation of the neurohormonal pathways effecting the gallbladder and sphincter of Oddi can induce biliary pain. In studies of sphincter of Oddi function, even small changes in sphincter tone (even within the normal range) have been known to trigger a sensation of pain.[1]

Pathology

Histologic evaluation of the gallbladder after cholecystectomy is required for all patients. Both the operative note and pathology report should document evidence of gallstones. Gallbladder sludge and/or gallstones should be absent in functional gallbladder disorder. In the management of postcholecystectomy syndrome, this process can guide further evaluation, particularly in the more common clinical presentation of cystic duct remnant stones or choledocholithiasis. In patients with a preoperative diagnosis of functional gallbladder disorder, histologic evidence of chronic inflammation is not consistent across studies and can be found in as many as 86% of patients.[11,12]

Gallbladder ejection fraction

A decreased gallbladder ejection fraction (<40%) is considered an objective measure of functional gallbladder disorder. Importantly, based on the Rome IV criteria, a low gallbladder ejection fraction supports the diagnosis of but is not required for the diagnosis of a functional gallbladder disorder. Repeated testing of gallbladder ejection fraction indicates that it is not static and is influenced by medications, radiotracer dose, and length of infusion.[11,13] In fact, Rose and colleagues[14] reported normal gallbladder ejection fraction in 53% of patients after retesting.

Concomitant diseases

Biliary dyskinesia is linked with multiple other disorders including irritable bowel syndrome, gastroesophageal reflux disease, chronic constipation, colonic inertia, and gastroparesis. Systemic diseases such as morbid obesity, rapid weight loss, and diabetes mellitus can alter gallbladder contractility. Steatohepatitis and end-stage liver disease are also associated with biliary dyskinesia.

EPIDEMIOLOGY

Biliary dyskinesia should be considered a diagnosis of exclusion and is a rare disorder. However, in the United States, 20% of cholecystectomies are performed for diagnosis of functional gallbladder disorder. The incidence of biliary dyskinesia outside the United States is 25 cases per million versus 85 cases per million in the United States. From 1991 to 2001, the incidence of biliary dyskinesia increased dramatically in the United States from 43 cases per million to 89 cases per million.[15] In the United States from 1997 to 2010, we have also witnessed a dramatic increase (700%) in the incidence of biliary dyskinesia among children.[16] The incidence of biliary dyskinesia varies by region in the United States with high incidence in the Southeast.[17] The wide adoption of CCK-CS testing by primary care providers has likely increased the frequency of positive tests and not necessarily increased the incidence of biliary dyskinesia.[11]

CLINICAL PRESENTATION AND EXAMINATION FINDINGS

A focused history is critical to establish a diagnosis of biliary dyskinesia given that it is a diagnosis of exclusion. What is the specific nature of the pain in relationship to food, bowel movements, duration, time of day, and previous treatment? Classic biliary colic symptoms are characteristic of biliary dyskinesia. These symptoms include postprandial pain in the right upper quadrant radiating to the flank, back, or right shoulder blade; fatty food intolerance; onset of pain in evening or awaking a person at night; bloating; nausea, and vomiting. Constant abdominal pain without tenderness, positive Murphy's sign, or jaundice is not likely due to a functional biliary disorder. Intermittent, crampy pain with periods of diarrhea or constipation would support an intestinal source or etiology such as irritable bowel syndrome. Alternative sources of pain are listed in **Box 4**. Symptoms consistent with a functional biliary disorder resolve within 6 hours. In observational cohort studies, symptoms attributed to biliary dyskinesia resolved without an invasive procedure in approximately 50% of patients.[11]

DIAGNOSTIC TESTING AND PROCEDURES

Diagnostic testing for biliary dyskinesia should focus on excluding more common and more likely diagnoses including malignancy, gallbladder microlithiasis or sludge, peptic ulcer disease, chronic pancreatitis, and musculoskeletal syndromes. Laboratory studies should be performed to evaluate liver function (serum aspartate aminotransferase, alanine aminotransferase, total bilirubin) and evidence of pancreatitis

---

Box 4
Alternative sources of right upper quadrant pain

Common abdominal pain syndromes mimicking biliary pain

Irritable bowel syndrome

Peptic ulcer disease

Chronic constipation

Gastroesophageal reflux disease

Cirrhosis/end stage liver disease

Coronary artery disease

Costochondritis/musculoskeletal disorder

(serum amylase and lipase). Although computed tomography is commonly performed to evaluate acute abdominal pain, it does not adequately evaluate gallbladder or biliary disease. Abdominal ultrasound should be the primary diagnostic test for biliary pain. MRI is a highly sensitivity diagnostic modality, but comes with significant expense and should be avoided as a primary study unless malignancy or biliary obstruction is suspected.

Ultrasound examination

Ultrasound examination is required during the evaluation of biliary colic. Although the sensitivity of ultrasound is excellent (>90%), it does have interobserver variability.[18-21] Very small stones and stones located at the infundibulum can be difficult to see. Endoscopic ultrasound examination is complementary, has increased diagnostic sensitivity for gallbladder disease, and provides an opportunity to evaluate the biliary tree and pancreas.[22,23]

Cholecystokinin–Cholescintigraphy

CCK-CS is an important diagnostic tool in evaluating patients for biliary dyskinesia; however, it requires proper patient preparation, data acquisition, and analysis.[7,24] Early studies evaluating gallbladder disease used oral administration of iodopanoic acid to opacify the gallbladder followed by the ingestion of a fatty meal to stimulate gallbladder contraction. In 1976, the first gallbladder tracer, Tc-99-labeled lidofenin, was reported.[25] The common name for Tc-99 lidofenin is hepatobiliary iminodiacetic acid. Although hepatobiliary iminodiacetic acid is commonly used in placed of CCK-CS, the specific radiotracer used for CCK-CS varies among institutions. In 1981, Krishnamurthy and colleagues[26] introduced gallbladder ejection fraction calculations.

CCK-CS requires fasting for more than 4 hours and the avoidance of any medications that can impact sphincter of Oddi function including narcotics, nitrates, and calcium channel blockers. After administration of the radiotracer, patients are monitored for the hepatic and gallbladder phases. CCK is administered and gallbladder ejection fraction is calculated by geometric measurement of gallbladder radioactivity after a specified period of time. Pain during CCK administration should be noted.

Multiple factors should be considered when obtaining and interpreting CCK-CS.[24] Patient selection is important. No studies have compared diagnostic accuracy of CS in the acute presentation versus the elective outpatient setting. Pain with biliary dyskinesia is not constant, but rather episodic. Certain medications (narcotics, nitrates, and calcium channel blockers) will impact the accuracy of CCK-CS. Therefore, the clinical presentation, setting, and timing of the test should be considered.

Pain at the time of CCK infusion during CS is frequently used as a confirmatory test in diagnosing biliary dyskinesia. However, the dose and duration of CCK infusion impact pain. A short, 3-utemin infusion has greater variability in patient-reported pain than a longer continuous infusion. The abnormal ejection fraction in Rome II criteria was less than 40%. However, other studies have suggested a variety of cutoffs ranging from 35% to 50%.[27,28] The ejection fraction is no longer required for a diagnosis of biliary dyskinesia, but remains an important supportive criteria. In a systematic review of 23 studies by DiBaise and Oleynikov,[27] gallbladder ejection fraction was reported as a useful diagnostic tool in predicting positive postoperative outcomes in the treatment of functional gallbladder disorder. However, the authors concluded that current available studies had poor study design preventing any standard recommendations.

MRI

MRI and magnetic resonance cholangiopancreatography are recommended in patients with suspected choledocholithiasis, biliary obstruction, or concern for malignancy. Magnetic resonance cholangiopancreatography provides excellent evaluation of the gallbladder and biliary system, as well as an evaluation of the pancreas, duodenum, and liver. With increased availability of gadoxetic acid-contrasted MRI (Eovist), functional studies of the gallbladder are now available.[29–31] Unlike gadolinium, which is excreted by the kidney, 50% of gadoxetic acid is excreted by the biliary system. In a small study of patients with suspected biliary dyskinesia, gadoxetic acid-contrasted MRI seemed to perform as well as CS.[32]

Endoscopic Retrograde Pancreaticocholangiography and Sphincter Manometry

ERCP and sphincter manometry should only be considered after cholecystectomy in patients with suspected functional biliary sphincter of Oddi disorder. The complication rate for ERCP is greater than that for laparoscopic cholecystectomy. Complications include perforation, acute pancreatitis, and delayed ampullary stenosis. In carefully selected patients, ERCP can provide critical imaging of the biliary and pancreatic ducts. Measurements of sphincter tone can then be obtained using manometry. Pressure in a normal sphincter of Oddi is less than 30 mm Hg. High pressure is defined as greater than 40 mm Hg. Manometry recordings are highly variable, time dependent, and susceptible to movement artifact. Medications, especially narcotics, can alter sphincter pressure and need to be avoided during any manometry readings. During manometry, sphincter of Oddi function can be evaluated using the basal sphincter pressure and the phasic wave amplitude, duration, frequency, and propagation pattern. However, baseline sphincter pressure is the standard measurement used clinically. Owing to the technical challenges associated with sphincter manometry, it is not widely available and should only be performed in a specialized center.

MANAGEMENT OPTIONS AND CLINICAL OUTCOMES

Laparoscopic cholecystectomy is standard treatment for biliary dyskinesia with an intact gallbladder. In the absence of the gallbladder, invasive procedures, such as ERCP with sphincterotomy or botulin toxin inject of the sphincter of Oddi, are more controversial. A management algorithm for biliary dyskinesia is provided in **Fig. 2**.

Nonoperative Management

Nonoperative management of bile dyskinesia is poorly studied. Observational studies indicate that symptoms can resolve with time and invasive procedures are not required.[11] The medical management of biliary dyskinesia particularly functional sphincter of Oddi dysfunction has been very limited.[33] Calcium channel blockers such as nifedipine have been evaluated with some potential improvement in pain, but with side effects of headache and tachycardia.[34]

Cholecystectomy

Cholecystectomy is considered the standard treatment of biliary dyskinesia. As highlighted in a Cochrane Review by Gurusamy and colleagues,[35] only 1 randomized controlled trial by Yap and colleagues[36] has been performed to evaluate the benefit of cholecystectomy. In this study, 91% of patients had symptomatic relief with mean follow-up of 34 months. Two metaanalyses and 1 systemic review have examined the effectiveness of surgical therapy for biliary dyskinesia.[37–39] Ponsky and colleagues[38] identified 5 studies including 274 patients with 98% of patients having

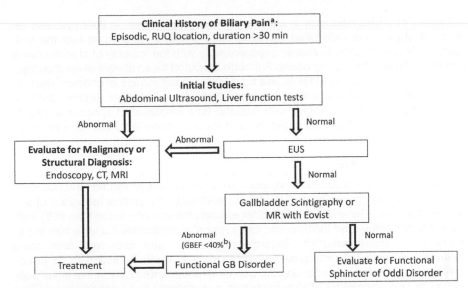

Fig. 2. Management recommendations for biliary dyskinesia. [a] Based on the Rome IV criteria. [b] If not all Rome IV criteria met, consider repeating gallbladder scintigraphy in 6 weeks. CT, computed tomography; EUS, endoscopic ultrasound; GBEF, gallbladder ejection fraction; RUQ, right upper quadrant.

symptomatic relief with surgery. Mahid and colleagues[37] identified 10 studies including 462 patients. Similarly, patients with no stones on ultrasound examination and a low gallbladder ejection fraction on CS benefited from cholecystectomy versus observation. Delgado-Aros and colleagues[39] reported in a systemic review of 9 studies involving 362 patients treated with cholecystectomy for biliary dyskinesia. In this study, they compared patients with normal gallbladder ejection fraction compared with abnormal gallbladder ejection fraction (<35%) to determine if CS could predict positive outcomes. Positive outcomes were experienced in both groups (odds ratio, 1.37; 95% confidence interval, 0.56–3.34; $P = .56$).

Studies of cholecystectomy are very promising, but can leave up to 20% patients with continued biliary pain.[40] By understanding the gallbladder–papillary reflex, we now understand that cholecystectomy can actually exacerbate functional sphincter of Oddi disorder. Therefore, patients should be counseled on this potential adverse outcome rather than proceeding with blind cholecystectomy.

Sphincterotomy

Sphincterotomy was once thought to be the optimal treatment for sphincter of Oddi dysfunction. Subtypes of sphincter of Oddi dysfunction (I, II, and III) have become outdated.[1] The EPISOD trial demonstrated no difference between sham sphincterotomy and sphincterotomy in type II sphincter of Oddi disorder.[4] Given unsatisfactory results and better recognition of procedure-related complications, sphincterotomy should only be performed for carefully selected patients at specialized centers well-versed in treating functional sphincter of Oddi disorder.

SPECIAL CONSIDERATIONS
The Pediatric Patient

Over the last decade, the number of children undergoing cholecystectomy for biliary dyskinesia has increased substantially.[16] Santucci and colleagues[41] evaluated the outcomes of cholecystectomy in children for biliary dyskinesia. In their systemic review, 31 studies were identified including 1833 children. All children had the gallbladder ejection fraction evaluated preoperatively with the majority of children being female (74%) and 48% being obese. Although the cutoff for an abnormal ejection fraction ranged from less than 35% to less than 50% among studies of children, the majority of studies used a cutoff of less than 35% for gallbladder ejection fraction. Outcomes were not encouraging with the long-term resolution of symptoms ranging from 34% to 100%. No prospective or randomized, controlled trials have been reported in children.

Hyperkinetic Gallbladder

CS (hepatobiliary iminodiacetic acid) reporting high gallbladder ejection fraction (over 80%) can be categorized as gallbladder hyperkinesia. The clinical relevance of this finding is unclear. Generally, a gallbladder ejection fraction of greater than 60% indicates normal gallbladder function and can support nonoperative management in patients with cholelithiasis.[42,43] Regardless, primary care providers and some gastroenterologists have interpreted a high gallbladder ejection fraction as abnormal. Very limited reports exist regarding the benefit of cholecystectomy in this small population. In a pediatric series of 12 patients with no gallstones and a gallbladder ejection fraction of greater than 80%, all patients were found to have histology consistent with chronic cholecystitis and 11 of the 12 patients were free of pain at postoperative follow-up (3–45 months).[44] In adults, Saurabh and Green[45] reported improvement in symptoms for 90% of patients undergoing cholecystectomy for hyperkinetic gallbladder.

SUMMARY

Biliary dyskinesia is defined as a functional disorder of the gallbladder or sphincter of Oddi with multiple potential underlying causative factors. CCK-CS demonstrating a low gallbladder ejection fraction facilitates diagnosis, but is not required. The diagnosis should be based on Rome IV criteria. Although a rare entity and diagnosis of exclusion, numerous retrospective studies indicate that it can be successfully treated with cholecystectomy. In the absence of the gallbladder, biliary dyskinesia is more challenging to treat and requires a specialized center with the capability of measuring sphincter manometry. The success of any invasive treatment for biliary dyskinesia is defined as absence of biliary pain more than 12 months after intervention. Unfortunately, prospective studies of biliary dyskinesia with patient-centered outcomes are lacking making evidence-based treatment recommends challenging.

REFERENCES

1. Cotton PB, Elta GH, Carter CR, et al. Gallbladder and sphincter of Oddi disorders. Gastroenterology 2016;150(6):1420–9.e2.
2. Corazziari E, Shaffer EA, Hogan WJ, et al. Functional disorders of the biliary tract and pancreas. Gut 1999;45(Suppl 2):II48–54.
3. Behar J, Corazziari E, Guelrud M, et al. Functional gallbladder and sphincter of Oddi disorders. Gastroenterology 2006;130(5):1498–509.
4. Cotton PB, Durkalski V, Romagnuolo J, et al. Effect of endoscopic sphincterotomy for suspected sphincter of Oddi dysfunction on pain-related disability following cholecystectomy: the EPISOD randomized clinical trial. JAMA 2014;311(20):2101–9.

5. You YN, Xing Y, Feig BW, et al. Young-onset colorectal cancer: is it time to pay attention? Arch Intern Med 2012;172(3):287–9.
6. Francis G, Baillie J. Gallbladder dyskinesia: fact or fiction? Curr Gastroenterol Rep 2011;13(2):188–92.
7. Krishnamurthy S, Krishnamurthy GT. Biliary dyskinesia: role of the sphincter of Oddi, gallbladder and cholecystokinin. J Nucl Med 1997;38(11):1824–30.
8. Thune A, Saccone GTP, Scicchitano JP, et al. Distension of the gall bladder inhibits sphincter of Oddi motility in humans. Gut 1991;32(6):690–3.
9. Westphal K. Muskelfunktion, Nervensystem and Patholgie der Gallenwege [German]. Ztscher F Klin Med 1923;96:22–150.
10. McGowan J, Butsch W, Walters W. Pressure in the common bile duct of man – its relation to pain following cholecystectomy. J Am Med Assoc 1936;106(26): 2227–30.
11. Bielefeldt K, Saligram S, Zickmund SL, et al. Cholecystectomy for biliary dyskinesia: how did we get there? Dig Dis Sci 2014;59(12):2850–63.
12. Patel NA, Lamb JJ, Hogle NJ, et al. Therapeutic efficacy of laparoscopic cholecystectomy in the treatment of biliary dyskinesia. Am J Surg 2004;187(2):209–12.
13. Ziessman HA. Functional hepatobiliary disease: chronic acalculous gallbladder and chronic acalculous biliary disease. Semin Nucl Med 2006;36(2):119–32.
14. Rose JB, Fields RC, Strasberg SM. Poor reproducibility of gallbladder ejection fraction by biliary scintigraphy for diagnosis of biliary dyskinesia. J Am Coll Surg 2018;226(2):155–9.
15. Preston JF, Diggs BS, Dolan JP, et al. Biliary dyskinesia: a surgical disease rarely found outside the United States. Am J Surg 2015;209(5):799–803.
16. Bielefeldt K. The rising tide of cholecystectomy for biliary dyskinesia. Aliment Pharmacol Ther 2013;37(1):98–106.
17. Bielefeldt K. Regional differences in hospitalizations and cholecystectomies for biliary dyskinesia. J Neurogastroenterol Motil 2013;19(3):381–9.
18. Hwang H, Marsh I, Doyle J. Does ultrasonography accurately diagnose acute cholecystitis? Improving diagnostic accuracy based on a review at a regional hospital. Can J Surg 2014;57(3):162–8.
19. Stone KS, Scholten DJ, Dean RE. Ultrasound as the initial diagnostic study in patients with suspected gallstones. Am Surg 1980;46(8):444–8.
20. Golea A, Badea R, Suteu T. Role of ultrasonography for acute cholecystic conditions in the emergency room. Med Ultrason 2010;12(4):271–9.
21. Davis CK, Schoffstall RO. Correlation of ultrasonic gallbladder studies with operative findings. South Med J 1981;74(7):781–4.
22. Somani P, Sunkara T, Sharma M. Role of endoscopic ultrasound in idiopathic pancreatitis. World J Gastroenterol 2017;23(38):6952–61.
23. Chantarojanasiri T, Hirooka Y, Kawashima H, et al. The role of endoscopic ultrasound in the diagnosis of gallbladder diseases. J Med Ultrason (2001) 2017; 44(1):63–70.
24. Richmond BK, Dibaise J, Ziessman H. Utilization of cholecystokinin cholescintigraphy in clinical practice. J Am Coll Surg 2013;217(2):317–23.
25. Loberg MD, Cooper M, Harvey E, et al. Development of new radiopharmaceuticals based on N-substitution of iminodiacetic acid. J Nucl Med 1976;17(7):633–8.
26. Krishnamurthy GT, Bobba VR, Kingston E. Radionuclide ejection fraction: a technique for quantitative analysis of motor function of the human gallbladder. Gastroenterology 1981;80(3):482.

27. DiBaise JK, Oleynikov D. Does gallbladder ejection fraction predict outcome after cholecystectomy for suspected chronic acalculous gallbladder dysfunction? A systematic review. Am J Gastroenterol 2003;98(12):2605–11.
28. DuCoin C, Faber R, Ilagan M, et al. Normokinetic biliary dyskinesia: a novel diagnosis. Surg Endosc 2012;26(11):3088–93.
29. Evoist B. Injection (safety information) 2018. Available at: https://www.radiologysolutions.bayer.com/products/mr/contrast/eovist-pi/?ecid=radiology:ps:de:psl:psl:42226:100197&gclid=CjwKCAjwxILdBRBqEiwAHL2R80L7hz0GdgP9nCQycPDrT6kixNaR5xGsxP3_1npvV03G5xrD_QtsdxoCtNcQAvD_BwE. Accessed September 18, 2018.
30. Schwope RB, May LA, Reiter MJ, et al. Gadoxetic acid: pearls and pitfalls. Abdom Imaging 2015;40(6):2012–29.
31. Palmucci S, Roccasalva F, Piccoli M, et al. Contrast-enhanced magnetic resonance cholangiography: practical tips and clinical indications for biliary disease management. Gastroenterol Res Pract 2017;2017. https://doi.org/10.1155/2017/2403012.
32. Lee JK, Kim Y, Lee S, et al. Hepatobiliary phase of gadoxetic acid-enhanced MR in patients suspected of having gallbladder dyskinesia: comparison with hepatobiliary scintigraphy. Clin Imaging 2015;39(1):66–71.
33. Bistritz L, Bain VG. Sphincter of Oddi dysfunction: managing the patient with chronic biliary pain. World J Gastroenterol 2006;12(24):3793–802.
34. Sand J, Nordback I, Koskinen M, et al. Nifedipine for suspected type II sphincter of Oddi dyskinesia. Am J Gastroenterol 1993;88(4):530–5.
35. Gurusamy KS, Junnarkar S, Farouk M, et al. Cholecystectomy for suspected gallbladder dyskinesia. Cochrane Database Syst Rev 2009;(1):CD007086.
36. Yap L, Wycherley AG, Morphett AD, et al. Acalculous biliary pain: cholecystectomy alleviates symptoms in patients with abnormal cholescintigraphy. Gastroenterology 1991;101(3):786–93.
37. Mahid SS, Jafri NS, Brangers BC, et al. Meta-analysis of cholecystectomy in symptomatic patients with positive hepatobiliary iminodiacetic acid scan results without gallstones. Arch Surg 2009;144(2):180–7.
38. Ponsky TA, DeSagun R, Brody F. Surgical therapy for biliary dyskinesia: a meta-analysis and review of the literature. J Laparoendosc Adv Surg Tech A 2005;15(5):439–42.
39. Delgado-Aros S, Cremonini F, Bredenoord AJ, et al. Systematic review and meta-analysis: does gall-bladder ejection fraction on cholecystokinin cholescintigraphy predict outcome after cholecystectomy in suspected functional biliary pain? Aliment Pharmacol Ther 2003;18(2):167–74.
40. Adams DB. Biliary dyskinesia: does it exist? if so, how do we diagnose it? is laparoscopic cholecystectomy effective or a sham operation? J Gastrointest Surg 2013;17(9):1550–2.
41. Santucci NR, Hyman PE, Harmon CM, et al. Biliary dyskinesia in children: a systematic review. J Pediatr Gastroenterol Nutr 2017;64(2):186–93.
42. Dauer M, Lammert F. Mandatory and optional function tests for biliary disorders. Best Pract Res Clin Gastroenterol 2009;23(3):441–51.
43. Pauletzki J, Althaus R, Holl J, et al. Gallbladder emptying and gallstone formation: a prospective study on gallstone recurrence. Gastroenterology 1996;111(3):765–71.
44. Lindholm EB, Alberty JB, Hansbourgh F, et al. Hyperkinetic gallbladder: an indication for cholecystectomy? Am Surg 2013;79(9):882–4.
45. Saurabh S, Green B. Is hyperkinetic gallbladder an indication for cholecystectomy? Surg Endosc 2018. https://doi.org/10.1007/s00464-018-6435-2.

Bile Metabolism and Lithogenesis: An Update

Austin R. Dosch, MD[a], David K. Imagawa, MD, PhD[a],
Zeljka Jutric, MD[a,b],*

KEYWORDS

• Bile acid synthesis • Lithogenesis • Gallstones • Bile metabolism • Cholelithiasis

KEY POINTS

• Bile is composed of multiple macromolecules, including bile acids, free cholesterol, phospholipids, bilirubin, and inorganic ions that aid in digestion, nutrient absorption, and disposal of the insoluble products of heme catabolism.

• The synthesis and release of bile acids is tightly controlled and dependent on feedback mechanisms that regulate enterohepatic circulation.

• Alterations in bile composition, impaired gallbladder relaxation, and accelerated nucleation are the principal mechanisms leading to biliary stone formation.

• Various physiologic conditions and disease states alter bile composition and metabolism, thus increasing the risk of developing gallstones.

INTRODUCTION

Biliary lithiasis is a common condition that leads to a significant health care burden nationwide, with an estimated 20 million Americans (10%–15% of the adult population) affected by gallstones.[1] As the incidence of obesity and advanced age have increased in the population, so has the frequency of cholelithiasis. With an annual cost of $6.5 billion, gallstones are among the most expensive disorders in the United States, having increased 20% over the last 3 decades. The development of biliary stones occurs when the careful balance between bile constituents is disturbed and can be precipitated by multiple conditions. This article discusses the synthesis and release of the components that comprise digestive bile and the diverse roles of bile in digestion, metabolism, and hormonal signaling within the gastrointestinal tract. It also examines the epidemiology of cholelithiasis, risk factors for developing gallstones, and the various chemical processes that underlie the pathophysiology of biliary stone disease.

Disclosure: The authors have nothing to disclose.
[a] Department of Surgery, University of California Irvine; [b] Hepatobiliary and Pancreas Surgery, Department of Surgery, University of California Irvine, Orange, CA, USA
* Corresponding author. Hepatobiliary and Pancreas Surgery, Department of Surgery, University of California Irvine, 333 City Blvd. West, Suite 1600, Orange, CA 92868.
E-mail address: zjutric@uci.edu

Surg Clin N Am 99 (2019) 215–229
https://doi.org/10.1016/j.suc.2018.12.003
0039-6109/19/© 2018 Elsevier Inc. All rights reserved.

Bile Metabolism

Chemical composition, synthesis, and excretion of bile

The chemical structure of bile is complex and depends on the diet, genetics, and gut microbiome present in each individual. The major constituents of bile are bile acids (BAs), phospholipids, cholesterol, and bilirubin, along with other trace metals and ions.[2] BAs comprise most of the bile substance and consist of a heterogeneous group of molecules that act as detergents to aid in food digestion and nutrient absorption. BAs are derived from cholesterol and contain a characteristic steroid nucleus (three 6-carbon rings, one 5-carbon ring) and are altered by the location and steric orientation of hydroxyl groups on this backbone.[3] Synthesis involves a multistep process that consists of 17 different enzymes. Of these, the most important and well characterized is cholesterol 7α-hydroxylase (cytochrome P 7A1 [CYP7A1]), a member of the cytochrome P450 superfamily of enzymes. CYP7A1 catalyzes the formation of 7α-hydroxycholesterol from steroid precursors, which is the initial and rate-limiting step in BA biosynthesis,[4] and 7α-hydroxycholesterol then undergoes a series of modifications during this multistep process, including ring modification, side chain oxidation, and conjugation of the final product to the amino acids glycine or taurine.[5,6] Conjugation is an important event in BA synthesis that increases the polarity of the molecule, thereby increasing its solubility and ability to form micelles in solution.[7,8]

BAs can be classified as either primary or secondary. Primary BAs are synthesized de novo in liver hepatocytes and consist of cholic acid and chenodeoxycholic acid. Secondary BAs are formed through a sequence of reactions (hydrolysis, dehydroxylation, epimerization) catalyzed by gut microbiota that alter primary BA structure and function.[9,10] These modifications result in a heterogeneous group of 15 to 20 secondary BA compounds, including deoxycholic acid (12%), ursodeoxycholic acid (9%), and lithocholic acid (0.4%).[11–14] Phosphatidylcholines are the predominant phospholipid present in bile and are synthesized by the liver expressly for secretion in biliary fluid.[8,15,16] Phosphatidylcholine and BAs act in concert to increase the solubility of cholesterol in bile, aiding in its secretion into the intestine.[17] Bilirubin, the waste product of heme catabolism, is the last major component of bile. Heme consists of an Fe^{2+} ion positioned at the center of the porphyrin ring, protoporphyrin-IX. Its breakdown is initiated in macrophages via activation of the enzyme heme oxygenase-1, eventually leading to its conversion to biliverdin after the processing of multiple intermediates. Biliverdin is further metabolized by the enzyme biliverdin reductase into unconjugated bilirubin, a product that is hydrophobic and toxic to normal tissues. Because it is poorly soluble, unconjugated bilirubin requires binding to albumin in order to transport it to the liver, where it is then transported on the sinusoidal surface of hepatocytes and undergoes conjugation via covalent attachment to glucuronic acid. This reaction is catalyzed by the enzyme uridinediphospho-glucuronosyltransferase 1A1 (UGT-1A1), which is functionally deficient in cases of Crigler-Najjar syndrome. The glucuronidation of bilirubin increases solubility and allows it to be excreted into the intestine, where it undergoes further processing by bacterial and intestinal brush border enzymes.[8,18]

The liver produces 600 to 750 mL of bile per day. Liver architecture and structure plays a key role in the secretion of bile. Hepatocytes show cellular polarity, with the basolateral (sinusoidal) membrane abutting the space of Disse and portal blood flow, whereas the apical (canalicular) membrane is in contact with the bile canaliculi. Bile canaliculi are formed through tight junctional complexes between adjacent hepatocytes and flow directly into the main biliary tree through the portal triad, countercurrent to hepatic artery and portal vein flow.[19] Secretion of bile requires both active and passive transport mechanisms. Hepatocytes actively secrete organic (BAs, glutathione) and inorganic ions (HCO_3^-, Cl^-) into canaliculi through multiple transmembrane channels, specifically the ATP-binding cassette (ABC)-transporter family of proteins. This process occurs against a high chemical gradient and is the rate-limiting step in BA secretion. Active transport of BAs and other solutes leads to passive movement of water across tight junctions because of the osmotic gradient formed in this process.[20]

In contrast with the hepatocyte-lined canaliculi, bile ducts and ductules are lined with specialized cells, known as cholangiocytes, which further process and alter bile composition as it is transported through the biliary tree. Gastrointestinal hormones, such as secretin, which is released from the S cells of the duodenum and functions in part to regulate the duodenal pH during digestion, exert their effects on the composition and flow of bile through binding to receptors on basolateral surface of these cells, thereby activating cyclic AMP (cAMP) response pathways within the cell. Intracellular accumulation of cAMP within cholangiocytes leads to a series of changes resulting in depolarization and the active extrusion of HCO_3^- across the canalicular membrane along with passive water movement, thus increasing biliary volume and flow.[21] Simultaneously, cholangiocytes continually alter bile composition by absorbing inorganic ions, BAs, glucose, and amino acids as it travels through the biliary tract.[22] These mechanisms are highly regulated and function to carefully adjust the molecular composition of bile fluid to meet physiologic demands.

Excess bile is stored in the gallbladder, a pear-shaped hollow organ that is connected directly to the common bile duct via the cystic duct. Gallbladder contraction and expulsion of additional bile during food consumption plays a vital role in meeting the physiologic demands of intraluminal fat digestion. The gallbladder receives its blood supply via the cystic artery, which usually originates from the right hepatic artery branch of the common hepatic artery, although anomalous cystic artery anatomy is common.[23] Although typically regarded as a reservoir for excess bile, the gallbladder plays an active role in adjusting the ratio of biliary components during storage. Because of their function as organic detergents, bile salts can be directly toxic to normal epithelial tissue. The mucosal lining of the gallbladder is shielded from potential damage because of the high level of prostaglandin E2, which stimulates the secretion of mucin within the lumen, which not only acts as a barrier but also neutralizes harmful free radicals present within bile salts, which are directly cytotoxic. The mucosal barrier is composed of a single layer of epithelial cells, which allow diffusion of ions and water across the membrane, a process that plays a key role in concentrating bile and aiding in the digestion of fats.[24,25] Biliary stone formation is heavily dependent on both the composition of bile and presence of mucin, making physiologic alterations in gallbladder function an important variable in the development of biliary lithiasis, which is discussed in further detail later in the article.

Digestive role of bile

Bile salts are amphipathic molecules and therefore invaluable in the solubilization of nonpolar compounds such as lipids and fat-soluble vitamins during digestion. Lipid metabolism and absorption is among the most important and well-studied functions of bile. After fats arrive in the stomach, emulsification begins. Emulsification is the process in which lipid droplets are mechanically suspended into an aqueous solution and acts to reduce the surface area of lipid droplets and allow them to interact with macromolecules that aid in digestion. This solution then enters the duodenum, where pancreatic lipase begins to initiate lipid hydrolysis. On entering the duodenum, cholecystokinin release is triggered from I cells of the duodenum and jejunum, which leads to gallbladder contraction, sphincter of Oddi relaxation, and release of bile into the intestinal lumen.[26] Bile plays a critical role in lipid digestion, principally interacting with luminal phospholipids to shield the nonpolar core of fatty acid emulsions by forming amphipathic molecules known as micelles. Micelle formation has 2-fold benefit. First, it allows dietary lipids to be dissolved in fluid and is the first step in preparing the emulsion for digestion. Second, the micelles formed by BAs (20–500 nm) are small enough to fit in between intestinal villae[27] and this aids in exposing lipids to brush border lipases, allowing them to be further processed for absorption.[28] When in close proximity to enterocytes, most digested lipids (monoglycerides, free fatty acids) can easily cross the plasma membrane. These lipids are then packaged in chylomicrons and shuttled into the systemic circulation through the portal lymphatics. In addition to lipid digestion, micelles aid in the absorption of cholesterol and fat-soluble vitamins (A, D, E, and K), which are contained within its hydrophobic core. To a lesser extent, bile participates in the digestion of proteins and carbohydrates as well.[29] However, bile is only indispensable for lipid metabolism and absorption. In cases in which BA production is insufficient (BA synthesis defects), biliary flow is obstructed (malignancy, impacted gallstone, intrahepatic cholestasis), or there is inadequate reabsorption of bile in the terminal ileum (inflammatory bowel disease, surgical resection, bacterial overgrowth), lipid metabolism is greatly inhibited. This inhibition results in steatorrhea, malabsorption, and deficiency in fat-soluble vitamins in affected patients.

Bile has pleotropic roles that extend beyond simple digestion, functioning extensively in both hormonal signaling and maintaining the microfloral composition of the gut. BAs mediate these effects largely through the nuclear farnesoid X receptor (FXR), which is expressed in hepatocytes, enterocytes, and even renal tubules, all of which play an important role in BA homeostasis.[30] FXR binds directly to BAs and initiates nuclear translocation, in which the FXR-ligand complex acts as a transcription factor through direct DNA binding.[31] This event has several important implications in the metabolism of multiple macromolecules. FXR activation lowers levels of plasma triglycerides, FFAs, and cholesterol and has also been shown to curtail hepatic steatosis in mouse models through induction of lipoprotein clearance from the bloodstream.[32–34] Glucose homeostasis is also regulated in part by FXR, with its activation stimulating cellular pathways that improve insulin sensitivity and inhibit hepatic gluconeogenesis.[35,36] FXR also plays an integral role in the regulation of BA biosynthesis, which is discussed in further detail later. In addition to its effects on the FXR, BA also modulates the host immune environment and overall gastrointestinal function through activation of a G-protein–coupled receptor, TGR5. TGR5 activation has numerous downstream functions, including regulating immune function and inflammation, influencing the composition of intestinal bacterial flora, altering intestinal motility, and stimulating macromolecule catabolism, further highlighting the diverse roles of BA.[34]

Enterohepatic circulation and the regulation of bile production

BAs are efficiently recycled during transit through the intestinal tract. Of the 2 to 4 g of BAs present in the body at any given time, roughly 5% to 10% are secreted daily in stool. The reuptake is remarkably efficient considering BA recycling occurs anywhere from 6 to 10 times per day between the ileum and liver.[34] The circulation of bile from intestines, through the portal vein, and back to the liver is known as enterohepatic circulation. After fulfilling their physiologic purposes and reaching the terminal ileum, the process of reabsorption and recirculation of luminal BAs begins. BAs are absorbed into enterocytes of the ileum via the apical sodium-dependent bile salt transporter

(ASBT) and extruded into the portal circulation through members of the organic anion transporter (OSTα/β) family.[37,38] They are then carried through the portal vein bound to albumin and enter the liver through hepatic sinusoids. Conjugated BA uptake by hepatocytes predominately occurs through the Na$^+$-taurocholate cotransporting polypeptide channel, whereas unconjugated bile can often be absorbed passively.[38,39] Within the hepatocyte, BAs may undergo processing and repair by a series of chemical reactions (oxidation, epimerization, hydroxylation, conjugation) before being resecreted into the bile canaliculi. This process is highly efficient, removing 50% to 90% of BAs from the portal system in its first pass.[38] New BAs are then synthesized from cholesterol to replenish those lost in stool or not extracted from the portal venous system.

On average, 500 mg/d of cholesterol is converted into new BAs to replace those lost during enterohepatic circulation. This amount represents nearly 90% of all cholesterol metabolism in the body, with the remainder reserved for synthesis of steroid hormones.[6] To ensure that a consistent amount of bile is available for digestion, the process of BA synthesis is tightly regulated and heavily dependent on feedback mechanisms triggered by gut BA absorption. The FXR in the ileal enterocyte acts as the initial gatekeeper in the regulation of BA homeostasis. On entry into the enterocyte, BA binds the FXR and initiates transcription of the hormone fibroblast growth factor 19 (FGF19). FGF19 signals through the receptor fibroblast growth factor receptor 4 (FGFR4) and its coreceptor β-Klotho on the cell surface of hepatocytes. Stimulation of the FGFR4-β-Klotho complex by FGF19 activates numerous downstream kinases, including ERK1/2, which culminates in transcriptional repression of CYP7A1, the rate-limiting enzyme in BA biosynthesis.[4,40] In this manner, BA reuptake by enterocytes of the ileum is able to directly repress the unnecessary transcription of new bile salts from cholesterol by signaling through the FXR-FGF19 axis (**Fig. 1**).

Bile acid sequestrants and lipid-lowering agents

Elucidation of the mechanisms controlling the regulatory pathway of BA synthesis has enabled the manipulation of BA levels in order to modulate metabolism in disease. BA sequestrants have been used as lipid-lowering medications for more than half a century. These agents, including cholestyramine, colestipol, and colesevelam, bind luminal BAs and block their absorption into the enterocyte, effectively depleting the pool of available BAs. This stimulates de novo synthesis of new BA from cholesterol by inducing CYP7A1 transcription. Because of the need for additional cholesterol, this results in lower plasma levels of lipoprotein carriers, such as low-density lipoproteins (LDLs), known culprits in the pathogenesis of ischemic heart disease.[41] The induction of CYP7A1 results in the release of systemic factors that also increase metabolic rates in peripheral tissues and reduce insulin sensitivity, further combating hypercholesterolemia and hyperglycemia. Although largely replaced by statins, these compounds are still used for select patients in the management of increased serum cholesterol levels.

Lithogenesis

Epidemiology and risk factors for the development of gallstones

Epidemiology and natural history Biliary lithiasis is a common medical problem and frequent cause of physician office visits and inpatient hospitalizations nationwide. The disease disproportionately afflicts women, with an estimated 14 million women affected annually compared with 6 million men.[42] Although highly prevalent in the population, only a minority of patients with gallstones (~20%) develop symptoms.[43] The risk of becoming symptomatic is 2% to 3% per year with a cumulative risk of 10% at

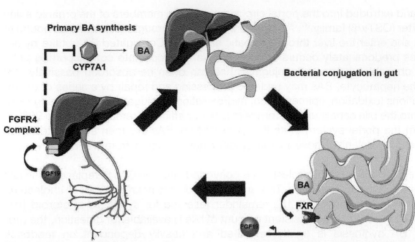

Fig. 1. Summary of enterohepatic circulation. New BAs are synthesized in the liver by a multistep process, with the rate-limiting enzyme CYP7A1 serving as a key regulatory step. Once synthesized, primary BAs are excreted into the duodenum through the biliary tree, where they undergo conjugation into secondary BAs by luminal bacteria. After circulating through the small intestine and aiding in digestion, BAs are absorbed into the enterocytes of the terminal ileum via the ASBT and extruded into the portal circulation through members of the OSTα/β family, where they are returned to the liver for further use. The process is highly efficient, with 90% to 95% of BAs reabsorbed through enterohepatic circulation each day. Synthesis of new BAs in the liver is regulated in part by the FXR on the surface of the ileal enterocyte. On arrival in the terminal ileum, free BAs bind FXR and initiate transcription of FGF19. FGF19 binds the FGF4-β-Klotho complex on the surface of hepatocytes, triggering the activation of numerous downstream pathways that result in transcriptional repression of CYP7A1 and the cessation of further BA synthesis.

5 years. A smaller percentage of these patients (1%–2% per year) develop choledocholithiasis or acute pancreatitis.

There seems to be both a strong genetic predisposition and environmental influence in the development of gallstone disease. According to population studies, the highest rate of biliary lithiasis is in patients of Native American heritage, with nearly two-thirds of the adult female population showing evidence of cholelithiasis by ultrasonography.[44] White Americans have a lower prevalence of stone disease, with 16.6% of women and 8.6% of men affected. Rates among Hispanic (5.4% men, 19.1% women) and black (5.3% men, 13.5% women) populations are similar to that of their white counterparts.[42,45]

Risk factors

Gender Women have a substantially higher rate of gallstone formation compared with men. This gender disparity narrows as age increases, particularly after women undergo menopause,[46] suggesting a role for female sex hormones in the pathogenesis of stone disease. Exogenous estrogen administration to postmenopausal women has been shown to increase the risk of biliary stones.[47,48] Multiple studies have defined the biological role of estrogen in regulating various cellular mechanisms that favor stone formation. The estrogen receptors ESR1 and ESR2 are both expressed in hepatocytes and receptor activation increases the secretion of cholesterol into bile. De novo synthesis of cholesterol through activation of the rate-limiting enzyme hydroxy-methylglutaryl coenzyme A reductase is promoted by estrogen binding, leading to enhanced synthesis of cholesterol and supersaturation of bile.[49,50] In addition to enhancing synthesis and excretion into bile, estrogen has been implicated in the development of cholesterol stones through enhanced expression of the sterol transporter Niemann-Pick type C 1 in intestinal cells, which increases gut absorption of cholesterol and contributes to systemic dyslipidemia.[51] These mechanisms also explain the increased incidence of biliary lithiasis in pregnant women, who have increased levels of circulating estrogens.

Metabolic syndrome Metabolic syndrome, defined as the constellation of insulin resistance, central obesity, and dyslipidemia, is a strong risk factor for the development of cholesterol gallstones.[52] This relationship is not caused by the increased prevalence of hypercholesterolemia in this population, as would be suggested by the high incidence of cholesterol stones in patients with metabolic syndrome. High levels of serum LDLs are poorly correlated with a risk of gallstone formation. It seems the more important factors are low levels of high-density lipoproteins and systemic hyperlipidemia, which contribute to lithogenesis rather than total cholesterol level alone.[53] Patients with metabolic syndrome frequently have increased levels of homocysteine, which can result in a proinflammatory state that is typically cited as a major risk factor for coronary artery disease but has also been shown to play a role in the formation of biliary stones.[54]

Rapid weight loss Extreme dieting, rapid weight fluctuations, and weight loss surgery have all been associated with an increased rate of cholelithiasis. In obese patients undergoing weight loss surgery, biliary sludge develops in nearly one-third of all patients.[55] A potential explanation for this phenomenon is enhanced hepatic secretion of cholesterol into bile caused by enhanced metabolism of lipid stores. In addition, fasting results in reduced gallbladder emptying and biliary stasis, which can also influence the development of cholesterol stones. For these reasons, consensus recommendation is to aim for weight loss of approximately 5% to 10% of starting weight in a 6-month period supplemented by a balanced diet and exercise regimen to avoid the risk of developing gallstones.[56]

Total parenteral nutrition and critical illness Although commonly associated with a risk of acalculous gallbladder disease, both total parenteral nutrition (TPN) and severe illness are risk factors for the development of microlithiasis and gallstones. Prospective studies surveying intensive care unit patients using ultrasonography have shown that stones form as early as 5 days after fasting.[57] Likewise, nearly all patients receiving prolonged TPN show evidence of gallbladder sludge after 6 weeks of therapy.[58] This increased risk is likely multifactorial, stemming from both biliary stasis caused by lack of dietary gallbladder stimulation and the systemic proinflammatory state induced by critical illness, which can be in itself lithogenic.[46]

Hepatic cirrhosis Gallstones occur in around one-third of patients with cirrhosis and is directly proportional to the severity of liver disease. The estimated cumulative incidence is 5.5 patients per 100 cirrhotic patients per year based on prospective studies.[59] In contrast with the general population, most biliary stones in cirrhotic patients are black pigment stones, indicating that the pathogenesis is more likely to be caused by disorders of hepatic bilirubin metabolism and excretion rather than imbalances in cholesterol.[60] The increased risk of biliary lithiasis in cirrhotic patients is caused by multiple factors, including impaired gallbladder contractility, reduced synthesis of BAs, and an increased rate of hypersplenism and red blood cell hemolysis.[61] The development of stones in this population can have disastrous consequences, because these patients are often poor operative candidates and may not tolerate cholecystectomy, leaving temporizing measures such as cholecystostomy tubes as the only suitable treatment option in certain cases.

Crohn disease Crohn disease, specifically affecting the terminal ileum (TI), can lead to impaired recycling of BAs, which exceeds the liver's capacity to produce additional BAs to solubilize cholesterol in bile and thus enhances cholesterol stone formation. Furthermore, pigmented stone formation may also be increased in patients with TI involvement because of enhanced reabsorption of bilirubin in the colon.[62] Overall, patients with Crohn disease have a 2 to 3 times higher rate of gallstones than the general population.[63]

Genetics Population studies suggest as high as a 30% genetic component in the development of gallstones. Genes controlling hepatic cholesterol metabolism have been associated with the pathway of gallstone formation in mouse models and in human subjects. Genes responsible for cholesterol absorption have also been studied in the development of gallstones caused by bile salt loss. Single-gene mutations that result in hemolysis cause an excess of unconjugated BAs that form polymerized calcium bilirubinate stones, and increase the incidence of black stones.[64]

Pathogenesis of biliary stones
Imbalances in the composition of bile, namely cholesterol or bilirubin, is the principal mechanism that leads to the formation of stones within the biliary tract. Stones are commonly classified into 3 types: cholesterol stones, black pigmented stones, and brown pigmented stones. Both cholesterol and black pigmented stones commonly form within the gallbladder and their formation is largely dependent on host lipid homeostasis and bilirubin metabolism. In contrast, brown pigmented stones are associated with infection of the biliary tract and typically form primarily within the bile duct, occurring only in the gallbladder rarely in cases of cholecystitis in which bacterial colonization has occurred.[65]

Cholesterol stones Almost all (90%) biliary stones are cholesterol stones.[66] Cholesterol supersaturation, accelerated nucleation, and gallbladder hypomotility are essential components that occur in concert during the initiation and propagation of cholesterol stones (**Fig. 2**). The initial step in the formation of cholesterol stones is sterol supersaturation in bile. Although very insoluble in an aqueous solution, the chemical properties of bile allow a high amount of cholesterol ($\sim$20 mM) to be dissolved in

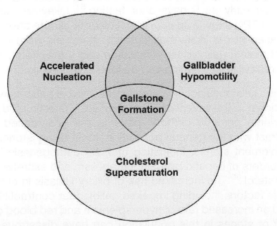

Fig. 2. Physiologic changes required for cholesterol stone formation.

fluid.[67] As outlined earlier, the major molecular mediators of cholesterol solubility in bile are bile salts and phospholipids, which form mixed micelles to stabilize free hydrophobic sterols. These amphipathic macromolecules allow cholesterol to dissolve in fluid by shielding sterols within a hydrophobic core, enabling transport and excretion into the intestine. Supersaturation refers to a chemical state in which the concentration of hydrophobic cholesterol molecules exceeds the capacity of these chaperone molecules to maintain its solubility in fluid. Cholesterol supersaturation can therefore occur when there is (1) hepatic hypersecretion of cholesterol, (2) reduced bile salt or phospholipid excretion by the liver, or (3) a combination of both cholesterol hypersecretion and reduced levels of bile salts or phospholipids necessary to solubilize sterols within micelles.[68] Increased secretion of cholesterol by the liver can occur through a variety of mechanisms. Hepatocytes contain receptors for nearly all lipoprotein classes, which enables the liver to uptake cholesterol from the systemic circulation for elimination in bile as either free cholesterol or through conversion into bile salts. Cholesterol derived from circulating lipoproteins provides most of the cholesterol that is secreted into bile. As such, systemic dyslipidemia and obesity are strong risk factors for the development of cholesterol gallstones.[69] After uptake from circulation, cholesterol is shuttled to the canalicular membrane by the Niemann-Pick type C 1 and 2 proteins, making it available for transport into the extracellular space. From there, cholesterol secretion into the bile canaliculi is mediated by multiple apical membrane transporters: ATPase class I type 8B member 1, ABCG5/ABCG8, Niemann-Pick C1-like protein 1, and SR-BI.[70] Dysregulation of these transport proteins can lead to an increase in the secretion of cholesterol into bile and an increased risk for the development of biliary stones. For example, the ABCG5/ABCG8 are transporters that are overactive in patients with insulin resistance because of upregulation of the FoxO1 transcription factor, which leads to an excess of biliary cholesterol and may partially account for the high rate of gallstones seen in the diabetic population.[71,72] Furthermore, secretion of cholesterol into bile is coupled to the transport of BAs (ABCB11) and phospholipids (ABCB4) to ensure that the delicate balance of bile constituents is not disturbed by cholesterol transport. These transporters are essential in the homeostasis of cholesterol solubility in bile and provide the BAs and phospholipids needed to shield cholesterol within micelles and prevent luminal precipitation. Genetic disorders resulting in dysfunctional ABCB11 or ABCB4 result in impaired secretion of BAs and phospholipids, respectively, and confer an increased risk for the development of gallstones caused by cholesterol supersaturation.[73] Variations in BA composition, which differ markedly among the population, can also influence this process. A higher composition of hydrophobic bile salts (chenodeoxycholate, deoxycholate) promotes cholesterol crystallization and gallstone formation.[65]

Nucleation refers to the process in which a new phase or structure is formed in a medium by self-assembly. This process depends on the thermodynamic and chemical properties of the system and differs depending on the surrounding microenvironment and concentration of solute within a fluid. For instance, at 0° (the freezing point) water begins to crystallize and form ice. However, at this exact temperature, the solution does not undergo instant, uniform change into a solid block of ice but requires sustained duration of exposure in order to completely solidify. Within the solution, there is spontaneous formation of ice crystals, which are continuously broken up and reformed. When enough molecules of water aggregate and the crystal reaches a critical mass, homogeneous nucleation may occur. Additional water molecules are recruited and eventually the whole solution turns to ice over time. Similarly, cholesterol stone formation cannot form from cholesterol supersaturation alone but requires the development of physiologic conditions that favor accelerated nucleation.[74] When cholesterol is supersaturated in a fluid and unable to be successfully shielded from its hydrophilic environment, it naturally adopts a conformation that favors its lowest energy state, which is referred to a vesicle. This vesicle can be stabilized by phospholipids within bile up to a certain point and prevents microscopic stone formation. However, when the capacity to stabilize the vesicle is exceeded, there is recruitment of additional cholesterol molecules, which eventually leads to the accumulation of cholesterol monohydrate crystals. Aided by pronucleating factors, these crystals promote further agglomeration of cholesterol and eventually progress into macroscopic stones. In humans, one major factor that facilitates nucleation and crystallization is the presence of mucin within the gallbladder. Mucin is an important physiologic glycoprotein that is secreted from the epithelial lining of the gallbladder and serves as a protective layer to shield the mucosa. At high concentrations, a phenomenon that is frequently present in patients with gallstones, mucin forms a viscous, gel-like substance within the gallbladder. Hydrophobic residues present in mucin are able to directly bind and stabilize free sterols in solution, as well as interacting with free calcium and bilirubin. This process forms a hydrophobic complex that has poor solubility in solution and favors nucleation and the development of stones. In murine models, disruption of mucin core protein (MUC1) expression confers resistance to stone formation, highlighting the importance of mucin in the pathogenesis of stone formation.[75] In contrast, conditions that are protective against cholesterol nucleation include reduced lipid concentrations (<3 g/dL), low concentration of hydrophobic BAs, low BA/lecithin and cholesterol/lecithin ratios, and reduced concentration of calcium ions in solution.[76]

Alteration in gallbladder contractility is the final contributor in the pathogenesis of cholesterol stones. In addition to altering the physical properties of bile to promote stone formation, prolonged exposure to supersaturated bile can directly impair gallbladder motility. Increased levels of cholesterol in bile leads to their excess absorption into the sarcoplasmic reticulum of smooth muscle cells within the gallbladder wall. Absorbed sterols are then converted into cholesterol esters within these organelles and stored in the mucosa and lamina propria of the gallbladder. This process leads to a loss of gallbladder wall elasticity, thereby impairing contractility and hindering relaxation. Poor gallbladder contractility leads to incomplete postprandial emptying and biliary stasis, thus promoting additional stone formation by fostering a microenvironment favoring the nucleation of cholesterol stones.[68,77] In addition, bile stasis within the gallbladder is a risk factor for chronic infection. Inflammation and direct enzymatic modifications resulting from bacterial colonization can independently alter bile composition and promote the nucleation of cholesterol and mixed-type gallstones.[78] Gallbladder dysmotility does not only result from cholesterol imbalances in bile but can also be a primary disorder (biliary dyskinesia) or occur secondarily in certain physiologic states (eg, diabetes, obesity, and pregnancy) caused by disruptions in metabolism and hormonal signaling. Genetic disorders, such as defects in the cholecystokinin 1 receptor, result in impaired gallbladder contractility and an increased risk for the development of gallstones, further highlighting the importance of gallbladder motility in preventing stone formation.

Pigmented (black and brown) gallstones Roughly 10% of biliary stones are brown or black pigmented stones and are not related to cholesterol imbalance within bile, but instead result from an excess of unconjugated bilirubin. Black pigment stones typically result from systemic overproduction of unconjugated bilirubin and are principally composed of calcium bilirubinate. Unconjugated hyperbilirubinemia commonly occurs in chronic hemolytic disorders such as sickle cell disease, thalassemia, or hereditary spherocytosis in which there is uncontrolled breakdown of heme from red blood cell products. Other chronic illnesses, such as ileal Crohn disease and cystic fibrosis, can also lead to systemic hyperbilirubinemia caused by enhanced absorption of bilirubin within the cecum. This condition occurs because of increased levels of bile salts within the cecum, which would normally be reabsorbed by a functional TI. Within the cecum, bilirubin is solubilized and reabsorbed into systemic circulation, thus increasing the risk for the development of black pigmented stones.[77]

Primary hepatolithiasis Unlike cholesterol and black pigmented stones, which are predominately formed within the gallbladder, pigmented brown stones are primary stones that form directly within the bile duct. The incidence of brown stones and intrahepatic stones tends to be much higher in East Asian countries, whereas they comprise a much lower percentage in the Western world.[46,79] The overall incidence of intrahepatic stones among all patients with lithiasis is approximately 2%. The cause of primary hepatolithiasis remains unknown in a high proportion of cases (70%–80%). Brown stones are commonly formed in instances of chronic biliary inflammation, biliary obstruction and stasis, concurrent bacterial colonization of the biliary tract, and changes in bile composition caused by nutrition and environmental factors. Anaerobic organisms, most commonly *Escherichia coli*, produce multiple enzymes, such as conjugated BA hydrolase, that chemically modify bilirubin within the bile duct. In this process, bilirubin glucuronide is converted into unconjugated bilirubin, which is insoluble and rapidly precipitates in solution. Free unconjugated bilirubin is then able to complex with calcium within the biliary tree, leading to nucleation and stone formation.[80] Chronic parasitic infection of the biliary tree (*Clonorchis sinensis*, *Opisthorchis viverrini*, or *Ascaris lumbricoides*) can also precipitate the development of brown stones through similar pathologic mechanisms.

Changes in bile composition can be a result of transporter proteins (multidrug-resistance proteins [MRPs]) in the bile canalicular membrane that are involved in secretion. MRP3 is involved in phospholipid secretion and therefore has a role in hepatolithiasis because it leads to changes bile composition. The presence of chronic biliary inflammation accelerates stone formation via increased secretion of MUCs. Bacterial lipopolysaccharide and lipoteichoic acid bind to Toll-like receptors on bile duct epithelial cell membranes, activating intracellular signal molecules that increase expression of MUCs and production of inflammatory cytokines from bile duct epithelium. The combination of these events is associated with stone formation and chronic proliferative cholangitis.[81]

SUMMARY

BA synthesis and regulation is a complex pathway that involves multiple organ systems and receptor-ligand crosstalk in order to ensure that the careful balance of bile constituents remains constant. Bile is essential in cholesterol homeostasis, elimination of the products of heme catabolism, and the maintenance of bacterial flora within the gut. Disorders of cholesterol or heme metabolism, impaired gallbladder motility, and infection of the biliary tract result in chemical alterations to bile that favor precipitation and macroscopic gallstone formation. There are numerous risk factors and disease states that predispose patients to stone formation and a detailed knowledge of these mechanisms is essential in caring for this population.

REFERENCES

1. Everhart JE, Ruhl CE. Burden of digestive diseases in the United States part III: liver, biliary tract, and pancreas. Gastroenterology 2009;136(4):1134–44.

2. Albers CJ, Huizenga JR, Krom RA, et al. Composition of human hepatic bile. Ann Clin Biochem 1985;22(Pt 2):129–32.
3. Holm R, Mullertz A, Mu H. Bile salts and their importance for drug absorption. Int J Pharm 2013;453(1):44–55.
4. Inagaki T, Choi M, Moschetta A, et al. Fibroblast growth factor 15 functions as an enterohepatic signal to regulate bile acid homeostasis. Cell Metab 2005;2(4): 217–25.
5. Falany CN, Johnson MR, Barnes S, et al. Glycine and taurine conjugation of bile acids by a single enzyme. Molecular cloning and expression of human liver bile acid CoA:amino acid N-acyltransferase. J Biol Chem 1994;269(30):19375–9.
6. Russell DW. The enzymes, regulation, and genetics of bile acid synthesis. Annu Rev Biochem 2003;72:137–74.
7. Small DM, Rapo S. Source of abnormal bile in patients with cholesterol gallstones. N Engl J Med 1970;283(2):53–7.
8. Reshetnyak VI. Physiological and molecular biochemical mechanisms of bile formation. World J Gastroenterol 2013;19(42):7341–60.
9. Lepercq P, Relano P, Cayuela C, et al. Bifidobacterium animalis strain DN-173 010 hydrolyses bile salts in the gastrointestinal tract of pigs. Scand J Gastroenterol 2004;39(12):1266–71.
10. Batta AK, Salen G, Arora R, et al. Side chain conjugation prevents bacterial 7-dehydroxylation of bile acids. J Biol Chem 1990;265(19):10925–8.
11. Dawson PA, Karpen SJ. Intestinal transport and metabolism of bile acids. J Lipid Res 2015;56(6):1085–99.
12. Hayakawa S. Microbiological transformation of bile acids. Adv Lipid Res 1973;11: 143–92.
13. Hylemon PB, Harder J. Biotransformation of monoterpenes, bile acids, and other isoprenoids in anaerobic ecosystems. FEMS Microbiol Rev 1998;22(5):475–88.
14. Sugita T, Amano K, Nakano M, et al. Analysis of the serum bile acid composition for differential diagnosis in patients with liver disease. Gastroenterol Res Pract 2015;2015:717431.
15. Alvaro D, Cantafora A, Attili AF, et al. Relationships between bile salts hydrophilicity and phospholipid composition in bile of various animal species. Comp Biochem Physiol B 1986;83(3):551–4.
16. Kawamoto T, Okano G, Akino T. Biosynthesis and turnover of individual molecular species of phosphatidylcholine in liver and bile. Biochim Biophys Acta 1980; 619(1):20–34.
17. Carey MC, Lamont JT. Cholesterol gallstone formation. 1. Physical-chemistry of bile and biliary lipid secretion. Prog Liver Dis 1992;10:139–63.
18. Fujiwara R, Haag M, Schaeffeler E, et al. Systemic regulation of bilirubin homeostasis: Potential benefits of hyperbilirubinemia. Hepatology 2018;67(4):1609–19.
19. Nathanson MH, Boyer JL. Mechanisms and regulation of bile secretion. Hepatology 1991;14(3):551–66.
20. Arrese M, Ananthananarayanan M, Suchy FJ. Hepatobiliary transport: molecular mechanisms of development and cholestasis. Pediatr Res 1998;44(2):141–7.
21. Strazzabosco M. New insights into cholangiocyte physiology. J Hepatol 1997; 27(5):945–52.
22. Tabibian JH, Masyuk AI, Masyuk TV, et al. Physiology of cholangiocytes. Compr Physiol 2013;3(1):541–65.
23. Ding YM, Wang B, Wang WX, et al. New classification of the anatomic variations of cystic artery during laparoscopic cholecystectomy. World J Gastroenterol 2007;13(42):5629–34.

24. Corradini SG, Elisei W, Giovannelli L, et al. Impaired human gallbladder lipid absorption in cholesterol gallstone disease and its effect on cholesterol solubility in bile. Gastroenterology 2000;118(5):912–20.
25. Behar J. Physiology and pathophysiology of the biliary tract: the gallbladder and sphincter of Oddi—a review. ISRN Physiol 2013;2013:15.
26. Chandra R, Liddle RA. Cholecystokinin. Curr Opin Endocrinol Diabetes Obes 2007;14(1):63–7.
27. Yi J, Knudsen TA, Nielsen AL, et al. Data for the size of cholesterol-fat micelles as a function of bile salt concentration and the physico-chemical properties of six liquid experimental pine-derived phytosterol formulations in a cholesterol-containing artificial intestine fluid. Data Brief 2017;10:478–81.
28. Hofmann AF, Borgstroem B. The intraluminal phase of fat digestion in man: the lipid content of the micellar and oil phases of intestinal content obtained during fat digestion and absorption. J Clin Invest 1964;43:247–57.
29. Shapiro H, Kolodziejczyk AA, Halstuch D, et al. Bile acids in glucose metabolism in health and disease. J Exp Med 2018;215(2):383–96.
30. Forman BM, Goode E, Chen J, et al. Identification of a nuclear receptor that is activated by farnesol metabolites. Cell 1995;81(5):687–93.
31. Calkin AC, Tontonoz P. Transcriptional integration of metabolism by the nuclear sterol-activated receptors LXR and FXR. Nat Rev Mol Cell Biol 2012;13(4): 213–24.
32. Watanabe M, Houten SM, Wang L, et al. Bile acids lower triglyceride levels via a pathway involving FXR, SHP, and SREBP-1c. J Clin Invest 2004;113(10):1408–18.
33. Zhang Y, Lee FY, Barrera G, et al. Activation of the nuclear receptor FXR improves hyperglycemia and hyperlipidemia in diabetic mice. Proc Natl Acad Sci U S A 2006;103(4):1006–11.
34. de Aguiar Vallim TQ, Tarling EJ, Edwards PA. Pleiotropic roles of bile acids in metabolism. Cell Metab 2013;17(5):657–69.
35. Cariou B, van Harmelen K, Duran-Sandoval D, et al. The farnesoid X receptor modulates adiposity and peripheral insulin sensitivity in mice. J Biol Chem 2006;281(16):11039–49.
36. Ma K, Saha PK, Chan L, et al. Farnesoid X receptor is essential for normal glucose homeostasis. J Clin Invest 2006;116(4):1102–9.
37. Balakrishnan A, Polli JE. Apical sodium dependent bile acid transporter (ASBT, SLC10A2): a potential prodrug target. Mol Pharm 2006;3(3):223–30.
38. Hofmann AF. The enterohepatic circulation of bile acids in mammals: form and functions. Front Biosci (Landmark Ed) 2009;14:2584–98.
39. Anwer MS. Cellular regulation of hepatic bile acid transport in health and cholestasis. Hepatology 2004;39(3):581–90.
40. Zhao Y, Meng C, Wang Y, et al. IL-1beta inhibits beta-Klotho expression and FGF19 signaling in hepatocytes. Am J Physiol Endocrinol Metab 2016;310(4): E289–300.
41. Ferrebee CB, Dawson PA. Metabolic effects of intestinal absorption and enterohepatic cycling of bile acids. Acta Pharm Sin B 2015;5(2):129–34.
42. Everhart JE, Khare M, Hill M, et al. Prevalence and ethnic differences in gallbladder disease in the United States. Gastroenterology 1999;117(3):632–9.
43. Gracie WA, Ransohoff DF. The natural history of silent gallstones: the innocent gallstone is not a myth. N Engl J Med 1982;307(13):798–800.
44. Everhart JE, Yeh F, Lee ET, et al. Prevalence of gallbladder disease in American Indian populations: findings from the Strong Heart Study. Hepatology 2002;35(6): 1507–12.

45. Maurer KR, Everhart JE, Ezzati TM, et al. Prevalence of gallstone disease in Hispanic populations in the United States. Gastroenterology 1989;96(2 Pt 1):487–92.
46. Shaffer EA. Gallstone disease: epidemiology of gallbladder stone disease. Best Pract Res Clin Gastroenterol 2006;20(6):981–96.
47. Uhler ML, Marks JW, Voigt BJ, et al. Comparison of the impact of transdermal versus oral estrogens on biliary markers of gallstone formation in postmenopausal women. J Clin Endocrinol Metab 1998;83(2):410–4.
48. Cirillo DJ, Wallace RB, Rodabough RJ, et al. Effect of estrogen therapy on gallbladder disease. JAMA 2005;293(3):330–9.
49. Wang HH, Afdhal NH, Wang DQ. Estrogen receptor alpha, but not beta, plays a major role in 17beta-estradiol-induced murine cholesterol gallstones. Gastroenterology 2004;127(1):239–49.
50. Coyne MJ, Bonorris GG, Chung A, et al. Estrogen enhances dietary cholesterol induction of saturated bile in the hamster. Gastroenterology 1978;75(1):76–9.
51. Duan LP, Wang HH, Ohashi A, et al. Role of intestinal sterol transporters Abcg5, Abcg8, and Npc1l1 in cholesterol absorption in mice: gender and age effects. Am J Physiol Gastrointest Liver Physiol 2006;290(2):G269–76.
52. Diehl AK. Cholelithiasis and the insulin resistance syndrome. Hepatology 2000; 31(2):528–30.
53. Petitti DB, Friedman GD, Klatsky AL. Association of a history of gallbladder disease with a reduced concentration of high-density-lipoprotein cholesterol. N Engl J Med 1981;304(23):1396–8.
54. Worthington HV, Hunt LP, McCloy RF, et al. Dietary antioxidant lack, impaired hepatic glutathione reserve, and cholesterol gallstones. Clin Chim Acta 2004; 349(1–2):157–65.
55. Shiffman ML, Sugerman HJ, Kellum JM, et al. Gallstone formation after rapid weight loss: a prospective study in patients undergoing gastric bypass surgery for treatment of morbid obesity. Am J Gastroenterol 1991;86(8):1000–5.
56. Jensen MD, Ryan DH, Apovian CM, et al. 2013 AHA/ACC/TOS guideline for the management of overweight and obesity in adults: a report of the American College of Cardiology/American Heart Association Task Force on Practice Guidelines and The Obesity Society. J Am Coll Cardiol 2014;63(25 Pt B):2985–3023.
57. Murray FE, Stinchcombe SJ, Hawkey CJ. Development of biliary sludge in patients on intensive care unit: results of a prospective ultrasonographic study. Gut 1992;33(8):1123–5.
58. Pitt HA, King W 3rd, Mann LL, et al. Increased risk of cholelithiasis with prolonged total parenteral nutrition. Am J Surg 1983;145(1):106–12.
59. Acalovschi M, Badea R, Pascu M. Incidence of gallstones in liver cirrhosis. Am J Gastroenterol 1991;86(9):1179–81.
60. Alvaro D, Angelico M, Gandin C, et al. Physico-chemical factors predisposing to pigment gallstone formation in liver cirrhosis. J Hepatol 1990;10(2):228–34.
61. Acalovschi M. Gallstones in patients with liver cirrhosis: incidence, etiology, clinical and therapeutical aspects. World J Gastroenterol 2014;20(23):7277–85.
62. Brink MA, Slors JF, Keulemans YC, et al. Enterohepatic cycling of bilirubin: a putative mechanism for pigment gallstone formation in ileal Crohn's disease. Gastroenterology 1999;116(6):1420–7.
63. Lapidus A, Bangstad M, Astrom M, et al. The prevalence of gallstone disease in a defined cohort of patients with Crohn's disease. Am J Gastroenterol 1999;94(5): 1261–6.
64. Chuang SC, Hsi E, Lee KT. Genetics of gallstone disease. Adv Clin Chem 2013; 60:143–85.

65. Carey MC. Pathogenesis of gallstones. Am J Surg 1993;165(4):410–9.
66. Schafmayer C, Hartleb J, Tepel J, et al. Predictors of gallstone composition in 1025 symptomatic gallstones from northern Germany. BMC Gastroenterol 2006; 6:36.
67. van Erpecum KJ. Biliary lipids, water and cholesterol gallstones. Biol Cell 2005; 97(11):815–22.
68. Lammert F, Gurusamy K, Ko CW, et al. Gallstones. Nat Rev Dis Primers 2016;2: 16024.
69. Tsai CJ, Leitzmann MF, Willett WC, et al. Central adiposity, regional fat distribution, and the risk of cholecystectomy in women. Gut 2006;55(5):708–14.
70. Dikkers A, Tietge UJ. Biliary cholesterol secretion: more than a simple ABC. World J Gastroenterol 2010;16(47):5936–45.
71. Biddinger SB, Haas JT, Yu BB, et al. Hepatic insulin resistance directly promotes formation of cholesterol gallstones. Nat Med 2008;14(7):778–82.
72. Wang J, Mitsche MA, Lutjohann D, et al. Relative roles of ABCG5/ABCG8 in liver and intestine. J Lipid Res 2015;56(2):319–30.
73. Pullinger CR, Eng C, Salen G, et al. Human cholesterol 7alpha-hydroxylase (CYP7A1) deficiency has a hypercholesterolemic phenotype. J Clin Invest 2002;110(1):109–17.
74. Small DM. Cholesterol nucleation and growth in gallstone formation. N Engl J Med 1980;302(23):1305–7.
75. Wang HH, Afdhal NH, Gendler SJ, et al. Targeted disruption of the murine mucin gene 1 decreases susceptibility to cholesterol gallstone formation. J Lipid Res 2004;45(3):438–47.
76. Wang HH, Portincasa P, Wang DQ. Molecular pathophysiology and physical chemistry of cholesterol gallstones. Front Biosci 2008;13:401–23.
77. Van Erpecum KJ. Pathogenesis of cholesterol and pigment gallstones: an update. Clin Res Hepatol Gastroenterol 2011;35(4):281–7.
78. Maurer KJ, Carey MC, Fox JG. Roles of infection, inflammation, and the immune system in cholesterol gallstone formation. Gastroenterology 2009;136(2):425–40.
79. Nakayama F, Soloway RD, Nakama T, et al. Hepatolithiasis in East Asia. Retrospective study. Dig Dis Sci 1986;31(1):21–6.
80. Lammert F, Sauerbruch T. Mechanisms of disease: the genetic epidemiology of gallbladder stones. Nat Clin Pract Gastroenterol Hepatol 2005;2(9):423–33.
81. Gerloff T, Stieger B, Hagenbuch B, et al. The sister of P-glycoprotein represents the canalicular bile salt export pump of mammalian liver. J Biol Chem 1998; 273(16):10046–50.

Gallstone Disease
Cholecystitis, Mirizzi Syndrome, Bouveret Syndrome, Gallstone Ileus

Farzad Alemi, MD[a],*, Natalie Seiser, MD, PhD[a],
Subhashini Ayloo, MD, MPH[b]

KEYWORDS

- Cholecystitis • Cholecystectomy • Mirizzi syndrome • Bouveret syndrome • Ileus

KEY POINTS

- Gallstones are most problematic when they cause luminal obstruction and can result in inflammation, cholestasis, or intestinal obstruction.
- The most common obstructive sequela of gallstones occurs in the cystic duct, which results in cholecystitis and usually requires a permanent drainage procedure (cholecystectomy) or temporizing drainage procedure (cholecystostomy tube).
- Gallstone ileus and Bouveret syndrome present with symptoms and sequelae of gastrointestinal obstruction such as dehydration, electrolyte abnormalities and hemodynamic instability. These issues have to be addressed and managed when deciding on the appropriate intervention for each individual patient.
- Mirizzi syndrome can lead to compression or erosion of gallstones into the common bile duct. Although imaging modalities and endoscopic retrograde cholangiopancreatography are useful, it requires careful management to avoid common bile duct injury.

 Video content accompanies this article at http://www.surgical.theclinics.com.

INTRODUCTION: NATURE OF THE PROBLEM

Gallstone disease is a leading cause of surgical intervention of the biliary tree in the United States. It is estimated that more than 700,000 cholecystectomies are performed annually to treat the more than 20 million people who harbor gallstones.[1,2] This burden is conservatively estimated to cost 6.5 billion dollars yearly for management and treatment in the United States.[1] Fortunately, the advent of improved

Disclosures: The authors have nothing to disclose.
[a] St Vincent Medical Center, Transplant & HPB Institute, 2200 West 3rd Street, Suite 200, Los Angeles, CA 90057, USA; [b] Rutgers, New Jersey Medical School, 185 South Orange Avenue, MSB G586, Newark, NJ 07102, USA
* Corresponding author.
E-mail address: FarzadAlemi@verity.org

diagnostic and treatment modalities has dramatically improved mortality rates of gallstone-related disease by 56% to 71%, the most among all common digestive diseases.[1]

Although gallstone disease is classically associated with the inflammatory sequela of cholecystitis, gallstones can also contribute to other, somewhat rarer, clinical presentations, such as gallstone ileus, Mirizzi syndrome, and Bouveret syndrome. This article explores the common–and uncommon—causes of surgical pathology owing to gallstones with an emphasis on clinical identification, diagnostics, and management options.

CHOLECYSTITIS

As its name implies, cholecystitis entails severe inflammation of the gallbladder. Typically, calculous cholecystitis develops when gallstones (and less often, biliary sludge) obstruct bile egress from the gallbladder, usually in the cystic duct. Acalculous cholecystitis may also occur in 5% to 10% of patients who present with cholecystitis, and typically these patients are critically ill.[3]

Clinical Presentation

Patients who develop cholecystitis classically present either with acute cholecystitis or chronic cholecystitis. In the acute setting, patients present with symptoms including severe, constant right upper quadrant pain lasting more than 6 hours with associated fevers, chills, nausea, or vomiting. This presentation is different from biliary colic, which is self-limited and not associated with systemic symptoms of infection such as fevers. In some patient populations (such as the elderly or diabetics), these classical symptoms are not present, because they may present with vague symptoms including anorexia, fatigue, or emesis. In these populations, a higher index of suspicion for cholecystitis is required because missing the diagnosis can have profound and dire consequences.

In the chronic setting, cholecystitis can be a result of repeated clinical or subclinical cycles of passage and clearance of stones throughout the biliary tree. These patients may have prolonged, less acute symptoms, which are usually present over weeks or months. As a result, this process increases the amount of scarring present in the gallbladder and biliary tree, typically leading to a shrunken, scarred, and thickened gallbladder over time.

Diagnostic Procedures

A patient presenting with suspected cholecystitis should undergo some or all of the following tests.

1. Physical examination: abdominal examination, especially peritoneal findings and Murphy's sign, harbor a sensitivity and specificity of 96% and 48%, respectively.[4]
2. Laboratory analysis: Specific attention should be paid to leukocytosis (especially left shifted), liver function tests/bilirubin, and lactate.[5]
3. Imaging
   a. Ultrasound examination: Assessment of gallbladder wall thickening of more than 5 mm, pericholecystic fluid, presence of gallstones, and sonographic Murphy's sign. Ultrasound examination harbors 88% sensitivity and specificity for diagnosis of cholecystitis.[6]
   b. Computed tomography (CT) scan: Although not a first-line assessment tool, oftentimes CT scans are the only imaging available when patients present emergently to the hospital or emergency department. Typical findings of gallbladder

wall thickening, pericholecystic fluid, and the presence of gallstones may be apparent, although typically most gallstones are isodense with bile.[7]

c. Magnetic resonance cholangiopancreatography (MRCP): MRCP allows for the assessment of gallbladder wall thickening, pericholecystic fluid, and the presence of gallstones in the biliary tree, especially cystic duct (sensitivity 100% vs 14% with ultrasound examination).[8]

d. Cholescintigraphy: For patients with equivocal signs, symptoms, and imaging, the absence of radionuclide within the gallbladder is diagnostic of cholecystitis. The study has a high sensitivity and specificity for acute disease at 97% and 90%, respectively.[9]

Management

The management of acute cholecystitis should encompass the goals of (1) relieving the inflamed gallbladder, (2) temporizing systemic illness, (3) preventing iatrogenic injury to the patient, and (4) preventing future occurrences of cholecystitis. Although each clinical situation and patient is unique, all 4 aspects need to be taken into account to provide patients with a treatment plan that is right for them (**Table 1**).

Supportive care

Treating a patient with acute or chronic cholecystitis with supportive care (intravenous hydration, pain control, antibiotics, and correction of electrolytes) oftentimes serves only as a temporizing measure to defer systemic illness before a definitive drainage procedure. Sometimes in very mild or questionable cases, antibiotics may be avoided.[10] However, antibiotics are indicated in more complicated cases such as with emphysematous changes or in patients who are diabetic or immunocompromised.[11]

When antibiotics are used as the only therapy, pain will usually recur and persist, as may infection or sepsis because the gallbladder is not drained. In one study of more than 10,000 patients who did not undergo cholecystectomy upon admission, the probability of an emergency room visit with 12 weeks of initial presentation was 19%.[12] Sometimes the rationale behind this treatment strategy alone includes the inability of the patient to tolerate surgical intervention owing to profound sepsis or comorbidities. In these situations, strong consideration must be made to drain the gallbladder using a cholecystostomy tube if indicated. Nevertheless, in high-risk patients a recent metaanalysis identified nonoperative management to be successful in 87% of patients with mortality of 0.5%. However, recurrent gallstone disease occurred in 22% of patients.[13]

Table 1 Different strategies to manage acute cholecystitis				
	Relieving Gallbladder Inflammation	Temporizing Systemic Illness	Preventing Iatrogenic Injury	Preventing Future Cholecystitis
Supportive care	+/−	+/−	+	+/−
Cholecystectomy	+	+	+/−	+
Subtotal cholecystectomy	+	+	+	+/−
Interval cholecystectomy	+/−	+/−	+/−	+
Cholecystostomy tube	+	+	+	+/−

+: optimal.
+/−: suboptimal.

The duration of antibiotics should be tailored to each patient's unique situation. For those managed purely with supportive care, the duration of therapy should be clinically judged. Typically, when patients are able to tolerate a diet, they can be transitioned to oral antibiotics and discharged.[14] For those patients who underwent uncomplicated surgical intervention, antibiotics can be discontinued postoperatively.[15]

Cholecystectomy
As a surgical intervention, removing the gallbladder and the offending obstructing gallstone in its entirety seems to be the most expeditious solution to a patient with cholecystitis. Most important, the causative factor of pain and systemic illness—the undrained fluid within the gallbladder—is removed in its entirety, which allows for a permanent cure of the index presentation and any future occurrences of cholecystitis. Cholecystectomy can be performed laparoscopically (the standard of care), robotically, or open.

However, the primary detractors to upfront surgery include the risks associated with operating in a severely inflamed field on an organ that is typically distended, friable, and possibly infected. In high-risk patients, cholecystectomy for acute presentations carries reported mortality rates as high as 19%.[16] Moreover, the rate of bile duct injuries increases daily as inflammation of the biliary tree increases.[17] Indeed, the timing of cholecystectomy for acute cholecystitis has been highly debated, but nevertheless consideration and prevention of iatrogenic bile duct injury or bile spillage is paramount in consideration of surgery in very early, early, or delayed presentations.

Subtotal cholecystectomy
Like cholecystectomy, subtotal cholecystectomy achieves the ability to drain the inflamed gallbladder but does not attempt to remove the organ in its entirety with the primary consideration being avoidance of bile duct injury. It is oftentimes necessary in the cases of the "difficult gallbladder," which can be predicted based on more than 72 hours of symptoms, a white blood cell count of greater than 18,000/mm^3, multiple comorbidities, and a palpable gallbladder on examination.[18]

Typically performed as either a fenestrating type (where the gallbladder is left open and the cystic duct maybe sutured internally) or reconstituting type (where the gallbladder partially resected, stones removed, and sutured closed),[19] this operative strategy harbors low morbidity with regard to hemorrhage, bile duct injury, and retained stones, but is associated with an 18% biliary fistula rate in the fenestrating type and 8% for reconstituting.[20] Nevertheless, these postoperative biliary fistulas are typically self-limiting and resolve with time and endoscopic biliary stenting. The recurrence rate of biliary events is lower after fenestrating versus reconstituting subtotal cholecystectomy (9% vs 18%), but may require a completion cholecystectomy more often (9% vs 4%).[21]

Interval cholecystectomy
The rationale for such an approach is the ability to temporize infection and inflammation with antibiotics, allowing the gallbladder time to "cool off," and operate after 4 to 6 weeks to decrease inflammation and risk for iatrogenic injury. This approach was historically favored up until recently, because many studies have demonstrated this approach comes with a failure rate of more than 20%, recurrent symptoms, and considerable patient morbidity during the interval period.[22] Moreover, mostly owing to increased rates of conversion to open procedure, operating time, and bile duct injury with interval operations,[23] this strategy has generally fallen out of favor for most acute presentations in lower risk patients.

Cholecystostomy tube

For those patients who are too ill (owing to severe sepsis or comorbidities) to undergo surgical intervention, placement of a cholecystostomy tube is a good temporizing measure. The tube allows for proper biliary drainage and relief of obstruction, and limits the iatrogenic injury that may occur with surgical intervention. Once the patient is clinically improved, either cholecystectomy can be performed or a tube study to identify cystic duct patency and tube removal. Some have also attempted percutaneous gallstone removal through the cholecystostomy tube, with success achieved in more than 80% of patients.[24] For those patients who do not undergo cholecystectomy, the risk of recurrent symptoms is approximately 20% within 1 year.[25]

However, dilemmas and variability of care regarding tube management arise. For those patients who improve clinically and can tolerate surgical intervention, the timing of tube removal can vary between 2 and 193 days.[26] In contrast, for those patients with severe comorbidities that will not improve with time, sometimes a cholecystostomy tube can become a prolonged fixture, which can lead to significant patient morbidity.

GALLSTONE ILEUS
Introduction and Epidemiology

Gallstone ileus is a rare complication in 0.3% to 0.5% of patients with cholelithiasis.[27] It usually occurs in the elderly (late 70–80s) and is more common in women than men with a ratio of 3.5 to 4.5:1.[28,29] It is the underlying etiology in 1% to 4% of patients with an intestinal obstruction, and most commonly results in a small bowel obstruction.[29] The average size of obstructing gallstones is 4 cm.[27,28] Gallstones may enter the intestine through a fistulous tract between the gallbladder and duodenum, stomach, or colon. They can also enter the duodenum after endoscopic retrograde cholangiopancreatography (ERCP) and endoscopic sphincterotomy. Most commonly, stones are impacted in the distal ileum and ileocecal valve (60%–75%).[30] Stones may traverse the ileocecal valve or enter the colon directly through a cholecystocolonic fistula, and cause obstruction of the sigmoid colon (4%).[31] The incidence of obstruction is higher if patients have colonic strictures from inflammation or diverticulitis. Proximal obstruction of the gastric outlet or duodenum occurs rarely (4%) and is eponymously known as Bouveret syndrome.[32]

Clinical Presentation

Patients usually present with the typical symptoms of a small bowel obstruction such as nausea, vomiting, abdominal distention, and crampy abdominal pain. Obstructive symptoms can be intermittent, indicating movement of the stones down the gastrointestinal tract. Sometimes, they experience symptoms of concomitant acute cholecystitis such fevers, chills, and right upper quadrant pain. Bowel obstruction may also be preceded by biliary symptoms. On physical examination patients are often tachycardic, have abdominal distention, and diffuse pain. If their gallstones ileus caused an intestinal perforation, they generally will have fevers and peritonitis.

Diagnosis

1. Abdominal radiograph: The classical signs of gallstone ileus include a partial or complete intestinal obstruction, pneumobilia or contrast in the biliary tree, and aberrant gallstone, which changes position on serial radiographs.[33,34]
2. CT scan: CT scanning harbors a sensitivity and specificity for detection of gallstone ileus as high as 93% and 100%, respectively. Findings of a small bowel obstruction, an aberrant gallstone, and an air–fluid filled gallbladder with an irregular wall

are diagnostic for a gallstone ileus. Multidetector CT scanners can identify the site of obstruction from aberrant stones and the presence and location of a cholecystoduodenal fistula.[35–37]

3. Ultrasound examination: Ultrasound examination can identify gallstones, choledocholithiasis, and a choledochoduodenal fistula. However, in the era of multidetector CT scans, the use of ultrasound examination is not needed for diagnosis.[38]

4. MRCP: MRCP can be used instead of CT scanning to evaluate for bowel obstruction if the patient has contraindications to CT scanning. Because MRCP is usually used to delineate the biliary tract, cholecystoenteric fistulas may be detected as well. Usually, there is no need for additional imaging if the CT scan is diagnostic.[39]

Management

The mainstay of treating gallstone ileus is removal of the gallstone. Because the majority of patients are elderly, have multiple comorbidities, and present with dehydration and electrolyte abnormalities, these issues should be addressed and managed before any intervention.[40–42] A nasogastric tube should be inserted and placed for suction to avoid vomiting and aspiration of enteric contents.

Surgery

There is no consensus on the best surgical approach in the literature, but a range of surgical procedures is used to treat gallstone ileus.

1. Exploratory laparotomy and enterolithotomy/bowel resection alone: Once the obstructing gallstone is identified, the bowel is opened longitudinally on the antimesenteric side proximal to the stone at an area of healthy appearing bowel, and the gallstone is extracted through the enterotomy. If the gallstone is large and bowel necrosis is suspected or visualized, a segmental bowel resection may be required. If gallstone ileus occurs in the sigmoid colon, the patient may require a sigmoid colectomy. The majority of authors recommend this procedure for sicker patients with a significant number of comorbidities (American Society of Anesthesiologists classes III and IV).[27,43,44] The concerns of enterolithotomy alone are recurrent gallstone ileus and cholangitis, which have been reported to be as high 33% and 60% respectively, depending on the type of cholecystoenteric fistula.[45]

2. Exploratory laparotomy and enterolithotomy/bowel resection, cholecystectomy and closure of cholecystoenteric fistula (1-stage procedure): In addition to enterolithotomy, an open cholecystectomy and fistula closure are performed. Most authors reserve this surgery for "healthier" patients (American Society of Anesthesiologists classes I and II), who are hemodynamically stable at the time of surgery. Although most authors cite a higher morbidity and similar mortality of the one stage procedure, Clavien and colleagues[27] found no difference in either when patients were matched for age and comorbidities.[28,43,45]

3. Exploratory laparotomy and enterolithotomy/bowel resection with delayed cholecystectomy and closure of cholecystoenteric fistula (2-stage procedure): Fewer cases of a staged procedure are reported in the literature, but morbidity and mortality of a 2-stage procedure seem to vary from much from enterolithotomy alone or a 1-stage procedure.[43]

4. Laparoscopy: Laparoscopic enterolithotomy, cholecystectomy, and fistula takedown have been reported for the management of gallstone ileus.[46] However, the number of cases are few and the conversion rate is approximately 50% in the literature.[29]

Endoscopy

Endoscopic intervention may be feasible for gastroduodenal or colonic gallstone obstructions. This intervention is discussed in more detail in the section on Bouveret syndrome, but case reports of successful combined lithotripsy and balloon enteroscopy or colonoscopy (or an obstructing stone in the sigmoid colon have been reported in the literature).[31,47-49]

Gallstone Ileus Summary

Gallstone ileus is generally a disease of the elderly, who have multiple comorbidities, and present with symptoms and sequelae of a bowel obstruction such as dehydration, electrolyte abnormalities, and hemodynamic instability. These issues have to be considered when deciding on the appropriate intervention for each individual patient.

BOUVERET SYNDROME

Introduction and Epidemiology

Bouveret syndrome is a rare (1%–4%) form of gallstone ileus, where the impacted stone leads to a gastric outlet obstruction. The stone enters the stomach though a cholecystogastric or cholecystoduodenal fistula before it gets impacted in the duodenum. The majority of patients are women over the age of 75 years.[42,50]

Clinical Presentation

The majority of patients present with nausea, vomiting (>85%), and abdominal pain (>70%). Patients may also experience upper gastrointestinal bleeding. On physical examination, they will show signs of dehydration such as tachycardia, low urine output, and abdominal pain and distention.[51]

Diagnosis

Abdominal CT scans and MRI are the main diagnostic imaging modalities, just as described for gallstone ileus. Rigler's triad, which includes pneumobilia, an aberrant gallstone in the duodenum, and a dilated stomach, are highly suggestive of Bouveret syndrome. MRCP can be useful in providing information about the cholecystogastric fistula tract. Endoscopy has not been proven to provide additional useful diagnostic information.[42,50,51]

Management

Endoscopy

In contrast with gallstone ileus in other locations of the gastrointestinal tract, endoscopic therapy has gained popularity recently. If possible, impacted gallstones are removed endoscopically with endoscopic nets and basket.[52] Stones, that are too large can undergo mechanical[53] or electrohydraulic lithotripsy.[54] Newer techniques for breaking up stones are laser[55] or extracorporeal shock wave lithotripsy.[56] Although there is great enthusiasm for endoscopic stone extraction, only 10% of stones can then be removed endoscopically.[57] Endoscopy can be used for recurrent Bouveret syndrome.

Surgery

If endoscopic therapy fails or does not allow complete clearance of all stones, surgery remains the main treatment option. Impacted gallstones can be removed through a gastrotomy or duodenotomy. Most authors recommend enterolithotomy alone. Enterolithotomy, cholecystectomy, and closure of concurrent fistula should be reserved for younger, healthier patients, where the risk of recurrence outweighs the surgical risk.[50,58] A laparoscopic approach has been shown to be successful in removing stones up to 5 cm.[59,60] In rare instances, after successful endoscopic treatment of a gastric outlet obstruction, a patient may develop a small bowel or colonic obstruction from a stone fragment that has traveled distally, requiring subsequent surgical intervention.[50]

Bouveret Syndrome Summary

Bouveret syndrome is a rare subset of gallstone ileus, leading to gastric outlet obstruction from a stone impacted in the duodenum or gastric antrum. Diagnosis and management are comparable with gallstone ileus, with the exception that endoscopic therapy has gained recent popularity.

MIRIZZI SYNDROME
Introduction and Epidemiology

Mirizzi syndrome is a rare complication of symptomatic cholelithiasis, which is most often found in women between ages 50 and 70 years.[61,62] The pathophysiology is believed to be due to a gallstone, which is impacted in the infundibulum, causing chronic inflammation of the gallbladder and pressure on the common bile duct. Over time, both can lead to erosion into the common bile duct, creating a cholecystobiliary fistula.[61,63,64]

There are multiple classification systems for Mirizzi syndrome, but the most recent was described by Csendes and validated by Beltran and colleagues.[61,65] A Csendes type I corresponds with external compression of the bile duct by and impacted gallstone in the infundibulum or cystic duct. Type II is a cholecystobiliary fistula from erosion of a gallstone into the common bile duct, involving less than one-third of the circumference of the bile duct. Type III consists of a cholecystobiliary fistula involving up to two-thirds of the bile duct circumference. Type IV is a cholecystobiliary fistula with complete destruction of the bile duct wall, with complete fusion of the gallbladder and bile duct wall. Type V consists of any type of Mirizzi syndrome with a cholecystoenteric fistula. Patients with a type Va fistula have gallstones and those with a type Vb fistula do not.

Clinical Presentation

The most common presentation of Mirizzi syndrome is obstructive jaundice, in the setting of gallstones disease. Patients may experience right upper quadrant pain and fevers. Laboratory data might show hyperbilirubinemia and elevated transaminases.[66] In the setting of acute cholecystitis, patients will have leukocytosis. Some authors reported a high carbohydrate antigen 19-9 level.[67]

Diagnosis

Preoperative diagnosis is crucial for the diagnosis of Mirizzi syndrome, because the incidence of common bile duct injury can be as high as 17% without it. Preoperative diagnosis, however, can be difficult and varies from 8% to 63%.[62,63]

1. Abdominal ultrasound examination may reveal an atrophic gallbladder with a gallstone impacted at the infundibulum, and hepatic ductal dilatation above the level of the obstruction. There might be signs of acute cholecystitis. The diagnostic accuracy of ultrasound examination is low at 27%. The sensitivity has been described as anywhere between 8% and 27%.[63,68]
2. CT: Although there are no specific CT findings for Mirizzi syndrome, they are useful to rule out portal or liver malignancies or other underlying reason for biliary obstruction.[68,69]

3. MRCP: MRCP is the preferred tool to noninvasively assess the biliary anatomy, and can reveal typical findings of Mirizzi syndrome such as extrinsic compression of the common hepatic duct with upstream dilatation, a normal common bile duct, and gallstones in the cystic duct. MRI is also used to assess inflammation around the gallbladder and rule out other reasons for bile duct obstruction such as choledocholithiasis. The diagnostic accuracy of MRCP is 50%.[63,70]

4. ERCP: ERCP is the gold standard for diagnosis and therapeutic intervention for Mirizzi syndrome. ERCP can identify extrinsic compression and the presence of a cholecystobiliary or cholecystoenteric fistula. Additionally, biliary obstruction can be relieved by placing a stent and stone retrieval. The diagnostic accuracy or ERCP for Mirizzi syndrome has been reported from 55% to 90% with a sensitivity from 76% to 100%.[71,72]

Management

Surgery

Open surgery Open surgery remains the standard of care for Mirizzi syndrome. Because Mirizzi syndrome is often diagnosed during surgery, optimal preoperative surgical planning is challenging. Beltran[63] recommends different surgical approaches depending on classification of Mirizzi syndrome. For type I Mirizzi syndrome, most investigators recommend an open classic cholecystectomy or subtotal cholecystectomy, if there is significant scaring in the triangle of Chalot. For a subtotal cholecystectomy the gallbladder is opened at the fundus and cleared of all stones. The cystic duct is identified from the inside of the gallbladder. Stones that can be removed easily will be removed. If the cystic duct is obliterated, it should be left alone. The gallbladder remnant should be closed with absorbable suture, although it may not need to be closed if the cystic duct is obliterated.[73,74] A subtotal cholecystectomy is also recommended for Mirizzi syndrome type II. Some authors have left a small remnant of gallbladder wall over the cholecystobiliary fistula, which can aid closure of the defect. The same approach can be used for the treatment of Mirizzi type III syndrome.[62,63] However, if the cholecystobiliary fistula is too large and the gallbladder is significantly inflamed, biliary enteric anastomosis such as a choledochoduodenostomy or Roux-en-Y hepaticojejunostomy is recommended. A bilioenteric anastomosis is also recommended for Mirizzi syndrome type IV. Mirizzi type V syndrome should be treated with division of the bilioenteric fistula, cholecystectomy, and closure of the fistula. If the patient has a gallstone ileus and Mirizzi syndrome (type Vb), many authors recommend addressing the gallstone ileus first with enterolithotomy, and delaying definite surgery for Mirizzi syndrome.[64]

Laparoscopy Although subtotal and simple laparoscopic cholecystectomy have been described for Mirizzi syndrome (Video 1), both can be challenging in the light of the acute inflammation in the porta, and the chance of a bile duct injury or conversion are as high as 22% and 30% to 100%, respectively.[75,76] Recently, robotic-assisted approaches have been described in the literature. Robotic surgery provides better 3-dimensional visualization and allows the surgeon for more precise, finer instrument control than laparoscopy. In the future, laparoscopy might provide a safe alternative to open surgery.[71,72,77,78]

Endoscopy

Although ERCP is mostly a diagnostic modality for Mirizzi syndrome, stent placement and sphincterotomy can facilitate surgery by relieving biliary obstruction and stone removal.[71,72,77]

Mirizzi Syndrome Summary

Mirizzi syndrome is a rare complication of cholelithiasis, leading to compression or erosion of a gallstone into the common bile duct. Although imaging modalities and ERCP are useful, Mirizzi syndrome is often diagnosed during surgery, and requires careful management to avoid common bile duct injury.

SUPPLEMENTARY DATA

Supplementary data related to this article can be found online at https://doi.org/10. 1016/j.suc.2018.12.006.

REFERENCES

1. Everhart JE, Ruhl CE. Burden of digestive diseases in the United States Part III: liver, biliary tract, and pancreas. Gastroenterology 2009;136(4):1134–44.
2. National Institute of Health Consensus Development Conference Statement on gallstones and laparoscopic cholecystectomy. Am J Surg 1993;165:390–8.
3. Fox MS, Wilk PJ, Weissmann HS, et al. Acute acalculous cholecystitis. Surg Gynecol Obstet 1984;159(1):13–6.
4. Singer AJ, McCracken G, Henry MC, et al. Correlation among clinical, laboratory, and hepatobiliary scanning findings in patients with suspected acute cholecystitis. Ann Emerg Med 1996;28(3):267–72.
5. Kurzweil SM, Shapiro MJ, Andrus CH, et al. Hyperbilirubinemia without common bile duct abnormalities and hyperamylasemia without pancreatitis in patients with gallbladder disease. Arch Surg 1994;129(8):829–33.
6. Shea JA, Berlin JA, Escarce JJ, et al. Revised estimates of diagnostic test sensitivity and specificity in suspected biliary tract disease. Arch Intern Med 1994; 154(22):2573–81.
7. Benarroch-Gampel J, Boyd CA, Sheffield KM, et al. Overuse of CT in patients with complicated gallstone disease. J Am Coll Surg 2011;213(4):524–30.
8. Park MS, Yu JS, Kim YH, et al. Acute cholecystitis: comparison of MR cholangiography and US. Radiology 1998;209(3):781–5.
9. Kiewiet JJ, Leeuwenburgh MM, Bipat S, et al. A systematic review and meta-analysis of diagnostic performance of imaging in acute cholecystitis. Radiology 2012;264(3):708–20.
10. Mazeh H, Mizrahi I, Dior U, et al. Role of antibiotic therapy in mild acute calculus cholecystitis: a prospective randomized controlled trial. World J Surg 2012;36(8): 1750–9.
11. Landau O, Kott I, Deutsch AA, et al. Multifactorial analysis of septic bile and septic complications in biliary surgery. World J Surg 1992;16(5):962–4 [discussion: 964–5].
12. de Mestral C, Rotstein OD, Laupacis A, et al. A population-based analysis of the clinical course of 10,304 patients with acute cholecystitis, discharged without cholecystectomy. J Trauma Acute Care Surg 2013;74(1):26–30 [discussion: 30–21].
13. Loozen CS, Oor JE, van Ramshorst B, et al. Conservative treatment of acute cholecystitis: a systematic review and pooled analysis. Surg Endosc 2017; 31(2):504–15.
14. Gomi H, Solomkin JS, Schlossberg D, et al. Tokyo guidelines 2018: antimicrobial therapy for acute cholangitis and cholecystitis. J Hepatobiliary Pancreat Sci 2018;25(1):3–16.

15. Regimbeau JM, Fuks D, Pautrat K, et al. Effect of postoperative antibiotic administration on postoperative infection following cholecystectomy for acute calculous cholecystitis: a randomized clinical trial. JAMA 2014;312(2):145–54.

16. Winbladh A, Gullstrand P, Svanvik J, et al. Systematic review of cholecystostomy as a treatment option in acute cholecystitis. HPB (Oxford) 2009;11(3): 183–93.

17. Blohm M, Österberg J, Sandblom G, et al. The sooner, the better? The importance of optimal timing of cholecystectomy in acute cholecystitis: data from the National Swedish Registry for Gallstone Surgery, GallRiks. J Gastrointest Surg 2017;21(1):33–40.

18. Hirota M, Takada T, Kawarada Y, et al. Diagnostic criteria and severity assessment of acute cholecystitis: Tokyo guidelines. J Hepatobiliary Pancreat Surg 2007;14(1):78–82.

19. Strasberg SM, Pucci MJ, Brunt LM, et al. Subtotal cholecystectomy-"fenestrating" vs "reconstituting" subtypes and the prevention of bile duct injury: definition of the optimal procedure in difficult operative conditions. J Am Coll Surg 2016;222(1): 89–96.

20. Elshaer M, Gravante G, Thomas K, et al. Subtotal cholecystectomy for "difficult gallbladders": systematic review and meta-analysis. JAMA Surg 2015;150(2): 159–68.

21. van Dijk AH, Donkervoort SC, Lameris W, et al. Short- and long-term outcomes after a reconstituting and fenestrating subtotal cholecystectomy. J Am Coll Surg 2017;225(3):371–9.

22. Papi C, Catarci M, D'Ambrosio L, et al. Timing of cholecystectomy for acute calculous cholecystitis: a meta-analysis. Am J Gastroenterol 2004;99(1):147–55.

23. Ackerman J, Abegglen R, Scaife M, et al. Beware of the interval cholecystectomy. J Trauma Acute Care Surg 2017;83(1):55–60.

24. Lim KH, Kim YJ. A novel technique of percutaneous stone extraction in choledocholithiasis after cholecystostomy. Hepatogastroenterology 2013;60(123):452–5.

25. Chou CK, Lee KC, Chan CC, et al. Early percutaneous cholecystostomy in severe acute cholecystitis reduces the complication rate and duration of hospital stay. Medicine (Baltimore) 2015;94(27):e1096.

26. Macchini D, Degrate L, Oldani M, et al. Timing of percutaneous cholecystostomy tube removal: systematic review. Minerva Chir 2016;71(6):415–26.

27. Clavien PA, Richon J, Burgan S, et al. Gallstone ileus. Br J Surg 1990;77(7): 737–42.

28. Ayantunde AA, Agrawal A. Gallstone ileus: diagnosis and management. World J Surg 2007;31(6):1292–7.

29. Halabi WJ, Kang CY, Ketana N, et al. Surgery for gallstone ileus: a nationwide comparison of trends and outcomes. Ann Surg 2014;259(2):329–35.

30. Reisner RM, Cohen JR. Gallstone ileus: a review of 1001 reported cases. Am Surg 1994;60(6):441–6.

31. Farkas N, Kaur V, Shanmuganandan A, et al. A systematic review of gallstone sigmoid ileus management. Ann Med Surg (Lond) 2018;27:32–9.

32. Haddad FG, Mansour W, Deeb L. Bouveret's syndrome: literature review. Cureus 2018;10(3):e2299.

33. Balthazar EJ, Schechter LS. Air in gallbladder: a frequent finding in gallstone ileus. AJR Am J Roentgenol 1978;131(2):219–22.

34. Rigler LG, Borman CN, Noble JF. Gallstone obstruction: pathogenesis and roentgen manifestations. JAMA 1941;117:1753–9.

35. Yu CY, Lin CC, Shyu RY, et al. Value of CT in the diagnosis and management of gallstone ileus. World J Gastroenterol 2005;11(14):2142–7.
36. Lassandro F, Gagliardi N, Scuderi M, et al. Gallstone ileus analysis of radiological findings in 27 patients. Eur J Radiol 2004;50(1):23–9.
37. Lassandro F, Romano S, Ragozzino A, et al. Role of helical CT in diagnosis of gallstone ileus and related conditions. AJR Am J Roentgenol 2005;185(5): 1159–65.
38. Ripollés T, Miguel-Dasit A, Errando J, et al. Gallstone ileus: increased diagnostic sensitivity by combining plain film and ultrasound. Abdom Imaging 2001;26(4): 401–5.
39. Pickhardt PJ, Friedland JA, Hruza DS, et al. Case report. CT, MR cholangiopan-creatography, and endoscopy findings in Bouveret's syndrome. AJR Am J Roentgenol 2003;180(4):1033–5.
40. DECKOFF SL. Gallstone ileus; a report of 12 cases. Ann Surg 1955;142(1):52–65.
41. Zaliekas J, Munson JL. Complications of gallstones: the Mirizzi syndrome, gallstone ileus, gallstone pancreatitis, complications of "lost" gallstones. Surg Clin North Am 2008;88(6):1345–68, x.
42. Nuño-Guzmán CM, Marín-Contreras ME, Figueroa-Sánchez M, et al. Gallstone ileus, clinical presentation, diagnostic and treatment approach. World J Gastrointest Surg 2016;8(1):65–76.
43. Doko M, Zovak M, Kopljar M, et al. Comparison of surgical treatments of gallstone ileus: preliminary report. World J Surg 2003;27(4):400–4.
44. Tartaglia D, Bakkar S, Piccini L, et al. Less is more: an outcome assessment of patients operated for gallstone ileus without fistula treatment. Int J Surg Case Rep 2017;38:78–82.
45. Warshaw AL, Bartlett MK. Choice of operation for gallstone intestinal obstruction. Ann Surg 1966;164(6):1051–5.
46. Moberg AC, Montgomery A. Laparoscopically assisted or open enterolithotomy for gallstone ileus. Br J Surg 2007;94(1):53–7.
47. Lübbers H, Mahlke R, Lankisch PG. Gallstone ileus: endoscopic removal of a gallstone obstructing the upper jejunum. J Intern Med 1999;246(6):593–7.
48. Heinzow HS, Meister T, Wessling J, et al. Ileal gallstone obstruction: single-balloon enteroscopic removal. World J Gastrointest Endosc 2010;2(9):321–4.
49. Zielinski MD, Ferreira LE, Baron TH. Successful endoscopic treatment of colonic gallstone ileus using electrohydraulic lithotripsy. World J Gastroenterol 2010; 16(12):1533–6.
50. Caldwell KM, Lee SJ, Leggett PL, et al. Bouveret syndrome: current management strategies. Clin Exp Gastroenterol 2018;11:69–75.
51. Cappell MS, Davis M. Characterization of Bouveret's syndrome: a comprehensive review of 128 cases. Am J Gastroenterol 2006;101(9):2139–46.
52. Zhao JC, Barrera E, Salabat M, et al. Endoscopic treatment for Bouveret syndrome. Surg Endosc 2013;27(2):655.
53. Afzal M, Ghosh D, Leigh T. Mechanical lithotripsy for Bouveret's syndrome. Gut 2007;56(5):733–4 [author reply: 734].
54. Makker J, Muthusamy VR, Watson R, et al. Electrohydraulic lithotripsy and removal of a gallstone obstructing the duodenum: Bouveret syndrome. Gastrointest Endosc 2015;81(4):1021–2.
55. Saldaña Dueñas C, Fernández-Urien I, Rullán Iriarte M, et al. Laser lithotripsy resolution for Bouveret syndrome. Endoscopy 2017;49(S 01):E101–2.
56. Hollowell JG, Roth RA, Beckmann CF. Radiologic technique to mark ureteral calculi for extracorporeal shock-wave lithotripsy. Urology 1987;30(2):127–9.

57. Baharith H, Khan K. Bouveret syndrome: when there are no options. Can J Gastroenterol Hepatol 2015;29(1):17–8.
58. Mavroeidis VK, Matthioudakis DI, Economou NK, et al. Bouveret syndrome-the rarest variant of gallstone ileus: a case report and literature review. Case Rep Surg 2013;2013:839370.
59. Malvaux P, Degolla R, De Saint-Hubert M, et al. Laparoscopic treatment of a gastric outlet obstruction caused by a gallstone (Bouveret's syndrome). Surg Endosc 2002;16(7):1108–9.
60. Newton RC, Loizides S, Penney N, et al. Laparoscopic management of Bouveret syndrome. BMJ Case Rep 2015;2015 [pii:bcr2015209869].
61. Beltran MA, Csendes A, Cruces KS. The relationship of Mirizzi syndrome and cholecystoenteric fistula: validation of a modified classification. World J Surg 2008;32(10):2237–43.
62. Chen H, Siwo EA, Khu M, et al. Current trends in the management of Mirizzi Syndrome: a review of literature. Medicine (Baltimore) 2018;97(4):e9691.
63. Beltrán MA. Mirizzi syndrome: history, current knowledge and proposal of a simplified classification. World J Gastroenterol 2012;18(34):4639–50.
64. Beltran MA, Csendes A. Mirizzi syndrome and gallstone ileus: an unusual presentation of gallstone disease. J Gastrointest Surg 2005;9(5):686–9.
65. Csendes A, Díaz JC, Burdiles P, et al. Mirizzi syndrome and cholecystobiliary fistula: a unifying classification. Br J Surg 1989;76(11):1139–43.
66. Yip AW, Chow WC, Chan J, et al. Mirizzi syndrome with cholecystocholedochal fistula: preoperative diagnosis and management. Surgery 1992;111(3): 335–8.
67. Robertson AG, Davidson BR. Mirizzi syndrome complicating an anomalous biliary tract: a novel cause of a hugely elevated CA19-9. Eur J Gastroenterol Hepatol 2007;19(2):167–9.
68. Lai EC, Lau WY. Mirizzi syndrome: history, present and future development. ANZ J Surg 2006;76(4):251–7.
69. Toscano RL, Taylor PH, Peters J, et al. Mirizzi syndrome. Am Surg 1994;60(11): 889–91.
70. Kim PN, Outwater EK, Mitchell DG. Mirizzi syndrome: evaluation by MRI imaging. Am J Gastroenterol 1999;94(9):2546–50.
71. Yonetci N, Kutluana U, Yilmaz M, et al. The incidence of Mirizzi syndrome in patients undergoing endoscopic retrograde cholangiopancreatography. Hepatobiliary Pancreat Dis Int 2008;7(5):520–4.
72. Yuan H, Yuan T, Sun X, et al. A minimally invasive strategy for Mirizzi syndrome type ii: combined endoscopic with laparoscopic approach. Surg Laparosc Endosc Percutan Tech 2016;26(3):248–52.
73. Bornman PC, Terblanche J. Subtotal cholecystectomy: for the difficult gallbladder in portal hypertension and cholecystitis. Surgery 1985;98(1):1–6.
74. Baer HU, Matthews JB, Schweizer WP, et al. Management of the Mirizzi syndrome and the surgical implications of cholecystcholedochal fistula. Br J Surg 1990; 77(7):743–5.
75. Kamalesh NP, Prakash K, Pramil K, et al. Laparoscopic approach is safe and effective in the management of Mirizzi syndrome. J Minim Access Surg 2015; 11(4):246–50.
76. Kwon AH, Inui H. Preoperative diagnosis and efficacy of laparoscopic procedures in the treatment of Mirizzi syndrome. J Am Coll Surg 2007;204(3): 409–15.

77. Lee KF, Chong CN, Ma KW, et al. A minimally invasive strategy for Mirizzi syndrome: the combined endoscopic and robotic approach. Surg Endosc 2014; 28(9):2690–4.
78. Magge D, Steve J, Novak S, et al. Performing the difficult cholecystectomy using combined endoscopic and robotic techniques: how I do it. J Gastrointest Surg 2017;21(3):583–9.

An Update on Technical Aspects of Cholecystectomy

Dominic E. Sanford, MD, MPHS

KEYWORDS

- Cholecystectomy • Laparoscopic cholecystectomy • Robotic cholecystectomy
- Critical view of safety • Laparoscopy • Robotic surgery

KEY POINTS

- Laparoscopic cholecystectomy (LC) is the standard of care for the treatment of symptomatic cholelithiasis.
- The Critical View of Safety should be the goal of dissection and should be confirmed before clipping or cutting cystic structures.
- Open cholecystectomy is most commonly performed when LC is converted to open or when LC is contraindicated.
- Most surgical trainees are graduating with insufficient experience in open cholecystectomy, which may change the role of converting to open during LC in the near future.
- Robotic cholecystectomy is safe with outcomes similar to LC, and should follow the same operative principles of LC, including the attainment of the Critical View of Safety.

INTRODUCTION

Carl Langenbuch of Germany performed the first open cholecystectomy (OC) in 1882.[1] Contrary to the belief that cholecystostomy was the treatment of choice at the time, he theorized that the gallbladder was the source of stone formation. This newly introduced operation was met with vehement opposition at first, but eventually became accepted as the standard of care for the treatment of symptomatic cholelithiasis. In 1985, Erich Muhe performed the first laparoscopic cholecystectomy (LC), also in Germany[2]; However, Muhe was met with harsh criticism from his German contemporaries. Eventually, the procedure was adopted by French gynecologist Philippe Mouret and modified by French surgeons F. Dubois and J. Perissat. J. Barry McKernan and William B. Saye performed the first LC in the United States in 1988; however, the dissemination and widespread adoption of LC can largely be credited to Eddie J. Reddick and Douglas O. Olsen,[3] who were the primary teachers of LC

The author has nothing to disclose.
Division of Hepatobiliary, Pancreatic, and Gastrointestinal Surgery, Washington University School of Medicine, 660 South Euclid Avenue Box 8109, St Louis, MO 63110, USA
E-mail address: sanfordd@wustl.edu

Surg Clin N Am 99 (2019) 245–258
https://doi.org/10.1016/j.suc.2018.11.005
0039-6109/19/© 2018 Elsevier Inc. All rights reserved.

technique in the United States at the time. Reddick and Olsen[3] organized structured courses to teach the technique to surgeons throughout the country and were largely responsible for the rapid spread of laparoscopy in the United States. Currently, more than 400,000 cholecystectomies are performed per year in the United States. LC is considered the gold standard for removing the gallbladder, with OC usually being performed when there is confusion over the anatomy or other intraoperative difficulties.[4] However, converting from LC to OC is not an intraoperative complication. On the contrary, conversion is usually an important and responsible decision made to maximize the safety of cholecystectomy often in hostile conditions, such as severe cholecystitis.

With the widespread adoption of LC in the late 1980s and early 1990s throughout the world, it soon became apparent that, in addition to the obvious benefits of the laparoscopic approach to most patients, there was unfortunately a higher incidence of bile duct injury as well.[5] In the early 1990s, Steven Strasberg and others[6–8] began studying how bile duct injuries occur during LC. In 1995, Strasberg and colleagues[7] described the Critical View of Safety (CVS), which has become the gold standard for ductal identification during LC. The goal of the CVS is to prevent bile duct injury by being protective against misidentification.[7]

Since the introduction of LC, many modifications have been attempted to further reduce the morbidity of the operation, such as the use of smaller-diameter trocars, single-incision cholecystectomy, and natural orifice transluminal endoscopic surgery (NOTES).[9,10] However, these techniques have not undergone widespread adoption, as they have largely failed to consistently demonstrate a benefit over conventional LC and often at the cost of making this procedure more cumbersome and/or difficult.[11,12] With the introduction of robotic surgical systems, LC is being increasingly being performed with the aid of robotics. The improved 3-dimensional visualization, magnification, tremor suppression, and degrees of freedom that the robotic platform offer, give robotic cholecystectomy (RC) theoretic advantages over the conventional laparoscopic approach. There is no demonstrable advantage to the robot in terms of patient outcomes when comparing RC with conventional LC, but the operative time and cost of the robotic approach are significantly higher.[13,14] As more surgeons begin to adopt the robot in their practice, performing LC with the use of a robotic platform is sometimes used as a way to familiarize surgeons with the robot and can serve as a bridge to performing more complex robotic procedures.[15]

INDICATIONS FOR CHOLECYSTECTOMY

- Symptomatic cholelithiasis
- Complicated cholelithiasis (acute calculous cholecystitis, choledocholithiasis, gallstone pancreatitis)
- Biliary dyskinesia (gallbladder ejection fraction <35% on cholecystokinin hepatobiliary iminodiacetic acid [HIDA] scan)
- Acalculous cholecystitis
- Gall bladder polyps (>1 cm)
- Concern for malignant or premalignant condition (gallbladder wall calcifications)

TECHNIQUES FOR PERFORMING CHOLECYSTECTOMY

- LC: Considered the gold standard.[4]
- OC: Usually performed when LC in converted to open, when LC in contraindicated, when there is concern for gallbladder malignancy, or as a part of a separate open abdominal procedure (such as pancreaticoduodenectomy).

- RC: becoming more frequently performed as an alternative to traditional LC. No clear advantage of RC over LC in terms of patient outcomes, but RC is associated with increased operative time and costs.[13,14]
- NOTES approach, most commonly transvaginal or transgastric: rarely performed today. This approach is reviewed elsewhere.[16]
- Single-incision LC: Benefits of traditional LC are unclear. Although single-incision LC offers perhaps better cosmetic results, it does so at the cost of a higher risk of hernia.[17] This approach is reviewed elsewhere.[16]

In this article, we review the steps of LC, OC, and RC. The latter 2 techniques are reviewed elsewhere.[16]

LAPAROSCOPIC CHOLECYSTECTOMY

LC is the gold standard for gallbladder removal. There are few absolute contraindications to LC besides the inability of a patient to tolerate CO_2 pneumoperitoneum and diffuse peritonitis with hemodynamic compromise.

Relative contraindications are often dependent on the surgeon's judgment and experience and include the following:

- Suspicion of gallbladder cancer
- Cirrhosis with portal hypertension
- Severe cardiopulmonary disease
- Bleeding disorders
- Multiple prior operations

The patient is usually positioned supine with arms out (American approach), and the surgeon stands on the patient's left side. Alternatively, the patient can be placed in a split leg position (French approach) with the surgeon standing between the legs. One or both arms can be tucked as needed to facilitate intraoperative cholangiogram if needed.

The usual equipment needed for a standard LC include the following:

- Laparoscopy equipment
  - Camera
  - Monitor
  - Light source
  - Insufflator
  - 4 trocars, typically two 5-mm trocars and two 12-mm trocars
  - A 30° 5-mm or 10-mm camera scope
- Laparoscopic instruments
  - Hook electrocautery
  - 2 atraumatic graspers, at least 1 of which is locking
  - Maryland dissector
  - Laparoscopic clip applier
  - Laparoscopic scissors
  - Laparoscopic retrieval bag

The steps for LC are described in the following sections (**Box 1**).

ACCESSING THE ABDOMEN

A 12-mm or 5-mm incision is made in the periumbilical region. This incision can be above or below the umbilicus depending on the patient's body habitus. For extremely

> **Box 1**
> **Steps of laparoscopic cholecystectomy**
>
> 1. Accessing the abdomen
> 2. Port placement
> 3. Initial dissection of adhesions
> 4. Dissection of hepatocystic triangle
> 5. Dissection of gallbladder off bottom one-third of cystic plate
> 6. Confirmation of the Critical View of Safety
> 7. Intraoperative cholangiogram (if indicated)
> 8. Division of cystic duct and cystic artery
> 9. Dissection of gallbladder off remainder of cystic plate
> 10. Gallbladder extraction and port closure

obese patients, the incision can be placed a few fingerbreadths cephalad and to the patient's right. Options for entering the peritoneal cavity include the following:

- Veress needle: Pneumoperitoneum is established with a Veress needle inserted into the peritoneal cavity, often in the left upper quadrant (ie, Palmer point). Once pneumoperitoneum to 15 mm Hg has been achieved, a trocar can be introduced into the peritoneal cavity in a blind fashion or using an optical viewing trocar.
- Open (Hasson) technique: The trocar is inserted directly into peritoneal cavity and pneumoperitoneum is established.
- Optical viewing trocar insertion: The trocar is inserted under direct visualization using a 0° camera scope inside the trocar.

TROCAR PLACEMENT

After the abdomen is insufflated to 15 mm Hg, a laparoscope is introduced and the abdominal cavity is inspected. The bed is adjusted so that the patient is in reverse Trendelenburg with the right side slightly elevated. Three additional trocars are placed in the following positions (**Fig. 1**):

- 5-mm trocar 2 to 3 fingerbreadths below the costal margin, in plane with the anterior axillary line.
- 5-mm trocar 2 to 3 fingerbreadths below the costal margin, in plane with the midclavicular line.

A locking, atraumatic grasper is then introduced from the far right lateral port and the fundus of the gall bladder is grasped and retracted toward the patient's right shoulder. It is important to do this step before placing the final trocar, so that the final location of the gallbladder (specifically, the cystic structures) is apparent when deciding how high to place the final trocar.

- 12-mm trocar (or 5-mm) in the epigastrium, near midline at a slight angle so that the trocar enters the peritoneum to the patient's right of the falciform ligament or through the right side of the falciform ligament.

INITIAL DISSECTION OF ADHESIONS

Adhesions from the duodenum, colon, or omentum are commonly encountered during LC. These can be taken down bluntly or sharply with the aid of traction and

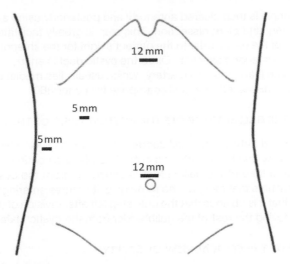

Fig. 1. LC port placement.

countertraction. Electrocautery is sometimes needed, but should be used with extreme caution so as not to injure adjacent viscera.

DISSECTION OF THE HEPATOCYSTIC TRIANGLE

With the fundus of the gallbladder retracted toward the patient's right shoulder via a locking atraumatic grasper from the far right lateral port, an atraumatic grasper, from the midclavicular port, then grasps the infundibulum of the gallbladder and provides traction laterally to the patient's right (**Fig. 2**). Hook electrocautery is used to divide just the peritoneum overlying the hepatocystic triangle, both anteriorly and posteriorly. This is continued cephalad along the neck of the gallbladder near the liver. Typically, it is safest to dissect from lateral to medial. The fibrofatty tissue within the

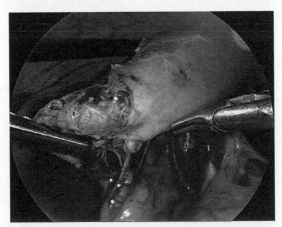

Fig. 2. Gallbladder retraction for dissection of the hepatocystic triangle. The gallbladder fundus is retracted cephalad and toward the patient's right shoulder while the infundibulum is retracted laterally.

hepatocystic triangle is then cleared anteriorly and posteriorly using a combination of hook electrocautery and blunt dissection. This step is greatly facilitated by retracting the infundibulum of the gallbladder to the patient's right for the anterior dissection and to the left for the posterior dissection. Once the cystic duct is encountered, a plane is developed between it and the cystic artery, which usually lies medial to the duct. The cystic duct is then dissected free of fibroadipose tissue for 360°.

DISSECTION OF THE GALLBLADDER OFF THE BOTTOM THIRD OF THE CYSTIC PLATE

A plane is developed between the gallbladder neck and the liver, while retracting the gallbladder anteriorly and to the patient's right. This plane is continued cephalad until at least the bottom third of the gallbladder is separated from the cystic plate of the liver. This step ensures that there are no remaining structures entering the gallbladder posteriorly, and that it is obvious that the only step left after division of the cystic structures will be removing the rest of the gallbladder from the cystic plate.[18]

CONFIRMATION OF THE CRITICAL VIEW OF SAFETY

Once a surgeon believes the cystic artery and cystic duct have been identified and are ready to divide, he or she should ensure that the 3 requirements of the CVS have been met: the hepatocystic triangle has been cleared of fibroadipose tissue, the gallbladder has been removed from the bottom third of the cystic plate, and 2 and only 2 structures are seen entering the gallbladder (**Box 2, Fig. 3**).[18] If any of these criteria are not present, the CVS has not been achieved, and further dissection may be needed. If the CVS cannot be safely met, such as in the case of severe inflammation, strong consideration should be given to performing a bailout procedure, such as open conversion or subtotal cholecystectomy.[19]

Subtotal cholecystectomy has 2 forms: fenestrating and reconstituting.[20] Subtotal reconstituting cholecystectomy closes off the lower end of the gallbladder, thus reducing the incidence of postoperative fistula, but it creates a remnant gallbladder. Subtotal fenestrating cholecystectomy involves the removal of the gallbladder wall and ablation of the mucosa. The cystic duct may be sutured shut from inside the gallbladder. Subtotal fenestrating cholecystectomy is more difficult to complete laparoscopically and may have a higher incidence of postoperative biliary fistula[21]; however, subtotal reconstituting cholecystectomy has a higher incidence of recurrent biliary events (ie, choledocholithiasis, pancreatitis, cholecystitis, and cholangitis).[21]

INTRAOPERATIVE CHOLANGIOGRAM (IF PERFORMED)

Whether or not intraoperative cholangiogram (IOCG) prevents bile duct injury is controversial, but it can recognize a bile duct injury intraoperatively.[22]

Box 2
Requirements of the critical view of safety[a]

1. Clearance of the hepatocystic triangle of all adipose and fibrous tissue

2. Removal of the gallbladder from the bottom one-third of the cystic plate of the liver

3. Two and only 2 structures seen entering the gallbladder: the cystic duct and cystic artery

   [a] If the critical view of safety cannot be obtained, strong consideration should be given to performing a bailout procedure, such as open cholecystectomy or subtotal fenestrating cholecystectomy.

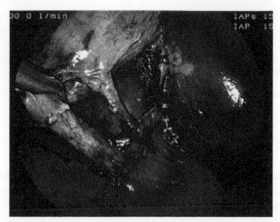

Fig. 3. Intraoperative photo of the CVS. The hepatocystic triangle has been completely cleared of fibrofatty tissue, the bottom third of the cystic plate is visible, and only 2 structures are entering the gallbladder.

Intraoperative cholangiogram is typically performed when

- The biliary anatomy is unclear
- There is concern for choledocholithiasis
- There is concern for bile duct injury

To perform IOCG, most commonly a clip is applied to the cystic duct, close to where it enters the gallbladder. A small ductotomy is then made on the anterior wall of the cystic duct, a few millimeters to the patient's left of the clip, and a cholangiocatheter is inserted for a few centimeters (**Fig. 4**). The cystic duct is then occluded using clips or a specialized clamp, and saline is injected to ensure there is no leakage. Contrast is then injected through the catheter while on table, fluoroscopy is performed. It is important that air bubbles be removed from the syringe before injection as these can mimic

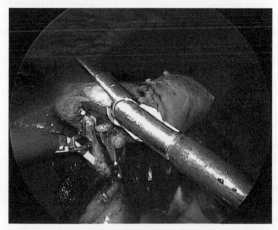

Fig. 4. Insertion of cholangiogram catheter. After a clip is placed on the cystic duct near its junction with the gallbladder, a small ductotomy is made on the anterior surface of the cystic duct and a cholangiogram catheter (*yellow*) is passed into the duct for a few centimeters.

choledocholithiasis. Alternatively, contrast can be injected directly into the gall-bladder, creating a cholecystogram; however, this method is not useful when the cystic duct is occluded by inflammation or stones.

Ultimately, the utility of IOCG is limited by the ability of the individual interpreting it. There are 3 requirements for a normal IOCG:

- Contrast is visualized in both the right hepatic duct (including the right anterior and right posterior sectoral ducts) and left intrahepatic duct above their confluence
- Lack of filling defects in the common bile duct
- Free flow of contrast into the duodenum

If any of these are not present, further investigation or intervention is needed. If chol-edocholithiasis is detected, laparoscopic or open common bile duct exploration can be performed. This procedure is reviewed elsewhere.[23]

DIVISION OF CYSTIC DUCT AND ARTERY

Once the CVS has been confirmed, the cystic duct and artery can be clipped and divided. Typically, the cystic duct is clipped in a medial to lateral fashion, with 2 clips placed on the remaining cystic duct stump. Similarly, the cystic artery is doubly clip-ped on the stay side with one clip on the specimen side. A laparoscopic scissors is then used to divide the structures. Alternatively, the duct can be ligated with the use of an Endoloop, a pre-tied suture, or intracorporal/extracorporal knot, especially when the cystic duct is of large diameter. However, surgeons should take pause if considering a stapling device for transection of the presumed cystic duct, as this may suggest a misinterpretation of the anatomy.

DISSECTION OF THE GALLBLADDER OFF THE CYSTIC PLATE

Once the cystic structures have been divided, the gallbladder is dissected off the cystic plate using hook electrocautery. To facilitate this, the infundibulum of the gall bladder is retracted anteriorly and slightly cephalad, while the fundus of the gall-bladder is retracted cephalad. Retraction of the infundibulum is alternated from right to left to facilitate adequate tension to expose the correct plane between the cystic plate and gallbladder. Sometimes this plane is absent, such as with severe inflamma-tion or cirrhosis, and this step can be difficult. If the gallbladder is perforated during this step, every effort should be made to limit the spillage of stones and bile by grasping, suturing, or clipping the site of a hole. Rarely, the posterior gallbladder wall can be left on the liver to avoid hemorrhage and the mucosa ablated.

GALLBLADDER EXTRACTION AND PORT CLOSURE

Typically, the gallbladder is placed within a laparoscopic extraction bag and removed. When the gallbladder is not distended or inflamed and the stones are of relatively small size, the gallbladder can be removed directly through the incision with little risk of wound infection and at reduced cost. Most commonly, the gallbladder is removed through the 12-mm periumbilical incision, but it also can be removed from a 12-mm subxiphoid port as well.

Before or after extraction of the gallbladder, the liver bed and clips should be checked one last time to ensure hemostasis and secure closure of the cystic duct. The port sites can then be anesthetized with local anesthetic and the lateral ports removed under direct visualization. The author routinely closes the fascial defect of the 12-mm periumbilical port, which is dilated during extraction of the gallbladder. If the epigastric port site is not dilated or used for specimen extraction, closure of the fascia is not necessary at this location, regardless of whether a 5-mm or 12-mm trocar is used.

2018 TOKYO GUIDELINES: SAFE STEPS DURING CHOLECYSTECTOMY FOR ACUTE CHOLECYSTITIS

The 2018 Tokyo Guidelines (TG18) was a consensus conference of more than 60 experts worldwide.[19] One of the goals of TG18 was to stratify acute cholecystitis by severity and recommend treatment based on severity. TG18's safe steps during cholecystectomy for cholecystitis include the following[19]:

- If the gallbladder is distended and interferes with view, it should be decompressed by needle aspiration.
- Effective retraction of the gallbladder to develop a plane in the Calot triangle area and identify its boundaries (countertraction).
- Starting dissection from the posterior leaf of the peritoneum covering the neck of the gallbladder and exposing the gallbladder surface above the Rouviere sulcus.
- Maintaining the plane of dissection on the gallbladder surface throughout LC.
- Dissecting the lower part of the gallbladder bed (at least one-third) to obtain the CVS.
- Creating the CVS.
- For persistent hemorrhage, achieving hemostasis primarily by compression and avoiding excessive use of electrocautery or clipping.

POSTOPERATIVE MANAGEMENT

- Oral analgesics are given as needed for pain control.
- Diet is resumed as tolerated.
- Patients are usually discharged home on the same or following day depending the patient's preoperative health status.

COMPLICATIONS

- Significant hemorrhage is rare during LC; however, occasionally the middle hepatic vein (or a large branch) runs immediately deep to the cystic plate and can cause quite impressive sudden bleeding when it is inadvertently injured, usually during removal of the gall bladder from the liver bed. Treatment involves direct pressure with a gauze and often requires placement of a suture, laparoscopically or open, or use of an advanced energy device.
- Superficial wound infection is uncommon during LC.
- Injury to nearby organs, especially colon and duodenum, can occur during LC.
- Bile leakage from the cystic duct stump, cystic plate/liver bed, or unrecognized bile duct injury can occur. This often presents within the first week as pain, fevers, chills, and occasionally jaundice. Treatment for cystic duct stump or ducts of Luschka leaks usually involves percutaneous drain placement within a biloma, antibiotics, and an endoscopic retrograde cholangiopancreatography with sphincterotomy and stent.
- Bile duct injury is rare (~0.3% of LC), but it is the most feared complication, as the consequences can be devastating. Treatment is predicated on the type of injury sustained and is reviewed elsewhere.[24]
- Retained stones can occur within the common bile duct and can present with abdominal pain, jaundice, and cholangitis.

- Spilled stones can cause chronic recurrent abscesses. The treatment is surgical removal; however, these stones can be notoriously difficult to locate intraoperatively. Note that spilled stones in an asymptomatic patient and discovered incidentally on imaging is not itself a reason for operative removal.

OPEN CHOLECYSTECTOMY

LC is the gold standard and thus OC is often performed due to conversion of LC, when LC is contraindicated, or as a part of or in conjunction with an open abdominal operation. In the era when LC was being developed and disseminated, OC was the gold standard and so surgeons could readily convert to open because they were more experienced with OC. The pendulum has now swung dramatically in the other direction in that most graduating chief residents perform very few OCs during their training and are much more comfortable with LC.[25] Therefore, conversion of LC to OC is not necessarily the best option for all surgeons when LC is not progressing or becomes unsafe.

Indications for conversion can include the following:

- Patients unable to tolerate pneumoperitoneum
- Difficulty identifying ductal anatomy, which is often due to inflammation
- Hemorrhage
- Concern for malignancy

Preoperative factors associated with conversion of LC to OC in acute cholecystitis:

- Male sex[a]
- Increasing age[a]
- Leukocytosis[a]
- Obesity
- Duration of symptoms
- Fever
- American Society of Anesthesiologists score
- Elevated C-reactive protein
- Hypoalbuminemia
- Transaminitis
- Pericholecystic fluid
- Impacted gallstone

The steps of OC are as follows:

- OC is performed with patient supine with arms out.
- A right subcostal incision is made 2 to 3 fingerbreadths below the ribs, the round ligament is divided, and a retractor is placed. A midline laparotomy can be performed in very thin patients. If an LC is converted to OC, the abdomen should be completely desufflated before incision, as the pneumoperitoneum distorts the abdominal wall anatomy and incisions made with the abdomen insufflated will often result in a subcostal incision that is too cephalad. Placement of sponges behind the liver to lift it forward is often helpful with exposure.
- The fundus of the gallbladder is retracted cephalad and toward the patient's right shoulder and the infundibulum is retracted laterally, similar to LC.

---

[a] Indicates factors most consistently shown in the literature to be associated with conversion to open during acute cholecystitis.[26]

- The peritoneum overlying the hepatocystic triangle is incised and the fibroadipose tissue within this space is swept toward the common bile duct using a combination of electrocautery and blunt dissection. A Yankauer suction or Kittner are useful in facilitating this maneuver.
- Once the presumed cystic duct and artery are identified, the gallbladder is dissected off the cystic plate of the liver in a top-down fashion. Once the gallbladder is free from the liver, 2 and only 2 structures should be remaining connected to the gallbladder, the cystic duct and artery, and this confirms the identity of these 2 structures. Of note, this dissection technique serves as the basis for identifying the cystic duct and artery when obtaining the CVS during LC.
- The cystic duct and artery are then divided between ties or clips.
- Hemostasis is confirmed and the abdominal fascia is closed in 2 layers followed by the skin.

ROBOTIC CHOLECYSTECTOMY

RC is a variation of LC and follows the same general principles of LC. Most RCs are performed using multiple ports with the DaVinci Xi Surgical Systems (Intuitive Surgical Inc., Sunnyvale, CA); as such, this technique is described. RC is associated with similar outcomes as traditional LC, but is associated with increased operative times and costs. RC also requires larger ports (8 mm) compared with the traditional 5-mm ports for 2 or 3 ports during LC. However, RC costs are decreasing with time, and robot docking time decreases with experience as well.[27] The technical benefits for the surgeon of RC over standard LC include improved visualization, full instrument wrist action, and improved ergonomics. RC also allows a safe and reliable method of training future surgeons with a shorter learning curve compared with LC.

The indications and contraindications for RC are the same as those for LC.

The 3 basic components of the DaVinci Surgical System are as follows:

- The surgeon console (SC) is located away from the operative field and contains the controls for the robotic arms and camera.
- The vision cart is located outside the sterile surgical field and provides the light source, energy source, and optical integration software. There is also usually a monitor on this cart with an interactive screen.
- The patient-side cart (PSC) is located within the operative field. The PSC is the component that contains the articulating robotic arms, which are docked to the ports. It is covered with sterile drapes.

The steps of RC are as follows:

- RC is performed with the patient supine. The right arm only or both arms can be tucked to more easily facilitate docking the robot; however, this is not absolutely necessary.
- The abdomen is accessed in the periumbilical region similar to LC, with the caveat that a 12-mm port (camera port) should be placed at least 15 cm from the target operative site. This often means that the incision should be placed infraumbilical (**Fig. 5**).
- After inspection of the abdomen, 2 additional 8-mm trocars are placed in the right upper quadrant in the plane with the midclavicular line and anterior axillary line at roughly 1 to 2 fingerbreadths above the level of the umbilicus. These ports should be approximately 8 to 10 cm apart.
- An 8-mm port should be placed in the left upper quadrant in the midclavicular line roughly 3 to 4 cm above the umbilicus.

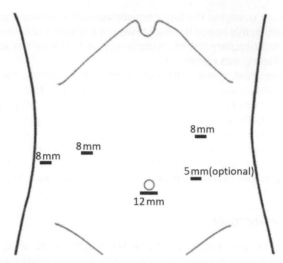

Fig. 5. RC port placement.

- An optional fifth trocar (assistant trocar) can be placed to the left of the umbilicus.
- The PSC is then moved into the surgical field from the patient's right (Xi) or from the patient's head (Si). The patient's bed may need to be rotated to facilitate this step. The robotic arms are then docked to the ports. The camera is first inserted through the periumbilical port followed by the robotic instruments (atraumatic graspers in the 2 right-sided ports and hook electrocautery in the left-sided port).
- The surgeon leaves the operative field and sits at the SC and assumes command of the robotic instruments and camera.
- The dissection technique for RC is essentially the same as that of LC.
- After the gallbladder is removed from the gallbladder bed, the robot is undocked, a 5-mm laparoscopic camera is inserted through the left-sided trocar, and the gallbladder is placed inside a laparoscopic retrieval bag and removed through the periumbilical trocar site.
- The 12-mm port site fascial defect is closed. The author does not routinely close the fascial defects of the 8-mm port sites if they were not dilated during the procedure.

The postoperative management and complications after RC are the same as those discussed previously for LC.

SUMMARY

LC is the gold standard for the treatment of symptomatic cholelithiasis. It is associated with a slightly higher incidence of bile duct injury compared with OC, and steps, such as routine use of the CVS, should be taken to reduce this risk. OC is usually performed when LC is converted to open, or when LC is contraindicated, but should be performed only with adequate training in OC. RC is a safe alternative to conventional LC with similar outcomes, but is associated with increased costs.

REFERENCES

1. Traverso LW. Carl Langenbuch and the first cholecystectomy. Am J Surg 1976; 132:81–2.

2. Reynolds W Jr. The first laparoscopic cholecystectomy. JSLS 2001;5:89–94.
3. Reddick EJ, Olsen DO. Laparoscopic laser cholecystectomy. A comparison with mini-lap cholecystectomy. Surg Endosc 1989;3:131–3.
4. Soper NJ, Stockmann PT, Dunnegan DL, et al. Laparoscopic cholecystectomy. The new 'gold standard'? Arch Surg 1992;127:917–21 [discussion: 21–3].
5. Gouma DJ, Go PM. Bile duct injury during laparoscopic and conventional cholecystectomy. J Am Coll Surg 1994;178:229–33.
6. Davidoff AM, Pappas TN, Murray EA, et al. Mechanisms of major biliary injury during laparoscopic cholecystectomy. Ann Surg 1992;215:196–202.
7. Strasberg SM, Hertl M, Soper NJ. An analysis of the problem of biliary injury during laparoscopic cholecystectomy. J Am Coll Surg 1995;180:101–25.
8. Strasberg SM, Sanabria JR, Clavien PA. Complications of laparoscopic cholecystectomy. Can J Surg 1992;35:275–80.
9. Horgan S, Meireles OR, Jacobsen GR, et al. Broad clinical utilization of NOTES: is it safe? Surg Endosc 2013;27:1872–80.
10. Rawlings A, Hodgett SE, Matthews BD, et al. Single-incision laparoscopic cholecystectomy: initial experience with critical view of safety dissection and routine intraoperative cholangiography. J Am Coll Surg 2010;211:1–7.
11. Marks JM, Phillips MS, Tacchino R, et al. Single-incision laparoscopic cholecystectomy is associated with improved cosmesis scoring at the cost of significantly higher hernia rates: 1-year results of a prospective randomized, multicenter, single-blinded trial of traditional multiport laparoscopic cholecystectomy vs single-incision laparoscopic cholecystectomy. J Am Coll Surg 2013;216: 1037–47 [discussion: 47–8].
12. Schwaitzberg SD, Roberts K, Romanelli JR, et al. The NOVEL trial: natural orifice versus laparoscopic cholecystectomy—a prospective, randomized evaluation. Surg Endosc 2018;32:2505–16.
13. Han C, Shan X, Yao L, et al. Robotic-assisted versus laparoscopic cholecystectomy for benign gallbladder diseases: a systematic review and meta-analysis. Surg Endosc 2018;32(11):4377–92.
14. Strosberg DS, Nguyen MC, Muscarella P 2nd, et al. A retrospective comparison of robotic cholecystectomy versus laparoscopic cholecystectomy: operative outcomes and cost analysis. Surg Endosc 2017;31:1436–41.
15. Herron DM, Marohn M. A consensus document on robotic surgery 2007. Available at: http://www.sages.org/publications/guidelines/consensus-document-robotic-surgery/. Accessed December 31, 2018.
16. Ferreres AR, Asbun HJ. Technical aspects of cholecystectomy. Surg Clin North Am 2014;94:427–54.
17. Haueter R, Schutz T, Raptis DA, et al. Meta-analysis of single-port versus conventional laparoscopic cholecystectomy comparing body image and cosmesis. Br J Surg 2017;104:1141–59.
18. Strasberg SM, Brunt LM. Rationale and use of the critical view of safety in laparoscopic cholecystectomy. J Am Coll Surg 2010;211:132–8.
19. Wakabayashi G, Iwashita Y, Hibi T, et al. Tokyo Guidelines 2018: surgical management of acute cholecystitis: safe steps in laparoscopic cholecystectomy for acute cholecystitis (with videos). J Hepatobiliary Pancreat Sci 2018;25:73–86.
20. Strasberg SM, Pucci MJ, Brunt LM, et al. Subtotal cholecystectomy-"fenestrating" vs "reconstituting" subtypes and the prevention of bile duct injury: definition of the optimal procedure in difficult operative conditions. J Am Coll Surg 2016;222: 89–96.

21. van Dijk AH, Donkervoort SC, Lameris W, et al. Short- and long-term outcomes after a reconstituting and fenestrating subtotal cholecystectomy. J Am Coll Surg 2017;225:371–9.
22. Ford JA, Soop M, Du J, et al. Systematic review of intraoperative cholangiography in cholecystectomy. Br J Surg 2012;99:160–7.
23. Verbesey JE, Birkett DH. Common bile duct exploration for choledocholithiasis. Surg Clin North Am 2008;88:1315–28, ix.
24. Winslow ER, Fialkowski EA, Linehan DC, et al. "Sideways": results of repair of biliary injuries using a policy of side-to-side hepatico-jejunostomy. Ann Surg 2009;249:426–34.
25. Dunham R, Sackier JM. Is there a dilemma in adequately training surgeons in both open and laparoscopic biliary surgery? Surg Clin North Am 1994;74: 913–21 [discussion: 23–9].
26. Panni RZ, Strasberg SM. Preoperative predictors of conversion as indicators of local inflammation in acute cholecystitis: strategies for future studies to develop quantitative predictors. J Hepatobiliary Pancreat Sci 2018;25:101–8.
27. Vidovszky TJ, Smith W, Ghosh J, et al. Robotic cholecystectomy: learning curve, advantages, and limitations. J Surg Res 2006;136:172–8.

Technical Aspects of Bile Duct Evaluation and Exploration: An Update

William Scott Helton, MD[a], Subhashini Ayloo, MD, MPH[b],*

KEYWORDS

- Common bile duct • Common bile duct exploration
- Technique of common bile duct exploration • Choledocholithiasis
- Robot-assisted common bile duct exploration • Lithotripsy • ERCP

KEY POINTS

- Choledocholithiasis is optimally addressed in a single setting at the time of cholecystectomy. Surgeons should be trained in laparoscopic common bile duct exploration and supported by a multidisciplinary team with technical resources.
- Bile duct evaluation involves review of preoperative imaging, visual inspection, palpation, intraoperative ultrasound, cholangiography, and choledochoscopy.
- Transcystic common bile duct exploration and stone clearance can be successfully in open or minimally invasive approach in most patients with small primary common bile duct stones.
- Patients with a dilated common bile duct, large or impacted stones, more than 5 stones, and primary/recurrent choledocholithiasis are best managed with minimally invasive choledochotomy.
- Primary closure of the common bile duct with endoluminal transpapillary or transcystic duct drainage is preferable to closure around a T-tube.
- Surgeons should be familiar with techniques to treat impacted common bile duct stones as well as ways to provide safe drainage of the common bile duct when stones cannot be removed in the operating room.

 Video content accompanies this article at http://www.surgical.theclinics.com.

INTRODUCTION: NATURE OF THE PROBLEM

The most common bile duct (CBD) diseases worldwide are choledocholithiasis (CD), cholangiocarcinoma, benign strictures, and biliary injury. Historically, these CBD

The authors have nothing to disclose.
[a] Virginia Mason Medical Center, Seattle, WA, USA; [b] Rutgers, New Jersey Medical School, 185 South Orange Avenue, MSB G586, Newark, NJ 07103, USA
* Corresponding author.
E-mail address: Ayloo.Sub@rutgers.edu

problems were managed primarily by general surgeons. However, advances in medical technology, imaging, interventional radiology, endoscopy, and minimally invasive surgery over the past 30 years have radically changed the evaluation and management of CBD diseases such that most conditions are now managed primarily by nonsurgical specialists. Particularly true for patients with CD, biliary strictures, and unresectable biliary duct (BD) cancer. However, the importance of general surgeon involvement in the multidisciplinary management of patients with BD diseases is very important given recent advances in surgical technologies, such as surgical robotics, which has increased a surgeon's ability to more safely and effectively operate on the CBD. General surgeons should be familiar with how to evaluate, prepare for, and carry out operations on the CBD. It is also important for surgeons to appreciate their role within a multidisciplinary setting for how to most safely and cost-effectively manage patients with BD pathologic condition. This article focuses on the technical aspects of surgical exploration of the CBD for CD.

Ten percent to 15% of patients with symptomatic cholelithiasis present with concurrent CD.[1] Cholecystectomy and intraoperative cholangiography (IOC) or intraoperative ultrasound (IOUS) are recommended as the first step in managing these patients so long as they are fit for surgery.[2] If CD is identified at operation, efforts to clear the BD are recommended during the same anesthetic. This single-stage approach to treat both cholelithiasis and CD is supported by internationally accepted consensus guidelines.[2–7] This recommendation is dependent upon surgeons' experience and competence to perform laparoscopic common bile duct exploration (LCBDE) and the presence of adequate hospital resources and technological support.[6,7] A 2-stage approach to managing cholelithiasis and CD by either preoperative/postoperative endoscopic retrograde cholangiography (ERC) and endoscopic sphincterotomy (ES) for CBD clearance, although equally effective to the single-stage approach, is more expensive, associated with longer hospital stay, and subjects patients to additional morbidity.[2,8,9]

Updates from the 2016 Guidelines on the Management of CBD Stones from the British Society of Gastroenterology[2] recommend the following

- Patients with suspected CD who have not been previously investigated should undergo ultrasound (US) and liver function tests (LFTs) followed by magnetic resonance cholangiopancreaticography (MRCP) or endoscopic ultrasound (EUS), unless patients proceed directly to cholecystectomy and IOC or IOUS. ERC should be reserved for patients in whom preceding assessment indicates a need for endoscopic therapy.
- Transcystic/transductal LCBDE is an appropriate technique for CD removal. There is no evidence of a difference in efficacy, mortality, or morbidity when LCBDE is compared with perioperative ERC, although LCBDE is associated with a shorter hospital stay and is more cost-effective.
- For difficult ductal stones, LCBDE and ERC (supplemented by endoscopic papillary biliary dilation with prior sphincterotomy, mechanical lithotripsy, or cholangioscopy where necessary) are highly successful in removing CD.
- Cholangioscopy-guided electrohydraulic lithotripsy (EHL)/laser lithotripsy (LL) is considered when other endoscopic treatment options fail to achieve duct clearance.
- Percutaneous radiological stone extraction and open CBD exploration should be reserved for patients in whom the above techniques fail or are not feasible.
- Patients with Roux-en-Y gastric bypass and CD should be referred to centers that are able to offer the advanced endoscopic/surgical treatment.

The above guidelines are specific to patients with primary CD and do not apply to patients with secondary or recurrent CD, or previous cholecystectomy. For these patients, choledochoduodenostomy or Roux-en-Y hepaticojejunostomy should be considered. For patients with recurrent CD, ERC with sphincterotomy can be considered. After that, any further recurrence strong consideration for a drainage procedure should be given, especially in the Asian population with higher incidence of recurrent CD.

SURGICAL TECHNIQUE
Preoperative Planning

Evaluation of suspected CBD disease starts preoperatively (**Fig. 1**). Surgeons should not operate on a patient without some knowledge of the clinical situation. Preoperative evaluation starts with a good history, examination, LFTs, and imaging to delineate biliary anatomy and other pathologic condition.

Consensus guidelines recommend US when CD is suspected followed by MRCP and/or EUS.[2] MRCP can demonstrate cystic duct anatomy and its variations, which provide a roadmap before surgical interventions.[10]

ERC should be considered preoperatively for patients with painless jaundice, suspected biliary strictures, recurrent stones, Mirizzi syndrome, resectable malignancy, patients with a hostile upper abdomen or significant inflammation of the porta hepatis, the presence of portal varices, and in those who are unfit for operation. Abdominal contrast computed tomography (CT) with intravenous (IV) contrast should be performed in patients with suspected malignant obstructive jaundice. In certain situations, preoperative cholangiography can be done indirectly via a previously placed cholecystostomy tube in patients with previous acute cholecystitis or via subhepatic drains placed in patients with biliary injury. In the latter situation, cholangiography is essential before operative repair of the BD injury.

Percutaneous transhepatic cholangiogram and percutaneous transhepatic biliary drainage (PTDB) are reserved for patients who are not candidates for or fail ERC.

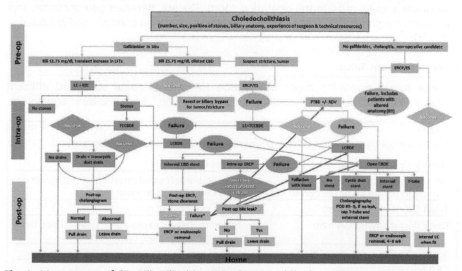

Fig. 1. Managment of CD. Bili, Bilirubin; CBD, Common bile duct; CBDE, Common bile duct exploration; ERCP, Endoscopic retrograde cholangiopancreatography; ES, Endoscopic sphincterotomy; IOC, Intraoperative cholangiogram; LC, Laparoscopic cholecystectomy; LCBDE, Laparoscopic common bile duct exploration; LFTs, Liver function test; PTBD, Percutaneous transhepatic biliary drainage; RDV, Rendezvous; RY, Roux-en-Y; TCCBDE, Transcystic common bile duct exploration.

The approach chosen by a surgeon to clear CD, whether preoperative, intraoperative, or postoperative, depends on the following: (1) past history of CD or prior biliary operations; (2) size, number, and location of stones; (3) size and anatomic course of the cystic duct; (4) size of CBD; (5) need for permanent biliary drainage procedure; (6) patient body habitus and ability to safely expose the CBD. Indications and contraindications for transcystic common bile duct exploration (TCCBDE) or direct common bile duct exploration (DCBDE) are listed in **Table 1**.

Preoperative Preparation for Common Bile Duct Exploration

Surgical team preparation is fundamental for safe, effective, and cost-efficient CBD clearance. Such preparation starts with the surgeon understanding the patient's BD pathologic condition and having a plan for unexpected or unusual findings.

In addition, the surgeon should be adequately trained in laparoscopic/open common bile duct exploration (CBDE) and ensure the availability of proper instruments/trained staff and hospital resources. When these basic elements are not met, surgeons should consider referring patients with common bile duct stones (CBDS) to specialized health facility and surgeons who are prepared and experienced to safely manage BD disease.

Preoperative antibiotic prophylaxis for gram-positive/-negative organisms should be administered to patients with suspected CD. Placement of a nasal or orogastric tube for decompression of stomach and a Foley catheter should be considered if the operation is expected to take more than 3 hours.

There is a wealth of resources to learn the skill set and knowledge to perform CBDE. These resources include posted videos on YouTube, professional society websites (American College of Surgeons/Clinical Robotic Surgery Association/Society of American Gastrointestinal and Endoscopic Surgeons), Webinars, and courses.[11–14] Simulation training facilities and models offer surgeons the opportunity to observe, learn, and practice skills outside the operating room. Recent literature demonstrates that simulation training in CBDE improves competency, surgeon comfort, and confidence in LCBDE.

Operating Room Setup

A large hybrid operating room with space to accommodate easy and efficient portable fluoroscopy, robot docking and undocking, and ancillary equipment,

Table 1
Indications for transcystic and direct approaches to common bile duct exploration

Transcystic CBDE	Direct CBDE
Nontortuous cystic duct: right-sided midinsertion of cystic duct on to CBD	Low and/or left-sided insertion of cystic duct on to CBD (intrapancreatic)
Small CBD stones (<10 mm)	Large stones (>10 mm)
Cystic duct diameter (>4 mm)	Failed transcystic exploration: small caliber, thin, or unable to dilate cystic duct
Stones distal to cystic duct/CBD junction	Stones proximal to cystic duct/CBD junction
CBD (<8 mm)	Dilated CBD (>8 mm)
Number of CBD stones (<5)	Multiple stones (>5) Recurrent stones Previous cholecystectomy Surgeon experience Available resources at the health care facility

IOUS/LL provides the safest, most efficient setting for managing CBDS with modern minimally invasive technologies. The surgeon and support staff should be familiar with equipment to perform CBDE and practice in a simulated environment. Such preparation promotes efficiency and success and reduces staff tension and complications. Nursing staff and surgical technician and biomedical engineering personnel should be available and competent to set up and troubleshoot all equipment used for CBDE.

The surgeon and scrub technician are best positioned to stand on the patient's left, and the fluoroscopy unit should come in from the patient's right. The surgeon and assistant should wear radiation-protective gowns instead of standing behind a shield, which impedes ergonomics for carrying out catheter exchanges and manipulation of the duct with laparoscopic instruments under real-time fluoroscopy.

Special Equipment/Tools/Staff Needed for Common Bile Duct Exploration

There are several commercial kits with all components to facilitate LCBDE.[15] Alternatively, the essential pieces of equipment necessary to perform LCBDE can be assembled individually from several companies. It is recommended that all equipment needed to perform CBDE should be stored in a common area or in a portable cart to facilitate efficiency.

- Sliding operating room table to facilitate fluoroscopy
- Flexible digital video choledochoscope/ureteroscope: <3 mm outer diameter, 1.2-mm working channel, ideally with 270° deflection of the distal tip, 90° angle of view, 50 cm length
- Silicone-padded laparoscopic grasping forceps for guiding choledochoscope[16]
- Two videoscopic cameras and light sources, a second monitor aligned next to the laparoscopic monitor or video switcher for split screen capability or picture in picture setup to simultaneously visualize laparoscopic and fluoroscopic and choledochoscopic views on the same screen
- Fogarty vascular embolectomy catheters (3, 4, 5 French) for LCBDE
- Biliary Fogarty 4 French for open CBDE
- Portable fluoroscopy unit
- Wearable protective radiation jacket
- Wire access: 125 cm long, 0.031/0.035-in diameter floppy-tipped hydrophilic coated guidewire
- Long 5-French pediatric feeding tubes/5 French ureteral catheter for cystic duct drain
- High-pressure pneumatic dilator, catheter with radiopaque markers for visualization of distal/proximal balloon ends, catheter 5 French/1.67 mm diameter, inflated 6 mm diameter, balloon/overall length 4/75 cm, respectively
- High-pressure LeVeen inflator 10-cc syringe with pressure gauge inflation
- Segura type retrieval baskets: 4-wire, flat, 2.4 French/0.8 mm diameter. Open basket 15 mm diameter, length 100 cm
- Stone forceps
- Laparoscopic microknife, straight, distendable, size 5 mm, length 31 cm, or Berci microknife, pointed, distendable, size 5 mm, length 31 cm[16]
- Mechanical lithotripter
- Holmium LL or EHL[17,18]
- 7 and 10 French, 5-cm endobiliary stents
- Laparoscopic needle drivers

- T-tube (sizes 12–18 French)[19–23]
- 14-gauge IV catheter for introduction of balloon catheters/baskets
- Absorbable clips

In addition, equipment and tools specific for robot-assisted CBDE include the following:

- Robotic graspers
- Vascular Fogarty (secondary to limitation of length with biliary Fogarty)
- Irrigation catheter and cannula
- Indocyanine green (ICG)
- Laparoscopic endobag

Patient Positioning

Open approach

- The patient is positioned supine ideally with both arms tucked to the sides to clear the side bars of the operating table for placement of retractors.
- If one arm needs to be adducted, tuck the right arm so that the portable fluoroscopic unit can easily access the patient. With modern sliding operating tables, it is no longer a challenge because these operating tables can slide cranially or caudally as required. The operating table should be able to rotate side to side and go into steep reverse Trendelenburg to facilitate exposure. A gel pad is put underneath the patient, a safety strap is put across the hips, and a foot board is used to prevent sliding while in steep reverse Trendelenburg.

Minimally invasive (laparoscopic/robotic) approach

- Supine or split leg position with all the pressure points well padded and with both arms tucked to the sides. The patient's final position would be reverse Trendelenburg with the robot docked cranially (Video 1). A liver retractor for laparoscopic or the third arm of the robot is used to retract the liver cranially with countertraction from gravity to retract the stomach/colon caudally, exposing the liver hilum.

SURGICAL APPROACH

The approach chosen by a surgeon to clear CD, whether TCCBDE or LCBDE, will depend on several factors, listed in **Table 1**. Relative contraindications to choledochotomy are (1) a hostile abdomen from previous surgery, radiation, severe acute inflammation; (2) the presence of portal varices; (3) intolerance to major upper abdominal surgery; (4) surgeon inexperience; and (5) small CBD (<8 mm). In these circumstances, endoscopic extraction should be considered first line.

SURGICAL PROCEDURE
Intraoperative Evaluation

All operations on the CBD begin with a thorough evaluation of the upper abdomen with a focus on the porta hepatis. Such evaluation should always involve inspection, palpation, IOUS, and cholangiography.

Inspection

The extrahepatic bile duct is readily identified in most patients as it courses up toward the hilar plate. Sometimes segment IV of the liver needs to be lifted upward and the duodenum retracted caudally in order to view its entire length (**Fig. 2**). Often the

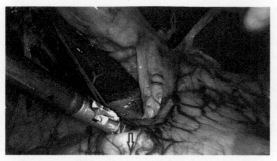

Fig. 2. Technique to expose CBD. The liver is retracted anteriorly by the gallbladder, and the duodenum is retracted inferiorly to straighten out the CBD and bring it anteriorly.

CBD is not seen because of significant inflammation in the porta hepatis and visceral fat. When the CBD cannot be identified visually, the surgeon needs to identify its depth, size, and course by other means, such as palpation, IOUS, fluoroscopic cholangiography, and/or near-infrared fluorescence imaging with ICG.

Palpation

Palpation of the porta hepatis is best done when the surgeon is on the patient's left side, placing their left index figure through the foramen of Winslow, and then pinching with their thumb, palpating up and down the CBD for masses and stones. The surgeon should get a general sense of whether there is inflammation and induration of the CBD. Bimanual palpation is valuable to identify the hepatic artery as it courses up toward the liver and to identify any accessory or replaced right hepatic artery, which typically runs posterior lateral at the 7 o'clock position to the CBD (**Fig. 3**).

Intraoperative Ultrasound

IOUS is a valuable tool for assessing size, course, and pathologic condition of the CBD when it cannot be visually seen or palpated. In skilled hands, IOUS is as good as cholangiography to detect CD. However, it is not easy to identify the course of the cystic duct from the gallbladder to the CBD. When the cystic duct cannot be identified because of inflammation or when it is surgically absent, IOUS can be used to guide needle placement for cholangiography (**Fig. 4**).

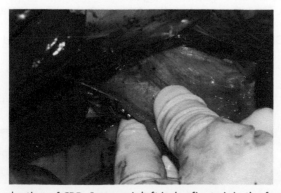

Fig. 3. Bimanual palpation of CBD. Surgeon's left index finger is in the foramen of Winslow, and thumb is on the CBD. Cystic duct stump ligated and clipped.

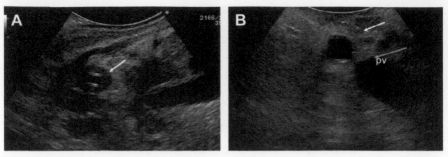

Fig. 4. Intraoperative US-guided identification of the CBD in patients with inflamed porta hepatis. (*A*) Thickened CBD wall with endoluminal plastic stent (*B*) IOUS shows thickened CBD wall in patients with cholangiocarcinoma. White arrow, thickened CBD; Blue arrow, loss of plan between CBD and portal vein (pv).

Cholangiography

It is imperative to perform cholangiography before opening the CBD to identify the anatomy and any biliary anomalies. Introduction of contrast media into the biliary system is usually achieved by cannulation of the cystic duct or directly into the gallbladder when the cystic duct is not able to be safely dissected. When this is not possible, direct injection with a 21- to 25-gauge needle into the CBD is considered (**Fig. 5**).

The point of insertion of the cystic duct into the common hepatic duct is highly variable. Most commonly it enters the common hepatic duct from the right lateral aspect about halfway between the hepatic confluence and ampulla of Vater. Important variations of cystic duct drainage that preclude TCDBDE are (1) low insertion of cystic duct, (2) parallel course of cystic duct with common hepatic duct, (3) anterior or posterior spiral course with medial insertion, (4) drainage of cystic duct to right or left hepatic duct, (5) aberrant or accessory intrahepatic ducts draining into cystic duct[24] (**Fig. 6**).

Near-Infrared Fluorescence Imaging

Adjunct imaging can be obtained by IV injection of 2.5 mg Indocyanine green about 45 minutes before the operation and visualized using near infrared systems such as the da Vinci Firefly system. Indocyanin green injection would show both the ductal and the vascular structures in the liver hilum and porta hepatis.[25]

Fig. 1 illustrates the various options surgeons can/should consider when managing patients with CD. The subsequent section addresses the different steps outlined with the algorithm.

If IOC shows CD (<3-mm stones, CBD diameter <4 mm), proceed to step 1.

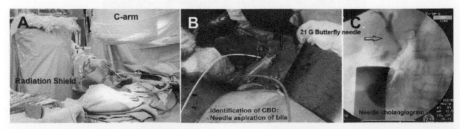

Fig. 5. Intraoperative cholangiogram. (*A*) Setup, (*B*) needle cholangiography of CBD, (*C*) fluoroscopic image of cholangiogram.

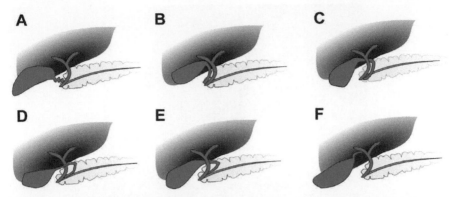

Fig. 6. Variations in the cystic duct precluding transcystic CBD exploration. (*A*) Insertion of cystic duct; (*B, C*) parallel cystic duct; (*D, E*) low left-sided insertions of cystic duct; (*F*) hepatic duct insertion of cystic duct.

Step 1: relaxing the sphincter of Oddi

1. IV glucagon (1 mg)
2. Flush CBD with warm saline and contrast under fluoroscopy. The authors suggest avoiding lidocaine injection of CBD because it could be hepatotoxic. If unable to clear stones, the surgeon evaluates length, tortuosity, and insertion of cystic duct into CBD and its size to determine candidacy for TCCBDE. If appropriate, proceed to step 2.
   a. If TCCBDE is not feasible, the surgeon proceeds to step 3a/b, 4 and considers draining the CBD via the cystic duct and postoperative ERC if necessary.

Step 2: transcystic common bile duct exploration[4,26]

1. A 5-mm trocar in the right lateral anterior axillary line allows parallel insertion of catheters, balloons, and biliary endoscope into the cystic duct.
2. For a normal size cystic duct, consider a second incision about a 1 cm from cystic duct junction with CBD to avoid traversing cystic duct valves.
3. A floppy-tipped 0.035-in guidewire is advanced via cystic duct into the duodenum under fluoroscopy.
4. A balloon dilating catheter is advanced over the guidewire into the CBD with the balloon positioned at the entrance of the cystic duct. A LeVeen syringe with pressure gauge is used to inflate the balloon for 5 minutes at 12 atm of pressure not to exceed 6 mm. Avoid damage if the ducts are thin and/or friable.
5. Choledochoscope/ureteroscope is passed into the CBD. Warm saline is flushed through the working channel with a pressure bag.
6. The wire Segura basket is passed under direct visualization to capture the stones.
7. Alternatively, a vascular Fogarty balloon catheter (4 and 5 French) is passed through the cystic duct under fluoroscopy to pull out stones. Care must be taken to avoid pulling the stone proximal to the cystic duct junction with mild compression on the hepatic duct with a grasper.
8. Small stones can be flushed distally into the duodenum or pushed with the scope beyond the ampulla (Videos 2 and 3).
9. A completion cholangiogram is performed.
10. If stones are unable to be dislodged or removed, consider EHL/LL[27] (**Fig. 7**) (Video 4).

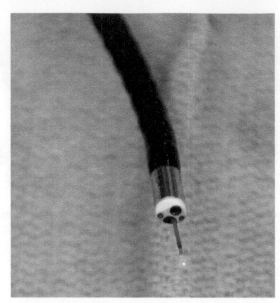

Fig. 7. Lithotripsy. A 2.8-mm choledochoscope with laser fiber for Holmium Yag laser.

11. Less preferable, when stones are not able to be flushed distally, gentle dilation of the ampulla to 3 or 4 mm over 3 minutes with the balloon catheter can be done. However, this maneuver can lead to pancreatitis and should be done only in rare circumstances.[28]

12. If completion cholangiography shows no residual stones, ligate the cystic duct with an endoloop and/or double clips to avoid bile leak from dilated cystic duct.

13. In an uncomplicated TCCBDE, with no significant edema or low probability of recurrent stones, primary closure without drainage is acceptable.

14. If unable to clear CBDS or edema/stricture of the distal duct, proceed to steps 3 and/or 4. Alternatively, if the choice is to clear the CBDS postoperatively, then provide external/internal drainage of the CBD, as discussed later (**Fig. 8**). This will allow decompression of the duct/prevent cholangitis/recurrent obstruction until the patient can undergo ERC.[29]

   a. TCCBDE[30] is preferred because it is quick and easy, provides decompression, and ensures postoperative access for subsequent imaging/intervention. If ERC stone extraction is required, the insertion of a guidewire through the transcystic ductal drain (TCDD) into the duodenum will provide a guaranteed access for ES and negates the need to perform endoscopy to remove an internal stent. TCDD can be done with a 5-French uretero catheter or a 5-French pediatric feeding tube with its tip cut off. The catheters are introduced into the abdomen through a peel-away introducer in the right costal position, advanced via the cystic duct into the CBD lumen 2 to 4 cm, secured to the cystic duct by a 12 mm absorbable Lapro-Clip[31] or 2 separate O-gauge chromic ties spaced a few mm apart while irrigating with saline to prevent overtightening and occlusion of the catheter. A loose loop of the catheter is left inside the abdomen before exiting on the right subcostal area, where it is secured to the skin with nylon sutures. A completion cholangiogram is performed to confirm the correct position of the catheter and to ensure free flow of contrast into the

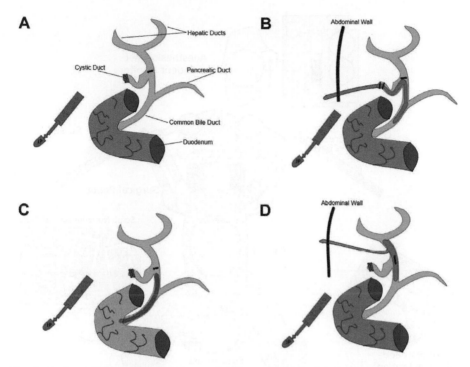

Fig. 8. Drainage options in the set-up of CBD exploration. (*A*) No drainage; (*B*) internal/external stent via cystic duct; (*C*) internal stent via cystic duct or choledochotomy; (*D*) T-tube. JP, Jackson-Pratt drain.

duodenal lumen. The catheters are left to dependent drainage into a bag (see management of catheters in the postoperative section).

  b. Deployment of a laparoscopic endobiliary 7- to 10-French stent across the ampulla.[29,32–35]

Step 3a: minimally invasive robotic common bile duct exploration

1. If considering a minimally invasive approach for CBDE, the positions of the trocars are of paramount importance.
2. Contrary to standard laparoscopy, the robotic platform offers a leeway in placement of the trocars secondary to higher degrees of freedom associated with the instruments.
3. The patient is positioned supine or in the split leg position, preferably with both arms tucked to the sides (**Fig. 9**).
4. A camera port is placed just right of the umbilicus; an 8-mm robotic trocar is placed at right lateral abdomen for surgeon's left arm, and an 8-mm robotic trocar is placed just left of umbilicus for the surgeon's right arm. An 8-mm robotic trocar is placed in the left lateral abdomen for the third arm of the robot. The ideal position for the first assistant port is between the camera port and the surgeon's left arm (Video 5).
5. A diagnostic laparoscopy is performed before docking the robot. The patient is positioned in reverse Trendelenburg to allow gravity to caudally retract the stomach and transverse the colon.

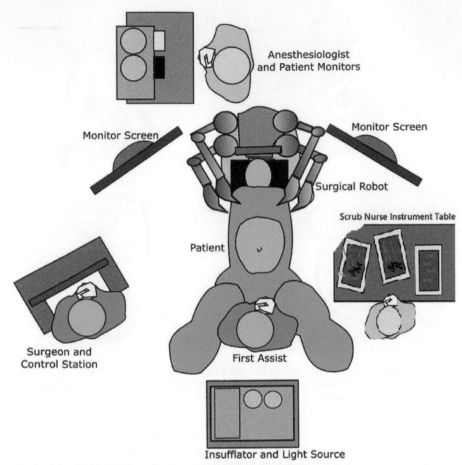

Fig. 9. Operating room setup for robot-assisted CBD exploration.

6. The robot is ideally docked cranially; another option would be to dock the robot from right shoulder of the patient.
7. The ideal position for the third arm of the robot is from the patient's left side of the abdomen.
8. If available, a Firefly camera is an asset in case ICG fluorescence is used to visualize the CBD and cystic duct.
9. A fenestrated bipolar grasper is used for the surgeons' left arm; a Cadiere grasper is used for the surgeon's right arm and in the third arm of the robot (Video 6).
10. If the procedure requires cholecystectomy, start with creating the critical view of safety first in the standard fashion. Leave the gallbladder fundus attached to the liver to provide retraction cranially using the third arm of the robot (Video 7).
11. Leave the distal cystic duct stump long and unclipped for passing a glide wire or to perform cholangiography. Address the cystic duct stump closure at the very end of the procedure because it could be used to drain the CBD postoperatively by leaving a percutaneous catheter through it.
12. Identification of CBD in addition to the above mentioned techniques involves following the cystic duct to its insertion on CBD. If available, use ICG

immunofluorescence to clarify CBD and cystic duct structures (Video 8) or direct aspiration of bile with a needle (Video 9).

13. Clear up the duct as safely as possible with minimal devascularization.

14. The advantage offered by the robotic camera involves magnified 3-dimensional (3D) stable vision, which can be switched from infrared vision to white light with ease. Furthermore, the proximity of the camera to the working field can be adjusted with ease to the extent that the camera can be used to visualize inside the duct far superiorly than with the laparoscopic camera.

15. Create a 1-cm vertical or transverse choledochotomy just above the duodenum (Video 10).

16. If necessary, place a stay suture and use the third arm to retract open the duct to facilitate exposure and CBDE (Video 11).

17. Use a Cadiere or a Prograf to probe the duct manually to pull out any obvious stones. Use the right arm instrument to milk the duct proximally or distally to dislodge any stones toward the choledochotomy.

18. Use a 4- to 5-French vascular Fogarty to pass distally and proximally until no more stones are extracted (Video 12).

19. Choledochoscopy is performed to visualize CBD up into liver and down to the papilla.

20. Undock the robot and partially move it cranially and bring in the fluoroscopic unit to perform cholangiogram.

21. If no more CBDS are identified and the contrast is seen freely entering the duodenum, proceed to close the choledochotomy.

22. If more CD are identified, repeat forceful irrigation. Use a long irrigating catheter that can be snaked into the intrahepatic duct and alternate with balloon sweep, and intraoperative basket retrieval.

23. Leave access to the CBD through cystic duct as discussed in step 3.

24. If no further stones are noted and completion cholangiogram is satisfactory, the authors prefer primary closure of the CBD without a T-tube or internal stent.

25. Alternatively, if there is worrisome downstream ductal inflammation, residual stone debris, pancreatitis, cholangitis, or ampullary disease, follow step 2, number 14a/b.

26. T-tube drainage should be considered the last resort for biliary drainage because it is associated with the highest morbidity, bile leak, and patient discomfort and must remain in place for 4 to 6 weeks before removal[19–23] (see placement of T-tube section).

Step 3b: laparoscopic common bile duct exploration

1. Although it is not always necessary, sometimes sharp and blunt dissection is necessary to clear fatty tissue on top of CBD above the duodenum for a distance of 2 cm. Bipolar cautery can be used to achieve hemostasis on small vessels running on top of the CBD.

2. Lift gallbladder and/or falciform superiorly to bring CBD anteriorly into view. Depress the first part of duodenum caudally, which will straighten the CBD.

3. When the CBD surface and edges are not clearly visualized because of severe inflammation or portal fat, consider IOUS to locate the 12 o'clock position on the duct before incision.

4. Alternatively, consider needle aspiration of the duct at the presumed 12 o'clock position. Leave needle in position as a guide for choledochotomy.

5. Distend the CBD with warm saline flushing via a cystic duct catheter.

6. Use a 5-mm laparoscopic BD knife, scissors, or needle point cautery (when inflamed and thickened) to open CBD.
7. A transverse supraduodenal incision between marginal vessels at 3 and 9 o'clock is acceptable/safe when the duct is greater than 1.5 cm (Video 13), but care must be taken not to injure either marginal vessel.[36]
8. For CBD less than 1.5 cm, consider vertical ductotomy 1 cm above the duodenum.
9. The ductotomy length is initially kept to less than 1 cm long, or to the diameter of the largest stone.
10. Stay sutures are not usually required but considered in thickened CBD at 3 to 9 o'clock; retract them via a suture passer through the abdominal wall.
11. Forceful irrigation with suction irrigator/catheter into duct in combination with gentle kneading with smooth graspers from both sides and behind usually dislodges large stones.
12. Balloon catheter extraction is followed by wire basket (extraction), blindly or preferably with fluoroscopic or choledochoscopic guidance (Video 14). If flexible choledochoscopy is not available and CBD is large, a rigid ureteroscope can be used from umbilical and subxiphoid ports.[37]
13. For impacted stones not able to be removed with the techniques discussed above, consider a small hand port to facilitate stone clearance by squeezing with thumb and forefinger and/or using open instruments through a 12-mm subxiphoid port before larger laparotomy, as discussed in step 4.

Step 4: open common bile duct exploration

1. Right subcostal incision with vertical midline extension provides the best exposure.
2. Self-retaining retractors provide optimal porta hepatis exposure.
3. Divide the falciform ligament. Laparotomy pads are placed above the liver to displace it caudally.
4. Retract segment IV cephalad, retract duodenum/antrum caudally.
5. Consider radiopaque retractors that do not need to be removed during cholangiography.
6. Visually inspect.
7. Bimanual palpation of porta to identify hepatic arteries/CBD.
8. IOUS to define duct pathologic condition and location.
9. Cystic duct cannulation/cholangiography.
10. If unable to use cystic duct, use needle aspiration to identify duct location (**Fig. 10**).
11. Consider pediatric needle cholangiogram before ductotomy.
12. Placement of anterior wall sutures to lift CBD or saline distension via cystic duct while performing choledochotomy with knife, fine scissors, or needle point cautery (**Fig. 11**).
13. Flush forcefully up and downstream with pediatric feeding catheter or 12-French red rubber or irrigator.
14. Pass balloon Fogarty proximally and distally.
15. Perform choledochoscopy.
16. Extract stones under direct vision.
17. Perform completion cholangiography.
18. If there are retained calculi and/or obstruction or high risk for obstruction, then drain CBD directly or indirectly as discussed in step 2, number 14a/b, T-tube or perform intraoperative rendezvous ERC.[38,39]

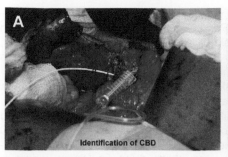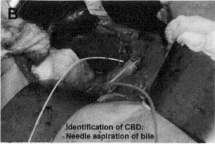

Identification of CBD

Identification of CBD:
Needle aspiration of bile

Fig. 10. Needle identification of CBD exploration. (*A*) Needle placement into BD; (*B*) aspiration of bile.

DRAINAGE AND CLOSURE OF THE COMMON BILE DUCT

Primary closure of the CBD without ductal drainage is considered safe so long as the following criteria are met:

- No cholangitis
- No pancreatitis
- No significant edema or inflammation of the ampulla
- No residual CBD debris or calculi
- The CBD is not flaccidly dilated
- The quality of the CBD tissues is good

When these criteria are not met, it is wise to drain the CBD with one of the approaches illustrated in **Fig. 8.**

Abdominal Drainage

The authors think a closed suction drain should be placed in the subhepatic space in all patients undergoing choledochotomy, regardless of the pathologic condition and integrity of the duct closure in order to provide site control for any postoperative bile leak that might occur. Uncomplicated patients who undergo successful TCCBD do not require closed suction drain.

Technique of Common Bile Duct Closure

1. Primary closure is preferred with a TCDD; or endoluminal transpapillary drain as discussed under step 2. TCDD is placed before CBD closure, and saline irrigation

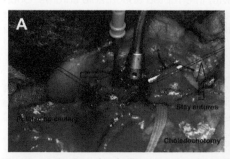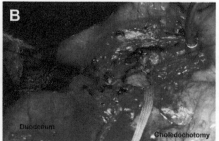

Stay sutures

Cautery

Choledochotomy

Duodenum

Choledochotomy

Fig. 11. Technique for fashioning the choledochotomy. (*A*) Stay sutures at 3 and 9 o'clock positions; (*B*) needle tip cautery and bullet tip suction used to create a controlled choledochotomy.

is done through it during closure of the choledochotomy to provide some distension and keep the surgical field clear. Primary closure of the choledochotomy in this manner without a T-tube greatly simplifies closure of the choledochotomy, because there is no tube just deep to the suture line. Hence, the technique is quicker and more precise (Videos 15 and 16).

2. Absorbable suture: 4-0 or 5-0, RB-1 or ski tip needle. Interrupted or running suture. Technique is left to the surgeon's discretion (Video 17).

3. There are techniques to overcome the difficulty of laparoscopic extracorporeal and intracorporeal knot tying in a tight space underneath the liver. A continuous 3-0 PDS II suture on a straight atraumatic needle suture can be used with an absorbable clip on the end that precludes the need to tie the first knot. Upon completing the suture closure, a second absorbable clip is placed followed by a metal clip to hold the suture taught against the BD.[40]

4. V-lock suture 180 (Covidien, Mansfield, MA, USA) is another good option for the laparoscopic approach because it also does not require intracorporeal knot tying. The barbed thread, which is another characteristic feature of the V-lock suture, may help to prevent loosening of the suture without the need for keeping continuous traction on the thread (which is usually performed by the assistant). As a result, the surgeon can suture laparoscopically without the assistant's help or the need for additional instrument in the field.

5. The authors have found that the surgical robot, because of its higher ergonomics, and 3D visualization greatly facilitate precise closure of choledochotomy, particularly when it is less than 1 cm in length and thin walled.

6. Completion cholangiogram is done via TCDD/T-tube under fluoroscopy.

Fashioning/Placement of a T-Tube

The T-tube is fashioned before being inserted into the abdomen (Video 18). It is then brought into the abdomen with a 5-mm grasper from the right lower abdomen trocar up through the 10-/12-mm epigastric trocar, grasping the 2 limbs of the horizontal limbs of the T-tube and then pulling the entire T-tube into the abdomen. An additional 5-mm trocar is inserted in the right upper quadrant in a position that allows the T-tube to be exteriorized in a straight line. It is important to reduce the pneumoperitoneum before choosing the exit site to avoid distortion of the catheter as it exits the abdominal wall relative to the costal margin. Once the trocar is inserted, full pneumoperitoneum can be again reestablished. A grasper is inserted via the right upper quadrant to grasp the long limb of the T-tube and then pull it through the anterior abdominal wall along with the trocar. The T-tube limbs are then inserted into the choledochotomy, using 2 fine graspers. The CBD is sutured closed with interrupted absorbable sutures. Cholangiography is performed via the T-tube to assess for any leaks. Should leakage occur around the T-tube, sutures should be removed and then replaced so as to afford a watertight closure (Video 19).

Rendezvous Laparoendoscopic Approach

If cholangiography demonstrates CD that are not able to be flushed out, a guidewire is passed via the cystic duct across the papilla, which serves as a safety guide for the endoscopists to cannulate the CBD, reducing the failure rate and post-ERC complications.[38,39]

Large Impacted Stones

Extraction of impacted stones can be facilitated with bimanual compression of the duct through a choledochotomy or forceful irrigation with saline (Video 20). If unsuccessful, consider biliary Fogarty catheter (4–5 French) or a Dormia basket under fluoroscopy or under direct vision with a choledochoscope,[41] through the cystic duct or more easily through the choledochotomy. The use of choledochoscopy significantly reduces the incidence of residual stones.[42] Choledochotomy also enables the use of larger and stronger mechanical lithotripters, or even stone forceps that are used in open CBDE placed through a laparoscopic 12-mm subxiphoid trocar.

In cases of large incarcerated CD, stone extraction can be difficult and unsuccessful. In these cases, consider fragmenting the stone first. Stone fragmentation can be performed mechanically with a stone fragmentation basket, EHL, or LL.[17,18,27]

Conversely, if the patient has already failed endoscopic attempts at fragmentation and is being referred for operative clearance, consider extracorporeal shock wave lithotripsy before operative CBDE. Extracorporeal shock wave lithotripsy before operative CBDE should only be undertaken with the presence of an endobiliary stent or PTDB in place. Operative CBDE can be performed electively any time thereafter so long as the CBD is decompressed. When operating on these patients, the surgeon needs to be prepared to use any one of the above technologies to attempt stone clearance. In addition, if the surgeon is not sufficiently experienced in lithotripsy, it is strongly recommended that they consult with and perhaps invite an experienced urologist or interventional endoscopist to assist them in the operating room.

LL (Holmium-Yag), although more expensive, is extremely easy to use and is safe and effective at fragmenting stones of any composition.[17,18,27] Stone fragments are removed with flushing, forceps, balloon catheters, and wire baskets as needed.

If a distally impacted stone cannot be dislodged or fractured, it is imperative to provide CBD drainage either by passing an endoscopic stent across the obstructing stone or to provide proximal decompression of the CBD by any of the methods[35] shown in **Fig. 8.**

Alternatively, the CBD could be decompressed by placement of a PTBD, either intraoperatively or postoperatively. Decompression of the duct proximally combined with friction between the stone and the PTDB catheter or endobiliary stent usually results in some shrinkage of the stone and resolution of edema over time. After a few weeks, repeat ERC is almost always successful at clearing the obstructing stone. Following this strategy avoids the extraordinarily rare need to perform transduodenal sphincteroplasty to relieve an impacted CD at the level of the ampulla.

Treatment of Hepatolithiasis

Many patients with CD also have primary or secondary hepatolithiasis, which may also be accompanied by intrahepatic/extrahepatic biliary strictures. Comprehensive management of these patients is beyond the scope of the current article. Briefly, such patients are managed with multiple ERC, PTBD, or wide drainage via biliary-enteric anastomosis. It is the authors' opinion that hepaticoduodenostomy is the best approach to manage these patients because a duodenal-biliary anastomosis provides easy repeated endoscopic access to the proximal biliary tree.[43]

Reoperative Biliary Surgery for Biliary Strictures

The workup and management of recurrent CBD strictures from recurrent hepatolithiasis or previous BD surgery are quite different from a de novo situation and will depend on the underlying condition and past treatments. Biliary strictures after previous CBDE are almost always successfully managed with endoscopic stenting. Should that fail and the patient develops problems of recurrent abdominal pain, cholangitis, or jaundice, operative repair is desirable with either a Roux-en-Y hepaticojejunostomy or choledochoduodenostomy or hepaticoduodenostomy.[43] This recommendation presumes that the patient is fit and willing to undergo operation (Videos 21–23).

For patients who are unfit or unwilling to undergo surgery and who have failed endoscopic stenting, PTDB with internal drainage can be performed.

POSTOPERATIVE MANAGEMENT AND FOLLOW-UP CARE
Immediate Postoperative Care

The usual practice of the authors in an uncomplicated CBDE without significant medical comorbidities is to manage the patient on a regular hospital floor after their recovery in the postanesthesia care unit. The nasal or orogastric tube is removed at the time of extubation. The Foley catheter is left in place to monitor the urine output overnight, and if satisfactory, removed as early as possible. There are no dietary or ambulation restrictions. On postoperative day 1 and 2, LFTs are obtained to be assured they are normalizing. Patients do not require antibiotics unless there is evidence of a bile leak, which is suspected to be contaminated in the setting of CD or the patient had cholangitis. Abdominal drains are put to gravity, not suction, and monitored daily for any evidence of bile. In patients who have no external TCDD or T-tube, if LFTs are normal and there is no evidence of bile in the drain, it is removed on postoperative day 2. The patient is sent home as soon as they meet discharge criteria with a follow-up in clinic within 7 days. Conversely, in any patient with a drain that shows evidence of bile leakage, the drain remains in place until the biliary system is interrogated by either a cholangiogram or a hepatobiliary iminodiacetic acid (HIDA) scan or until the drain turns clear and LFTs normalize.

TCDD and T-tubes are left to gravity drainage for the first 2 postoperative days. Cholangiography is performed on postoperative day 2. If LFTs are normal, there is good passage of contrast into the ampulla with gravity cholangiogram, and there is no leak or bile duct stricture, the T-tube and TCDD are clamped and the abdominal drains are removed. Contrast is instilled into a syringe connected to the T-tube held no higher than 20 cm above the abdominal wall as a means to avoid causing postcholangiogram febrile reactions and cholangitis and postprocedure chills.[44]

Conversely, if LFTs do not decline postoperatively, then there is the possibility of a biliary leak, hemobilia, and/or bile duct blockage from remnant stone debris, CBD or ampullary edema, or stenosis at the site of choledochotomy closure. Abdominal drains should remain in place, and cholangiography is performed if the patient has an external biliary tube. If no external biliary drainage was placed, a HIDA scan should be considered to rule out biliary obstruction and/or leakage. An HIDA scan is a better option than ERC while trying to evaluate for bile leak due to ERC-associated pancreatitis and cost.

If no external/internal duct drainage was established intraoperatively, and there is evidence of postoperative bile leak by bile in the drain, as long as the patient is clinically stable and has no signs of bile peritonitis/fluid collection by US/CT, there is no need to perform an ERC on an emergent basis because the leak may subside over the course of a few days.

However, if the Jackson-Pratt drain shows a large amount of bile drainage (>100 cc/d) and persists for more than a few days, then ERC should be strongly considered because an endoscopically placed plastic or covered metal stent almost always controls the bile leak. If ERC is unsuccessful, unavailable, and/or not advisable for technical/patient-related reasons, then PTDB can be used to proximally divert bile and help control internal bile spillage.

Postoperative Cholangiography

Patients with T-tubes, TCDD, or PTDB should receive a postoperative cholangiogram before their removal. If no postoperative biliary tube decompression was established intraoperatively, then the patient should have normalized LFTs and no bilious output from abdominal drain before removal.

If any concern exists regarding patency of the CBD or an intra-abdominal bile leak might exist, obtain an HIDA scan.

If the HIDA scan is normal, it is safe to remove the abdominal drain.

If there are concerns for leak or biliary obstruction after HIDA, consider ERC or PTDB cholangiography.

If cholangiography shows no flow, leak, or stenosis, leave the BD decompressed via its external drain because sometimes obstruction/stenosis is due to suture line edema and resolves over time. Repeat cholangiography should be done in a week. If it still shows a problem, then strongly consider ERC with endoscopic stent and/or refer the patient to a specialized center. Most stenosis can be successfully treated endoscopically with stenting and will resolve over time. If there is a bile leak, endoscopic stenting with a covered stent can be useful. Leave the abdominal drain in place if any type of leak exists.

When to Pull a Percutaneous Transhepatic Biliary Drainage?

If the patient had a preoperative PTDB, it can be left in place at operation either proximal to or traversing the closure of the choledochotomy or biliary-enteric anastomosis. The PTBD will enable postoperative biliary drainage and cholangiography. It can be left in place until the surgeon is confident there is no biliary leak or stricture. The authors' practice is to clamp the PTBD catheter on postoperative day 2, if the postoperative cholangiogram looks satisfactory and LFTs are normal. If the patient remains on a stable clinical course with normal LFTs, an additional cholangiogram is done in 2 weeks' time in the interventional radiology suite. If the biliary tree is well healed and there are no strictures, the PTDB is pulled, and the patient is given a follow-up in 1 to 2 weeks.

When to Pull a Transcystic Duct Catheter?

If a TCDD was placed, and the original postoperative cholangiogram shows no problems, it should be clamped, left in place, and removed at a later date. Although these drains can usually be removed in the clinic as early as 4 days postoperatively,[31] they are more safely removed in the radiology suite under fluoroscopic control a couple of weeks postoperatively.[30] A final cholangiogram can be obtained at that time, to ensure there is no leak or biliary extravasation as the catheter is removed.

When to Pull a T-Tube?

T-tubes are clamped when there is no evidence of bile leak, recurrent stones, and good flow by cholangiography into the duodenum. Patients must be instructed how to protect and care for the tube and avoid dislodgment. In the absence of any clinical concern, a follow-up cholangiogram is performed 6 weeks postoperatively in the radiology suite. If normal, the tube is removed under fluoroscopic control to ensure there is no bile leak upon its removal. If a biliary stricture or recurrent stone is found on cholangiography, the T-tube is left in place to facilitate CBD clearance and endoscopic stenting if necessary.

REHABILITATION AND RECOVERY

- For LCBDE, the patient's recovery and discharge from hospital are short and usually on postoperative day 1 or 2 unless there are problems related to biliary leakage.
- In the absence of any drains, return to full activity should occur similar to any patient undergoing uncomplicated laparoscopic cholecystectomy.
- For patients with transabdominal drains of biliary catheters, return to full activity will depend on when they have their catheters removed. Patients with T-tubes have the most prolonged return to full activity and should not engage in strenuous activity for fear of dislodging the T-tube.[19–23]
- For open laparotomy, recovery is similar to any other major laparotomy and will depend on the absence of any complication, particularly wound infection and biliary leak.

CLINICAL RESULTS IN THE LITERATURE

- Mortality from CBDE when performed electively should be less than 1%.
- Laparoscopic TCCBDE is successful 80% of the time.[6,19,26,28,42]
- Laparoscopic choledochotomy is successful in more than 90% to 95% of patients.[3,19]
- Complication rates following the use of the T-tubes (16%) are substantially higher than primary CBD closure (4%).[19–23,45]
- Primary closure of CBD is associated with a shorter operative time and hospital stay.[46–48]
- The use of choledochoscopy significantly reduces the incidence of residual stones.[42]
- The laparoendoscopic rendezvous approach is associated with higher success rates (95.6% vs 80%), shorter hospital stay (4.3 vs 8 days), and lower cost (USD 3613.64 vs 4897.38), compared with the 2-stage procedure to clear CBDS.[38,39]
- Robotic surgery in CBD exploration is safe and feasible. The superior ergonomics with better visualization offers a stable platform for easier primary closure of the choledochotomy.[9,49–54]
- Transverse choledochotomy is as safe as vertical choledochotomy in an enlarged CBD.[31]
- The most frequent early complications after LCBDE are biliary leaks and deep space infections.
- The most worrisome late complications are biliary stricture resulting in obstructive jaundice, recurrent CBDS, and cholangitis. If not properly addressed, they can result in secondary biliary cirrhosis.[45,47,55]
- Randomized control trials show that successful clearance of CBDS with the one- and 2-stage approaches are comparable, although primary LCBDE is associated with shorter hospital stay and superior cost-effectiveness.[56,57]
- The European Association for Endoscopic Surgery recommends that TCCBDE be limited to stones that are smaller than the size of the cystic duct.[58]
- Choledochoscopic-assisted LL is safer/more effective than EHL.[17]

SUMMARY

General surgeons should be trained to perform and then practice LCBDE in a simulated environment to gain familiarity and efficiency with procedure-specific tools.

Prepare and anticipate the unexpected or worst case scenarios with a well-thought-out intraoperative plan and a backup plan for multiple difficult scenarios. Enlist the help of urologists, gastroenterologists, and/or interventional radiologists who are experienced in lithotripsy for impacted difficult stones. Surgeons should be familiar with techniques to treat impacted CBD stones as well as ways to provide safe drainage of the CBD when stones cannot be removed in the operating room.

ACKNOWLEDGMENTS

The authors thank Dr John Armstrong for assistance in the illustrations. Special acknowledgement for their contribution to Dr. Sergio Bustos, Mendoza, Argentina for video 13, 15 and 16; Dr. John B. Martinie, Carolinas Medical Center, Charlotte, NC for video 22; Dr. Thomas Biehl, Virginia Mason Medical Center, Seattle, WA & Dr. Rose Bart, University of Alabama, Birmingham, AL for video 23.

SUPPLEMENTARY DATA

Supplementary data related to this article can be found online at https://doi.org/10.1016/j.suc.2018.12.007.

REFERENCES

1. Verbesey JE, Birkett DH. Common bile duct exploration for choledocholithiasis. Surg Clin North Am 2008;88(6):1315–28, ix.
2. Williams E, Beckingham I, El Sayed G, et al. Updated guideline on the management of common bile duct stones (CBDS). Gut 2017;66(5):765–82.
3. Perissat J, Huibregtse K, Keane FB, et al. Management of bile duct stones in the era of laparoscopic cholecystectomy. Br J Surg 1994;81(6):799–810.
4. Phillips EH. Laparoscopic transcystic duct common blle duct exploration–outcome and costs. Surg Endosc 1995;9(11):1240–2.
5. Williams EJ, Green J, Beckingham I, et al. Guidelines on the management of common bile duct stones (CBDS). Gut 2008;57(7):1004–21.
6. Clinical application of laparoscopic biliary tract surgery. Avaialble at: https://www.sages.org/publications/guidelines/guidelines-for-the-clinical-application-of-laparoscopic-biliary-tract-surgery/. Accessed August 27, 2018.
7. Haggerty SRW, Santos B, Fanelli R, et al. Laparoscopic common bile duct exploration 2017. Avaialble at: www.SAGES.org. Accessed August 27, 2018.
8. Pan L, Chen M, Ji L, et al. The safety and efficacy of laparoscopic common bile duct exploration combined with cholecystectomy for the management of cholecysto-choledocholithiasis: an up-to-date meta-analysis. Ann Surg 2018; 268(2):247–53.
9. Almamar A, Alkhamesi NA, Davies WT, et al. Cost analysis of robot-assisted choledochotomy and common bile duct exploration as an option for complex choledocholithiasis. Surg Endosc 2018;32(3):1223–7.
10. Sarawagi R, Sundar S, Gupta SK, et al. Anatomical variations of cystic ducts in magnetic resonance cholangiopancreatography and clinical implications. Radiol Res Pract 2016;2016:3021484.
11. Sanchez A, Otano N, Rodriguez O, et al. Laparoscopic common bile duct exploration four-task training model: construct validity. JSLS 2012;16(1):10–5.
12. Sanchez A, Rodriguez O, Benitez G, et al. Development of a training model for laparoscopic common bile duct exploration. JSLS 2010;14(1):41–7.

13. Kemp Bohan PM, Connelly CR, Crawford J, et al. Early analysis of laparoscopic common bile duct exploration simulation. Am J Surg 2017;213(5):888–94.

14. Teitelbaum EN, Soper NJ, Santos BF, et al. A simulator-based resident curriculum for laparoscopic common bile duct exploration. Surgery 2014;156(4):880–7, 890-883.

15. Cook Medical. Avaialble at: https://www.cookmedical.com/data/IFU_PDF/C_T_FCC_REV4.PDF. Accessed July 5, 2018.

16. Storz K. Instruments for intraoperative video choledochoscopy. Avaialble at: exhibitors.globalcastmd.com/files/download/df132b9297ba557. Accessed August 27, 2018.

17. Varban O, Assimos D, Passman C, et al. Video. Laparoscopic common bile duct exploration and holmium laser lithotripsy: a novel approach to the management of common bile duct stones. Surg Endosc 2010;24(7):1759–64.

18. Petersson U, Johansen D, Montgomery A. Laparoscopic transcystic laser lithotripsy for common bile duct stone clearance. Surg Laparosc Endosc Percutan Tech 2015;25(1):33–6.

19. Martin IJ, Bailey IS, Rhodes M, et al. Towards T-tube free laparoscopic bile duct exploration: a methodologic evolution during 300 consecutive procedures. Ann Surg 1998;228(1):29–34.

20. Gurusamy KS, Koti R, Davidson BR. T-tube drainage versus primary closure after laparoscopic common bile duct exploration. Cochrane Database Syst Rev 2013;(6):CD005641.

21. Yin Z, Xu K, Sun J, et al. Is the end of the T-tube drainage era in laparoscopic choledochotomy for common bile duct stones is coming? A systematic review and meta-analysis. Ann Surg 2013;257(1):54–66.

22. Dong ZT, Wu GZ, Luo KL, et al. Primary closure after laparoscopic common bile duct exploration versus T-tube. J Surg Res 2014;189(2):249–54.

23. Podda M, Polignano FM, Luhmann A, et al. Systematic review with meta-analysis of studies comparing primary duct closure and T-tube drainage after laparoscopic common bile duct exploration for choledocholithiasis. Surg Endosc 2016;30(3):845–61.

24. Vezakis A, Davides D, Ammori BJ, et al. Intraoperative cholangiography during laparoscopic cholecystectomy. Surg Endosc 2000;14(12):1118–22.

25. Daskalaki D, Aguilera F, Patton K, et al. Fluorescence in robotic surgery. J Surg Oncol 2015;112(3):250–6.

26. Carroll BJ, Fallas MJ, Phillips EH. Laparoscopic transcystic choledochoscopy. Surg Endosc 1994;8(4):310–4.

27. Healy K, Chamsuddin A, Spivey J, et al. Percutaneous endoscopic holmium laser lithotripsy for management of complicated biliary calculi. JSLS 2009;13(2):184–9.

28. Carroll BJ, Phillips EH, Rosenthal R, et al. Update on transcystic exploration of the bile duct. Surg Laparosc Endosc 1996;6(6):453–8.

29. Gomez D, Cox MR. Laparoscopic transcystic stenting and postoperative ERCP for the management of common bile duct stones at laparoscopic cholecystectomy. Ann Surg 2018;267(5):e86–8.

30. Hensman C, Crosthwaite G, Cuschieri A. Transcystic biliary decompression after direct laparoscopic exploration of the common bile duct. Surg Endosc 1997; 11(11):1106–10.

31. Wei Q, Hu HJ, Cai XY, et al. Biliary drainage after laparoscopic choledochotomy. World J Gastroenterol 2004;10(21):3175–8.

32. Gersin KS, Fanelli RD. Laparoscopic endobiliary stenting as an adjunct to common bile duct exploration. Surg Endosc 1998;12(4):301–4.

33. DePaula AL, Hashiba K, Bafutto M, et al. Results of the routine use of a modified endoprosthesis to drain the common bile duct after laparoscopic choledochotomy. Surg Endosc 1998;12(7):933–5.
34. Fanelli stent set: a video resource. Avaialble at: https://www.cookmedical.com/surgery/fanelli-stent-set-a-video-resource/. Accessed July 5, 2018.
35. Rhodes M, Nathanson L, O'Rourke N, et al. Laparoscopic antegrade biliary stenting. Endoscopy 1995;27(9):676–8.
36. Lezoche E, Paganini AM, Carlei F, et al. Laparoscopic treatment of gallbladder and common bile duct stones: a prospective study. World J Surg 1996;20(5): 535–41 [discussion: 542].
37. Sardiwalla II, Koto MZ, Kumar N, et al. Laparoscopic common bile duct exploration use of a rigid ureteroscope: a single institute experience. J Laparoendosc Adv Surg Tech A 2018;28(10):1169–73.
38. Morino M, Baracchi F, Miglietta C, et al. Preoperative endoscopic sphincterotomy versus laparoendoscopic rendezvous in patients with gallbladder and bile duct stones. Ann Surg 2006;244(6):889–93 [discussion: 893–6].
39. Tricarico A, Cione G, Sozio M, et al. Endolaparoscopic rendezvous treatment: a satisfying therapeutic choice for cholecystocholedocolithiasis. Surg Endosc 2002;16(4):585–8.
40. Lezoche E, Paganini A, Feliciotti F, et al. Laparoscopic suture technique after common bile duct exploration. Surg Laparosc Endosc 1993;3(3):209–12.
41. Topal B, Aerts R, Penninckx F. Laparoscopic common bile duct stone clearance with flexible choledochoscopy. Surg Endosc 2007;21(12):2317–21.
42. Berthou J, Dron B, Charbonneau P, et al. Evaluation of laparoscopic treatment of common bile duct stones in a prospective series of 505 patients: indications and results. Surg Endosc 2007;21(11):1970–4.
43. Rose JB, Bilderback P, Raphaeli T, et al. Use the duodenum, it's right there: a retrospective cohort study comparing biliary reconstruction using either the jejunum or the duodenum. JAMA Surg 2013;148(9):860–5.
44. Dellinger EP, Kirshenbaum G, Weinstein M, et al. Determinants of adverse reaction following postoperative T-tube cholangiogram. Ann Surg 1980;191(4): 397–403.
45. Thompson MH, Tranter SE. All-comers policy for laparoscopic exploration of the common bile duct. Br J Surg 2002;89(12):1608–12.
46. Kanamaru T, Sakata K, Nakamura Y, et al. Laparoscopic choledochotomy in management of choledocholithiasis. Surg Laparosc Endosc Percutan Tech 2007; 17(4):262–6.
47. Alhamdani A, Mahmud S, Jameel M, et al. Primary closure of choledochotomy after emergency laparoscopic common bile duct exploration. Surg Endosc 2008; 22(10):2190–5.
48. Jameel M, Darmas B, Baker AL. Trend towards primary closure following laparoscopic exploration of the common bile duct. Ann R Coll Surg Engl 2008;90(1): 29–35.
49. Alkhamesi NA, Davies WT, Pinto RF, et al. Robot-assisted common bile duct exploration as an option for complex choledocholithiasis. Surg Endosc 2013; 27(1):263–6.
50. Gilbert A, Doussot A, Ortega-Deballon P, et al. Robot-assisted choledochoduodenostomy: a safe and reproducible procedure for benign common bile duct obstruction. Dig Surg 2017;34(3):177–9.
51. Jayaraman S, Davies W, Schlachta CM. Robot-assisted minimally invasive common bile duct exploration: a Canadian first. Can J Surg 2008;51(4):E93–4.

52. Ji WB, Zhao ZM, Dong JH, et al. One-stage robotic-assisted laparoscopic chole-cystectomy and common bile duct exploration with primary closure in 5 patients. Surg Laparosc Endosc Percutan Tech 2011;21(2):123–6.

53. Magge D, Steve J, Novak S, et al. Performing the difficult cholecystectomy using combined endoscopic and robotic techniques: how i do it. J Gastrointest Surg 2017;21(3):583–9.

54. Sanchez A, Rodriguez O, Davila H, et al. Robot-assisted laparoscopic common bile duct exploration: case report and proposed training model. J Robot Surg 2011;5(2):145–8.

55. Decker G, Borie F, Millat B, et al. One hundred laparoscopic choledochotomies with primary closure of the common bile duct. Surg Endosc 2003;17(1):12–8.

56. Urbach DR, Khajanchee YS, Jobe BA, et al. Cost-effective management of com-mon bile duct stones: a decision analysis of the use of endoscopic retrograde cholangiopancreatography (ERCP), intraoperative cholangiography, and laparo-scopic bile duct exploration. Surg Endosc 2001;15(1):4–13.

57. Rogers SJ, Cello JP, Horn JK, et al. Prospective randomized trial of LC+LCBDE vs ERCP/S+LC for common bile duct stone disease. Arch Surg 2010;145(1): 28–33.

58. Paganini AM, Guerrieri M, Sarnari J, et al. Thirteen years' experience with laparo-scopic transcystic common bile duct exploration for stones. Effectiveness and long-term results. Surg Endosc 2007;21(1):34–40.

An Update on Iatrogenic Biliary Injuries

Identification, Classification, and Management

Joshua T. Cohen, MD, Kevin P. Charpentier, MD, Rachel E. Beard, MD*

KEYWORDS

- Iatrogenic biliary injury • Common bile duct injury • Cholecystectomy

KEY POINTS

- Common bile duct injury occurs in 0.1% to 0.6% of cholecystectomies. Initially, rates of injury were significantly more common in laparoscopic cholecystectomies compared with open cholecystectomy. Contemporary reports now demonstrate more equivalent occurrences.
- Diagnosis is established with ultrasound or CT scan to identify a possible injury. If a biloma is identified, then percutaneous drainage or hepatobiliary iminodiacetic acid (HIDA) scan can confirm a leak. Percutaneous transhepatic cholangiography (PTC), magnetic resonance cholangiopancreatography, and/or endoscopic retrograde cholangiopancreatography can be used to define the anatomy of the injury.
- The priority of initial treatment is managing sepsis and establishing source control with PTC and biliary drainage, in cases of cholangitis, and with percutaneous drainage, in cases of intra-abdominal biloma or abscess.
- Injuries without total duct occlusion or transection can often be managed with endoscopic techniques. When occlusion or transection is present, operative management is required.
- Common bile duct injury results in significant morbidity, mortality, and cost.

INTRODUCTION

Disease of the hepatobiliary system is an extremely common reason for referral to general surgery, with approximately 750,000 cholecystectomies performed annually in the United States.[1–4] Although a vast majority of operations go well, with patients having straightforward recoveries and satisfactory outcomes, dire and severe

---

The authors have nothing to disclose.
Department of Surgery, Rhode Island Hospital, 2 Dudley Street, Suite 370, Providence, RI 02905, USA
* Corresponding author. Division of Hepatobiliary and Pancreatic Surgery, Rhode Island Hospital, The Lifespan Cancer Institute, Alpert Medical School of Brown University, 2 Dudley Street, Suite 370, Providence, RI 02905.
E-mail address: rbeard@usasurg.org

Surg Clin N Am 99 (2019) 283–299
https://doi.org/10.1016/j.suc.2018.11.006
0039-6109/19/© 2018 Elsevier Inc. All rights reserved.

complications are possible. Perhaps the most feared complication in both open and laparoscopic cholecystectomy is iatrogenic injury to the common bile duct (CBD).[1,4,5]

Incidence of CBD injury is widely reported at 0.4% to 0.6% in laparoscopic cholecystectomy.[4–9] Despite increasing experience and familiarity with laparoscopic surgery over the course of the past 3 decades, the incidence of iatrogenic CBD injury with laparoscopic cholecystectomy remains 2 times to 3 times elevated over that of open cholecystectomy (0.2%–0.3%).[4,10,11] Recent reports, however, have begun to demonstrate similar rates of CBD injury with open and laparoscopic approaches.[5–7,12,13]

Injuries to the CBD result in significant patient morbidity and mortality, requiring complex and costly management.[2,6,7,14–17] There is a 126% cost increase in patients requiring operative intervention for CBD injury compared with a straightforward laparoscopic cholecystectomy.[7,12,18] Fong and colleagues'[6] recent retrospective chart review of 809,827 patients undergoing laparoscopic cholecystectomy reported that 84% of patients with CBD injury required operative intervention with an average 1-year cost of more than $60,000.[18] Patients with CBD injury have an increase in all-cause mortality to 7.2% and 14.5% at 1 year and 5 years, respectively.[6,7,12,13,19] Published long-term mortality data demonstrate an 8.8% increase in all-cause mortality compared with age-matched controls undergoing laparoscopic cholecystectomy without CBD injury.[1,2]

This article reviews the diagnosis, classification, treatment, and outcome of iatrogenic bile duct injury, a costly and morbid complication of cholecystectomy.

ANATOMY

Bile drainage from the liver is accomplished via the left and right hepatic ducts, the confluence of which forms the common hepatic duct (CHD). Bile stored in the gallbladder is drained by the cystic duct, which joins with the CHD to form the CBD. Depending on the point at which the cystic duct joins the CHD, the length of CBD ranges from 5 cm to 15 cm. The normal diameter of the CBD is 6 mm, with an additional 1 mm added for every decade of life past 60 years of age.[1,5] The CBD then courses posterior to the duodenum and head of the pancreas, joining the main pancreatic duct to form the ampulla of Vater, which drains into the second portion of the duodenum. Drainage is mediated by the sphincter of Oddi.[1,3,20,21]

Blood supply to the CBD is variable but generally includes branches of the superior mesenteric artery (most consistently posterior superior pancreaticoduodenal artery), which supply the marginal arteries running at 3-o'clock and 9-o'clock positions and ultimately feed the epicholedochal plexus.[22]

PATHOGENESIS

Iatrogenic CBD injury occurs when surgeons fail to appropriately avoid the CBD and its blood supply during cholecystectomy dissection. Beyond cholecystectomy, any surgery requiring dissection in the right upper quadrant (RUQ) puts the CBD at risk. Injury to the CBD is a known, albeit rare, complication of total and partial gastrectomy as well as hepatectomy.[10,11,23]

In the first 3 decades of laparoscopic surgery, there was a 2-fold to 3-fold increase in CBD injury during laparoscopic cholecystectomy compared with open surgery.[4,7,18,24] More modern data sets have begun demonstrating equivalent risk of CBD injury in laparoscopic and open surgery.[5–7,23–28] One such retrospective review of 156,958 patients undergoing laparoscopic cholecystectomy demonstrated a decline in CBD injury to 0.08% at present, a vast improvement over previously published rates of 0.4% to 0.6% in laparoscopic cholecystectomy and 0.2% to 0.3% in open cholecystectomy.[2,4]

Failure to definitively identify the cystic duct intraoperatively, prior to clipping or dividing, is an independent risk factor for CBD injury.[12,13,25,26] Performing an adequate dissection and achieving the critical view of safety are widely believed to decrease the risk of CBD injury in laparoscopic cholecystectomy. The critical view of safety, as initially described by Strasberg, consists of 3 components[14,15,25–27,29]:

1. Clearance of the cystohepatic triangle (commonly referred to as the triangle of Calot)
   - Liver edge superiorly
   - Cystic duct inferolaterally
   - Hepatic duct medially
2. Cystic plate exposure by removal of the lower one-third of the gallbladder from the gallbladder fossa
3. Confirmation that 2, and only 2, structures are entering the gallbladder (the cystic duct and cystic artery)

Operating for acute cholecystitis doubles the risk of CBD injury compared with all other indications for cholecystectomy, likely due to obscured tissue planes secondary to inflammation. This risk quadruples in severe cholecystitis (as defined by Tokyo guidelines TG13).[7,12,18,24–27,30] Additional independent risk factors are anatomic variations in the anatomy of biliary tree, choledocholithiasis, urgent surgery, and baseline anemia.[12,19,27] One small case-control study in a single Canadian hospital identified a 5-fold increase in CBD injury in emergent operations compared with elective cases.[13]

Data are mixed regarding how an operating surgeon's level of experience affects CBD injury in laparoscopic cholecystectomy. Moore and Bennett initially reported in 1995 that 90% of CBD injuries occurred in the first 30 laparoscopic cholecystectomies a surgeon performed.[1,31] There Occurences were in the early days of laparoscopic surgery, however, where a majority of surgeons did not have laparoscopic techniques taught during residency training. Newer publications demonstrate fewer CBD injuries with surgeons who were trained in laparoscopic techniques during residency.[5] A study of 150,938 patients from 2000 to 2014 in New York demonstrated that there was no association of CBD injury in laparoscopic cholecystectomy with low cumulative volume surgeons (<103 total cases) and low annual volume surgeons (<19/y total cases). There was, however, an association between low annual volume surgeons and low cumulative volume surgeons for 30-day readmission, length-of-stay, and overall cost.[20]

DIAGNOSIS
Clinical Presentation

Iatrogenic injuries to the biliary tree can be difficult to recognize, with only approximately one-third of injuries identified at the time of operation.[26,27] A majority of these unrecognized injuries involve bile leaks from the cystic duct and rarely small ducts of Luschka in the liver bed that are in continuity with the biliary tree. True partial injury or transection of the CBD (Strasberg type E [**Table 3**]) are recognized at the time of operation in 70% to 80% of cases.[7,18,19,24]

When not recognized at the time of injury, signs and symptoms of iatrogenic bile duct injury can be vague and the diagnosis can be challenging. Presenting signs and symptoms are related to bile stasis and bile leakage (**Table 1**).[23–28] The most common symptoms at presentation are abdominal pain (89%), tenderness (81%), fever (74%), and nausea/emesis (43%).[23]

Table 1 Presenting signs and symptoms of iatrogenic bile duct injury	
Symptoms	Signs
Vague RUQ and epigastric pain	Peritonitis
Hiccups	Cholangitis
Fevers and chills	Sepsis
Ileus	Biloma
Nausea and emesis	Bile in surgical drains
	Cutaneous fistula

On laboratory evaluation, patients can present with leukocytosis and bandemia due to inflammation and infection secondary to bile in the peritoneal cavity or developing cholangitis. Clinical jaundice is present in approximately 30% to 50% of patients with associated hyperbilirubinemia and elevated alkaline phosphatase.[25,26] Hyperbilirubinemia results from obstruction in cases of CBD occlusion and can be associated with concomitant transaminitis as well as signs and symptoms of cholangitis. In cases of bile leak, hyperbilirubinemia can also be noted secondary to systemic reabsorption of bile by peritoneal surfaces and can be associated with biloma, cutaneous fistula, and peritonitis.[25–27]

Imaging

Diagnosis of iatrogenic CBD injury can be challenging both intraoperatively and post-operatively. Only one-third of Strasberg types A through D injuries are identified intra-operatively, with that number reaching 70% to 80% with Strasberg type E injuries (see **Table 3**).[7,18,24] Signs and symptoms are often nonspecific or, in the case of minor injuries, vague.[24–27] Intraoperatively, a CBD injury should be considered any time more than a single duct is ligated or divided. The operating surgeon should never assume extranumerary ducts are simply accessory, and ideally, further investigation, such as an intraoperative cholangiogram (IOC), should be undertaken when the anatomy is unclear and prior to clipping or division of any ducts.[27] If, intraoperatively, bile is observed to be leaking from the area of the porta hepatis and hepatoduodenal ligament, then concern should certainly be raised for a CBD injury.

If a bile duct injury is suspected postoperatively, a variety of diagnostic tests and procedures are available for work-up. The initial imaging study of choice is typically dictated by presenting signs and symptoms. For patients presenting with peritonitis and hemodynamic instability, prompt emergent operative exploration without further diagnostic imaging should be considered.

For stable patients presenting with RUQ pain and tenderness, the imaging study of choice is an abdominal ultrasound, which may visualize an extrahepatic fluid collection consistent with a biloma.[19,23,28,32] Ultrasound also allows for accurate assessment of CBD diameter, which is enlarged in distal occlusive injuries.[19,33] The addition of Doppler imaging can aid in diagnosis of concomitant vascular injury.[27,34] Patients with an uncontained bile leak after a CBD injury may present with uncontrolled sepsis as well as diffuse abdominal pain and tenderness. In these patients, contrast-enhanced CT scan should be the test of choice. CT can also demonstrate a biloma as well as ascites, abscess, and inflammation. Because these findings are nonspecific, they must be interpreted in the appropriate clinical context.[19,23,27,28,32,35–38]

If an RUQ ultrasound is concerning for CBD injury, a contrast-enhanced CT should be pursued. Confirmatory tests can include magnetic resonance cholangiopancreatography (MRCP) and hepatobiliary iminodiacetic acid (HIDA) scan. HIDA has increased sensitivity compared with MRCP for bile leak and demonstrates extraluminal extravasation of the nuclear tracer.[23,28,36,39] HIDA can be used to detect an ongoing bile leak after identification of a biloma or in the early postoperative period, whereas CT and ultrasound are more difficult to interpret. If a fluid collection suspicious for biloma is detected on CT or ultrasound, percutaneous drainage of bile also is diagnostic and therapeutic. MRCP, by contrast, has a lower degree of sensitivity for active bile leak but delineates ductal anatomy and locates injury with more accuracy. Unlike invasive diagnostic techniques, which are limited by a CBD disruption or occlusion, MRCP allows for delineation of the anatomy proximal and distal to the injury, which can be crucially important in determining a management approach.[40,41] Furthermore, MRI can also help elucidate the presence of a concomitant vascular injury (**Fig. 1**). Invasive techniques, such as endoscopic retrograde cholangiopancreatography (ERCP), allow for accurate assessment of the biliary tree anatomy only distal to an injury but have the added benefit of intervention at the time of diagnosis[19,23,35] (**Fig. 2**).

Patients with cholangitis at presentation and in whom a CBD occlusion is suspected based on imaging should undergo emergent percutaneous transhepatic cholangiography (PTC) with bile duct drain placement, which allows for therapeutic drainage of the biliary tree with better delineation of the resulting anatomy.

Routine Use of Intraoperative Cholangiogram

Since the introduction of laparoscopic cholecystectomy and the subsequent increase in CBD injuries, investigators have been studying intraoperative techniques for prevention and early identification of CBD injury. IOC is performed by the injection of radiopaque contrast dye through a catheter placed in a cystic ductotomy with fluoroscopic evaluation.[9,35] The routine use of IOC has long been proposed to avoid and identify CBD injury, but it remains controversial.

Several retrospective reviews have identified decreased rates of CBD injuries when IOC was used routinely; however, most were not limited to laparoscopic surgeries and were conducted before the development of the critical view of safety. Notably, in 2003, Flum and colleagues[9] published a retrospective review of 1,570,361 Medicare patients undergoing cholecystectomy with 7911 CBD injuries. They demonstrated a significant increase in CBD injuries from 0.39% to 0.58% (relative rate 1.51; 95% CI,

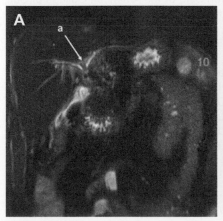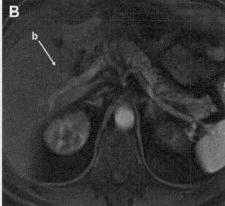

Fig. 1. (A) MRI demonstrating discontinuity of the left and right hepatic ducts at the bifurcation, compatible with injury in this location (*arrow* a). (B) A diminutive left portal vein raises concern for a concomitant vascular injury (*arrow* b).

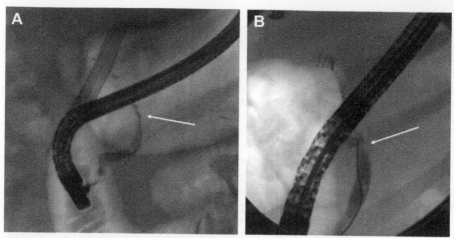

Fig. 2. (*A* and *B*) ERCP images demonstrating occluded CBDs secondary to surgical clips across the ducts (clips identified with *arrows*).

1.44–1.58) when IOC was not used. Only 21.5% of surgeons included in the study, however, routinely used IOC. Rates of CBD injury actually increased when IOC was used by surgeons who perform IOC in less than 25% of their cholecystectomies. A meta-analysis by Wysocki[41] in 2016 demonstrated that all included studies, including Flum and colleagues',[9] identified IOC as a marker for disease severity, and choice of surgical technique thus cannot be used to justify routine use of IOC.

Several more recent retrospective reviews, all specific to laparoscopic cholecystectomy and all after development of the critical view of safety, have not identified an associated benefit with routine IOC in preventing CBD injury.[42–45] The largest review included 111,815 patients and found no difference in CBD injury rate (0.25 vs 0.26%) with surgeons who routinely used IOC compared with those who only selectively used it. There was a slightly increased rate of overall complication in the routine IOC group (7.3 vs 6.7%).[43] As it stands currently, a majority of surgeons in the United States do not routinely perform IOC, a trend likely to continue as CBD injury rates continue to decrease. In a survey of 3992 members of the American College of Surgeons, with a 44% response rate, only 27% of all surgeons and 15% of academic surgeons performed IOC routinely.[46] American surgeons have numbers of routine IOC usage comparable to those of surgeons in Great Britain, where 31% of all surgeons report routinely using IOC.[47]

IOC is a useful tool in the general surgeon armamentarium when the anatomy of the biliary tree is difficult to discern, either due to inflammation or aberrant anatomy. Arguably, however, the greatest advantage with IOC is not the prevention of CBD injury but the ability to intraoperatively recognize an injury that has occurred. IOC does require a cystic ductotomy to perform; thus, if the CBD is mistaken for the cystic duct, a partial injury still occurs; however, a transection injury potentially is avoided. If a CBD injury does occur, IOC can help to delineate the level of injury through both retrograde and anterograde filling, thereby guiding both intraoperative and postoperative management.

Classification Systems

Multiple classification systems have been devised to describe iatrogenic bile duct injuries with the Bismuth (**Table 2**)[33] and Strasberg (**Table 3**)[32] classifications systems

Table 2 Bismuth classification system	
Type	**Criteria**
I	Transection ≥2 cm from the confluence of the hepatic ducts
II	Transection <2 cm from the confluence of the hepatic ducts
III	Transection involving the confluence of the hepatic ducts with continued right and left ductal communication
IV	Transection resulting in the destruction of the hepatic confluence (disruption of the confluence ceiling)
V	Aberrant right hepatic duct stricture ± CHD stricture

All defined as nearest available healthy mucosa.

the most commonly used.[27,35,36] The Strasberg classification system encompasses and expands on the original Bismuth classification system and was developed in an attempt to better characterize bile duct injuries in the laparoscopic era.[36]

The McMahon classification system is a less widely used system dividing bile duct injuries more simply into major injuries (laceration >25% of bile duct diameter, transection of CHD or CBD, or postoperative CBD stricture) and minor injuries (laceration of <25% of CBD diameter or tear at the junction of the cystic duct and CBD).[37] Stewart and Way[34] described a classification system based on a retrospective review of 88 patients with bile duct injuries. Their system divided patients into 4 classes based primarily on injury mechanism. Class I injuries involve mistaking the CBD for the cystic duct but realizing it before complete transection. Class II results from a cautery injury or misplaced clip resulting in strictures and fistula. Class III results from the same misidentification of the CBD as the cystic duct but results in complete transection. Finally, class IV is an injury to the right hepatic duct during overly vigorous dissection.[34]

The Neuhaus classification system was introduced to fill the relative paucity of data regarding the morbidity in bile duct injuries associated with simultaneous right hepatic artery injuries (**Table 4**).[38] This is the only classification system that draws a correlation with type of operative repair required and predicts recurrent cholangitis based on

Table 3 Strasberg classification system	
Type	**Criteria**
A	Leakage from the cystic duct or minor duct in gallbladder fossa
B	Occlusion of aberrant hepatic duct
C	Transection of aberrant hepatic duct (without concomitant occlusion)
D	Injury to the common hepatic or CBD lateral wall without transection
E1	Transection ≥2 cm from the confluence of the hepatic ducts
E2	Transection <2 cm from the confluence of the hepatic ducts
E3	Transection involving the confluence of the hepatic ducts with continued right and left ductal communication
E4	Transection resulting in the destruction of the hepatic confluence (and no communication between left and right hepatic ducts)
E5	Aberrant right hepatic duct injury and CHD injury

Table 4 Neuhaus classification system			
Type	**Description**	**Subtype**	**Description**
A	Peripheral bile leak	1	Cystic duct leak
		2	Leak in the gallbladder fossa
B	Main bile duct occlusion without injury	1	Incomplete occlusion
		2	Complete occlusion
C	Injury is tangential to CBD	1	<5-mm injury
		2	>5-mm injury
D	Bile duct transection	1	Without ductal defect
		2	With ductal defect
E	Main bile duct stricture	1	Short stricture <5 mm
		2	Longitudinal stricture >5 mm
		3	Stricture at hepatic duct confluence
		4	Stricture at segmental bile duct

injury pattern.[35] Despite the expanded scope of the Neuhaus classification system, it fails to describe the location of an injury in relation to the hepatic duct confluence, which is helpful both in operative planning and in describing injuries. The Hanover criteria is the most recent classification system to be published with the highest degree of granularity in describing injury patterns.[35] Bektas and colleagues[35] proposed that planning for surgical intervention and prognosis would require information regarding both vascular damage and the level of injury. In a retrospective review of 74 patients performed in Hanover, Germany, 21 injury patterns were described (**Table 5**). A correlation was made with each injury pattern and the operative approach required, including need for liver resection, resection of the confluence of the hepatic duct, and need for peripheral hepaticojejunostomy, was noted. This system failed to predict recurrent cholangitis based on injury pattern.[35]

MANAGEMENT OPTIONS

The management of CBD injuries first and foremost entails controlling sepsis, followed by re-establishing bile flow from the biliary tree to the alimentary canal. A search for simultaneous vascular injury is critically important because this can result in hepatic necrosis, abscess, intrahepatic bile duct ischemia, bile duct stricturing, and hepaticojejunostomy stenosis. Although an awareness of these potential complications is essential, the benefits of arterial reconstruction are not clear[48] (**Fig. 3**).

Timing of Repair and Need for Referral

Timing of iatrogenic bile duct repair can be challenging and remains controversial. Repair often involves complex multidisciplinary management involving interventional radiology, gastroenterology, and hepatobiliary surgeons, and thus referral to a tertiary care center is the standard of care when an injury is identified.[49–52] Late referral (>72 hours after injury) is associated with significantly more intra-abdominal abscesses and longer length of ICU stays.[49] Moreover, repair by nonhepatobiliary surgeons is associated with a significant increase in the rate of strictures, reoperation, and overall morbidity.[50]

Type	Description	Subtype	Description
Table 5			
Hanover classification system			
Type	Description	Subtype	Description
A	Peripheral bile leak in continuity with the main system	1	Cystic duct leak
		2	Leak in the gallbladder fossa
B	Main bile duct occlusion[a] without injury	1	Incomplete occlusion
		2	Complete occlusion
C[b]	Injury is tangential to CBD	1	<5-mm injury
		2	>5-mm injury below hepatic duct confluence
		3	>5-mm injury at the level of the hepatic duct confluence
		4	>5-mm injury above hepatic duct confluence
D[b]	Bile duct transection	1	Below confluence of hepatic duct
		2	Below confluence of hepatic duct with ductal defect
		3	At confluence of hepatic duct
		4	Above confluence of hepatic duct (±defect))
E	Main bile duct stricture	1	Short stricture <5 mm
		2	Longitudinal stricture >5 mm
		3	Stricture at hepatic duct confluence
		4	Stricture at segmental bile duct

[a] Main bile duct: right hepatic duct, CHD, and CBD.
[b] Vascular lesion modifiers: c: cystic artery; d, right hepatic artery; p, proper hepatic artery or common hepatic artery; pv, portal vein; and s, left hepatic artery;

Although a majority of bile duct injuries are identified postoperatively, the same recommendation for early referral to a tertiary center applies when injuries are identified intraoperatively. Should an injury occur at a tertiary center, an intraoperative consult should be called to a surgical colleague. In a review by Flum and colleagues[53] of all Medicare beneficiaries with iatrogenic bile duct injury, they identified an 11% increase in mortality if the surgeon causing the injury was the one to repair it. Published data on success of primary repair by the initial operative surgeon is dismal, with long-term success rates ranging between 17% and 27%.[49] If an injury is identified intraoperatively

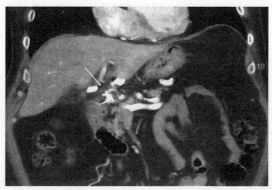

Fig. 3. CT demonstrating a ligation of the right hepatic artery with discrete cutoff at the location of surgical clips (clips identified by *arrow*). Two surgical drains are also visualized.

and a hepatobiliary surgeon is not readily available, the operative field should be widely drained to prevent sepsis, and transfer to a facility with a hepatobiliary surgeon should be promptly initiated.[54-66]

Some investigators have suggested that delaying operative intervention for at least 6 weeks, with temporizing drain placement for source control, allows inflammation to decrease and results in a less hostile operative field; however, this is controversial and the reported outcomes are mixed. Earlier reports indicated an increase in leaks, stricture, and death when CBD injuries are fixed within the first 6 weeks; however, this time frame has been challenged in more recent reports.[57] A retrospective chart review published in 2010 by Sahajpal and colleagues[54] evaluated 69 patients with primarily Strasberg type E injuries and investigated optimal timing of repair. It was demonstrated that repairs performed early, within 72 hours of injury, or late, more than 6 weeks after the injury, had significantly fewer long-term strictures compared with intermediate repairs (between 72 hours and 6 weeks after initial injury). This series had limited number of concomitant vascular injuries, however, and cannot determine if this has an impact on structuring. Careful consideration should be given to immediate repair in the setting of arterial injury.

The type of surgeon may influence the impact of timing of repair on outcomes. Two retrospective reviews show when hepatobiliary surgeons perform the repair there is no difference in recurrent cholangitis, stricture formation, need for reoperation, and overall morbidity when the repair is performed early (within 14 days or 21 days of injury) compared with late (after 14 days or 21 days of injury). When repair was performed early by the initial operative surgeon, however, outcomes were significantly worse in all categories.[50,55] Additionally, cost analysis demonstrates that early repair by a hepatobiliary surgeon results in a 29% cost decrease compared with delayed repair and a 39% decrease compared with repair by the primary surgeon.[58]

Percutaneous and Endoscopic Management

Nonoperative management of CBD injury can be used as either a temporizing measure prior to operative repair or as definitive management. In patients presenting with sepsis, urgent CT-guided or ultrasound-guided drain placement should be pursued when a discrete abscess or biloma is present to obtain source control.[54-56] If cholangitis is present secondary to an obstructing CBD injury, an urgent decompression of the biliary tree is mandatory and can be accomplished with PTC and placement of external drainage tubes. PTC further allows for accurate delineation of the remaining biliary tree anatomy for eventual operative repair in 85% of cases.[59]

For injuries that do not result in CBD occlusion or complete transection, ERCP can be used as definitive management. In a retrospective review of 71 patients with postcholecystectomy bile leaks, 83.33% of patients presented with Strasberg type A injuries, which are amenable to definitive ERCP management. Another 98.59% of patients had successful cannulation of the CBD, and 92% of patients were definitively managed with a single ERCP and endoscopic sphincterotomy either stent placement (64 of 66 patients), sphincterotomy alone (1 patient), or stent placement alone (1 patient). Only a minority of patients (7.5%) required repeat ERCP, and 1.5% of patients ended up requiring operative intervention. Furthermore, 3 of the 4 of patients in the study with a CBD injury were definitively managed with ERCP, sphincterotomy, and stent placement.[60]

Several additional studies have demonstrated excellent clinical outcomes after definitive endoscopic management of patients with Strasberg type A injuries.[61] In a study of 99 patients, no significant difference was found in definitive management of bile leaks when comparing sphincterotomy with stenting to sphincterotomy alone in patients with a bile leak from the cystic duct. The sphincterotomy-only group had fewer ERCPs overall because they did not require subsequent stent removal. A majority of patients (82%) with bile duct injury but without transection were managed definitively with ERCP, sphincterotomy, and stenting.[62] In the case of postcholecystectomy CBD stricture, 80% of patients can be definitively managed with ERCP, endoscopic balloon dilation, and stent placement.[48,62] Recently, there are sporadic reports of patients with significant operative risk factors and complete transection of the CBD, and without tissue defect, effectively treated with rendezvous techniques combining PTC and ERCP with stent placement, although this is far from routinely used.[63]

Operative Management

Operative management remains the gold standard for repair of iatrogenic biliary injury and is required in situations where injury cannot be managed with ERCP. Complete CBD transections and occlusions mandate operative repair with extraordinarily rare exceptions. A variety of approaches to operative repairs exist, including ligation of leaking duct, primary ductal repair, end-to-end bile duct anastomosis, biliary enteric anastamosis, transplantation, and partial hepatectomy. The preferred operative repair depends on the injury pattern.[61,64,65]

When the appropriate expertise is available, laparoscopic primary bile duct repair and placement of T tube is possible.[64] Although ERCP and sphincterotomy (with or without stenting) are quickly replacing the need for operative intervention for Strasberg type A procedures, open or laparoscopic clipping a leaking cystic duct or accessory duct can be an effective means of repair, especially if endoscopic options are not available.[61,64,66,67] Transection of small (<3 mm) ducts draining a single hepatic segment can be safely ligated.[68]

Simple repair
Simple repair over a T tube or with placement of a transcystic drain is appropriate for nonelectrocautery injuries involving less than 50% of the diameter of the CBD.[69] For small injuries to the lateral sidewall, a T tube can be placed through the iatrogenic choledochotomy. Larger injuries require a separate choledochotomy to be made for T-tube insertion, with subsequent closure of the injury over the T tube.[68] Simple repair is typically carried out with 4-0 to 7-0 absorbable monofilament suture.[64,70]

End-to-end bile duct anastomosis
End-to-end ductal anastomosis are common in adult liver transplantation but used less often in iatrogenic bile duct injuries due to the frequency of tissue defects. In sharp transection injuries without significant tissue loss or involvement of the hepatic duct confluence, a tension-free primary anastomosis is possible.[70] The advantage of primary anastomosis is a return to a more physiologic regulation of bile flow compared with hepaticojejunostomy, potentially resulting in better postoperative weight gain and fewer duodenal ulcers.[70,71] Overall, primary end-to-end CBD anastomosis has fewer early postoperative complications. There is a trend toward higher postoperative bile duct stricture rates; however, more than 90% of patients are stricture-free at long-term follow-up.[71] When strictures do develop, they can be initially managed with endoscopic dilation in two-thirds of patients, with a durable response rate of 80%.[72] The benefit of T tubes in end-to-end anastomosis remains unclear. Data are mixed, with some studies reporting higher rates of stenosis and lower rates of biliary fistula without T-tube placement.[70]

Biliary enteric anastomosis
The gold standard for repair of iatrogenic bile duct injury is the Roux-en-Y biliary-enteric anastomosis. Alternatively, the duodenum has been used in repairs to all levels

of bile duct injury.[25] Loss of hepatic duct confluence often necessitates a Roux-en-Y hepaticojejunostomy, but this injury can be repaired successfully with a hepaticoduodenostomy, although other injuries can also be reconstructed using this technique.[16,26,73]

Preoperatively, the placement of PTCs is helpful in defining and identifying the hepatic ducts for anastomosis. Typically, a right subcostal incision, sometimes with a left subcostal or vertical extension, is used and provides excellent exposure of the porta hepatis. Biliary and vascular anatomy is then defined, and necrotic tissue is débrided. There are varying techniques for performing a hepaticojejunostomy, but in general a Roux limb is created by dividing the jejunum 30-cm to 70-cm distal to the ligament of Treitz with a subsequent hand-sewn or stapled jejunojejunostomy. A hand-sewn single layer end-to-side hepaticojejunostomy is then created 2-cm to 3-cm distal to the end of the jejunal stump on the antimesenteric surface of the jejunum using 4-0 to 6-0 sutures, in an interrupted or running fashion, depending on surgeon preference or size of the duct. For small-caliber ducts, a Hepp-Couinaud technique can be performed in which an incision is extended from the cut surface of the CHD onto the extrahepatic segment of left hepatic duct to widen the anastomosis. If PTCs are present, they can either be left in place or withdrawn and replaced with a larger-diameter 5-French pediatric feeding tube or Hobbs stent left across the anastomosis prior to completion of the anastomosis, again depending on surgeon preference.[16,26,27,74,75] Rates of anastomotic strictures are reported in the range of 4% to 38% of hepaticojejunostomy. Although the majority are effectively managed with transhepatic dilation, rates of revision of hepaticojejunostomy are as high as 20% to 25%.[75]

Partial hepatectomy
Partial hepatectomy in patients with iatrogenic bile duct injuries should be avoided when possible. A small retrospective review reported a 60% morbidity and a 10% mortality when hepatectomy is required.[76] There are, however, instances in which hepatectomy cannot be avoided. Immediate postinjury period hepatectomy is indicated for control of peritonitis or sepsis in patients with liver necrosis, bile duct necrosis, significant liver abscess, or persistent bile leakage from segmental bile ducts not amenable to reconstruction. The likelihood of any of these complications is increased in the setting of a significant concomitant vascular injury. In delayed presentation, recurrent cholangitis refractory to nonoperative management is an indication for partial hepatectomy.[77]

Delayed presentation of biliary stricture can result in biliary cirrhosis and liver atrophy from long-term cholangitis. Furthermore, concurrent vascular injury may result in hepatic necrosis. Lesions proximal to the hepatic duct confluence and right hepatic artery injury are significant risk factors, with 72.7% of patients requiring hepatectomy when both injuries are present. In the most drastic situations, patients may present in acute liver failure requiring transplantation.[76]

CLINICAL OUTCOMES IN THE LITERATURE

Complications after operative repair of bile duct injuries are common, with reported rates exceeding 40%. The most common complications include wound infection, cholangitis, intra-abdominal abscess, anastomotic leaks, stricture, and an overall 30-day postoperative mortality of approximately 2%.[4,25] Published rates of stricture formation range from 10% to 19%, with development of chronic liver disease ranging from 6% to 22%.[27]

Published long-term mortality in patients with bile duct injury has been reported to exceed 20% at 5 years. A large review by Fong and colleagues[6] compared mortality in patients with major bile duct injury to those with straightforward cholecystectomy and found that 1-year and 3-year all-cause mortality rates increased to 7.2% compared with 1.3% and to 15.4% compared with 4.8%, respectively. When outcomes after endoscopic and operative management were compared, endoscopic management had significantly worse 1-year and 5- year all-cause mortality rates, with 15% compared with 6.0% and 31.9% compared with 12.4% reported, respectively.

Dageforde and colleagues[58] looked at the cost of repair per quality-adjusted life year and found that immediate repair by a hepatobiliary surgeon is the most cost-effective means of repair, with a reduction in cost per quality-adjusted life year of 60% compared with repair by the primary surgeon and 35% over delayed repair by a hepatobiliary surgeon. In 1 study that evaluated 1584 patients, operative repair at 1 year cost $60,539 compared with $118,245 in endoscopically managed patients.[6]

SUMMARY

Bile duct injury is a feared complication of cholecystectomy and results in significant morbidity, mortality, and health care spending. The clinical presentation can be vague and nonspecific, and the diagnosis can be challenging. Management is best accomplished by a coordinated multidisciplinary effort and frequently involves percutaneous, endoscopic, and surgical techniques.

REFERENCES

1. Moore KL, Dalley AF. Clinically oriented anatomy. 5th edition. Baltimore (MD): Lippincott Williams & Wilkins; 2006.
2. Halbert C, Altieri MS, Yang J, et al. Long-term outcomes of patients with common bile duct injury following laparoscopic cholecystectomy. Surg Endosc 2016; 30(10):4294–9.
3. Netter FH. Atlas of human anatomy. In: Hansen JT, Benninger B, Brueckner JK, et al, editors. Atlas of human anatomy. 5th edition. Philadelphia: Elsevier inc; 2011. p. 240–330.
4. Ismael HN, Cox S, Cooper A, et al. The morbidity and mortality of hepaticojejunostomies for complex bile duct injuries: a multi-institutional analysis of risk factors and outcomes using NSQIP. HPB (Oxford) 2017;19(4):352–8.
5. Halbert C, Pagkratis S, Yang J, et al. Beyond the learning curve: incidence of bile duct injuries following laparoscopic cholecystectomy normalize to open in the modern era. Surg Endosc 2015;30(6):2239–43.
6. Fong ZV, Pitt HA, Strasberg SM, et al. Diminished survival in patients with bile leak and ductal injuries: management strategy and outcomes. J Am Coll Surg 2018; 226(4):568–76.e1.
7. Barrett M, Asbun HJ, Chien H-L, et al. Bile duct injury and morbidity following cholecystectomy: a need for improvement. Surg Endosc 2017;32(4):1683–8.
8. Murray AC. An observational study of the timing of surgery, use of laparoscopy and outcomes for acute cholecystitis in the USA and UK. Surg Endosc 2018; 32(7):3055–63.
9. Flum DR, Dellinger EP, Cheadke A, et al. Intraoperative cholangiography and risk of common bile duct injury during cholecystectomy. JAMA 2003;289:1639–44.
10. Dixon JA, Morgan KA, Adams DB. Management of common bile duct injury during partial gastrectomy. Am Surg 2009;75(3):719–21.
11. Fragulidis G, Marinis A, Polydorou A, et al. Managing injuries of hepatic duct confluence variants after major hepatobiliary surgery: an algorithmic approach. World J Gastroenterol 2008;14(19):3049.

12. Kohn JF, Trenk A, Kuchta K, et al. Characterization of common bile duct injury after laparoscopic cholecystectomy in a high-volume hospital system. Surg Endosc 2018;32(3):1184–91.
13. Kholdebarin R, Boetto J, Harnish JL, et al. Risk factors for bile duct injury during laparoscopic cholecystectomy: a case-control study. Surg Innov 2008;15(2):114–9.
14. Conrad C, Wakabayashi G, Asbun HJ, et al. IRCAD recommendation on safe laparoscopic cholecystectomy. J Hepatobiliary Pancreat Sci 2017;24(11):603–15.
15. Pucher PH, Brunt LM, Fanelli RD, et al. SAGES expert Delphi consensus: critical factors for safe surgical practice in laparoscopic cholecystectomy. Surg Endosc 2015;29(11):3074–8.
16. Bobkiewicz A, Krokowicz Ł, Banasiewicz T, et al. Iatrogenic bile duct injury. a significant surgical problem. Assessment of treatment outcomes in the departments own material. Pol Przegl Chir 2015;86(12):576–83.
17. Sinha S, Hofman D, Stoker DL, et al. Epidemiological study of provision of cholecystectomy in England from 2000 to 2009: retrospective analysis of hospital episode statistics. Surg Endosc 2012;27(1):162–75.
18. Tornqvist B, Stromberg C, Persson G, et al. Effect of intended intraoperative cholangiography and early detection of bile duct injury on survival after cholecystectomy: population based cohort study. BMJ 2012;345(1):1–10.
19. Jabłońska B, Lampe P. Iatrogenic bile duct injuries: etiology, diagnosis and management. World J Gastroenterol 2009;15(33):4097.
20. Abelson JS, Spiegel JD, Afaneh C, et al. BiliaryEvaluating cumulative and annual surgeon volume in laparoscopic cholecystectomy. Surgery 2017;161(3):611–7.
21. Keplinger KM, Bloomston M. Anatomy and embryology of the biliary tract. Surg Clin North Am 2014;94(2):203–17.
22. Strasberg SM, Helton WS. An analytical review of vasculobiliary injury in laparoscopic and open cholecystectomy. HPB (Oxford) 2011;13(1):1–14.
23. Copelan A, Bahoura L, Tardy F, et al. Etiology, diagnosis, and management of bilomas: a current update. Tech Vasc Interv Radiol 2015;18(4):236–43.
24. Lillemoe KD, Martin SA, Cameron JL, et al. Major bile duct injuries during laparoscopic cholecystectomy. Ann Surg 1997;225:459–71.
25. Sicklick JK, Camp MS, Lillemoe KD, et al. Surgical management of bile duct injuries sustained during laparoscopic cholecystectomy. Ann Surg 2005;241(5):786–95.
26. Maddah G, Mashhadi MTR, Mashhadi MP, et al. Iatrogenic injuries of the extrahepatic biliary system. J Surg Res 2015;213:215–21.
27. McPartland KJ, Pomposelli JJ. Iatrogenic biliary injuries: classification, identification, and management. Surg Clin North Am 2008;88(6):1329–43.
28. Barkun AN, Rezieg M, Mehta SN, et al. Postcholecystectomy biliary leaks in the laparoscopic era: risk factors, presentation, and management. McGill Gallstone Treatment Group. Gastrointest Endosc 1997;45(3):277–82.
29. Strasberg SM, Hertl M, Soper NJ. An analysis of the problem of biliary injury during laparoscopic cholecystectomy. J Am Coll Surg 1995;180:101–25.
30. Törnqvist B, Waage A, Zheng Z, et al. Severity of acute cholecystitis and risk of iatrogenic bile duct injury during cholecystectomy, a population-based case–control study. World J Surg 2015;40(5):1060–7.
31. Moore MH, Bennett CL. The learning curve for laparoscopic cholecystectomy. The Southern Surgical Club. Am J Surg 1995;170(1):55–9.

32. Hogan NM, Dorcaratto D, Hogan AM, et al. Iatrogenic common bile duct injuries: increasing complexity in the laparoscopic era: a prospective cohort study. Int J Surg 2016;33(Part A):151–6.

33. Bismuth H, Majno PE. Biliary strictures: classification based on the principles of surgical treatment. World J Surg 2001;25:1241–4.

34. Stewart L, Way LW. Bile duct injuries during laparoscopic cholecystectomy. Arch Surg 1995;130:1123–9.

35. Bektas H, Schrem H, Winny M, et al. Surgical treatment and outcome of iatrogenic bile duct lesions after cholecystectomy and the impact of different clinical classification systems. Br J Surg 2007;94(9):1119–27.

36. Chun K. Recent classifications of the common bile duct injury. Korean J Hepatobiliary Pancreat Surg 2014;18(3):69.

37. McMahon AJ, Fullarton G, Baxter JN, et al. Bile duct injury and bile leakage in laparoscopic cholecystectomy. Br J Surg 1995;82(3):307–13.

38. Schmidt SC, Settmacher U, Langrehr JM, et al. Management and outcome of patients with combined bile duct and hepatic arterial injuries after laparoscopic cholecystectomy. Surgery 2004;135(6):613–8.

39. Bujanda L, Calvo MM, Cabriada JL, et al. MRCP in the diagnosis of iatrogenic bile duct injury. NMR Biomed 2003;16(8):475–8.

40. Ragozzino A, De Ritis R, Mosca A, et al. Value of MR cholangiography in patients with iatrogenic bile duct injury after cholecystectomy. AJR Am J Roentgenol 2004; 183(6):1567–72.

41. Wysocki AP. Population-based studies should not be used to justify a policy of routine cholangiography to prevent major bile duct injury during laparoscopic cholecystectomy. World J Surg 2016;41(1):82–9.

42. Hamad MA, Nada AA, Abdel-Atty MY, et al. Major biliary complications in 2,714 cases of laparoscopic cholecystectomy without intraoperative cholangiography: a multicenter retrospective study. Surg Endosc 2011;25(12):3747–51.

43. Ragulin-Coyne E, Witkowski ER, Chau Z, et al. Is routine intraoperative cholangiogram necessary in the twenty-first century? a national view. J Gastrointest Surg 2013;17(3):434–42.

44. Kumar A, Kumar U, Munghate A, et al. Role of routine intraoperative cholangiography during laparoscopic cholecystectomy. Surg Endosc 2015;29(9):2837–40.

45. Altieri MS, Yang J, Obeid N, et al. Increasing bile duct injury and decreasing utilizationof intraoperative cholangiogram and common bile duct exploration over 14 years: an analysis of outcomes in New York State. Surg Endosc 2017;32(2): 667–74.

46. Massarweh NN, Devlin A, Elrod JAB, et al. Surgeon knowledge, behavior, and opinions regarding intraoperative cholangiography. J Am Coll Surg 2008; 207(6):821–30.

47. Halawani HM, Tamim H, Khalifeh F, et al. Impact of intraoperative cholangiography on postoperative morbidity and readmission: analysis of the NSQIP database. Surg Endosc 2016;30(12):5395–403.

48. Sikora SS. Management of post-cholecystectomy benign bile duct strictures: review. Indian J Surg 2011;74(1):22–8.

49. Fischer CP, Fahy BN, Aloia TA, et al. Timing of referral impacts surgical outcomes in patients undergoing repair of bile duct injuries. HPB (Oxford) 2009;11(1):32–7.

50. Felekouras E, Petrou A, Neofytou K, et al. Early or delayed intervention for bile duct injuriesfollowing laparoscopic cholecystectomy? a dilemma looking for an answer. Gastroenterol Res Pract 2015;1–10.

51. de Reuver PR, Grossmann I, Busch OR, et al. Referral pattern and timing of repair are risk factors for complications after reconstructive surgery for bile duct injury. Ann Surg 2007;245(5):763–70.
52. Kirks RC, Barnes TE, Lorimer PD, et al. Comparing early and delayed repair of common bile duct injury to identify clinical drivers of outcome and morbidity. HPB (Oxford) 2016;18(9):718–25.
53. Flum DR, Cheadle A, Prela C, et al. Bile duct injury during cholecystectomy and survival in medicare beneficiaries. JAMA 2003;290(16):2168–73.
54. Sahajpal AK, Chow SC, Dixon E, et al. Bile duct injuries associated with laparoscopic cholecystectomy: timing of repair and long-term outcomes. Arch Surg 2010;145(8):757–63.
55. Perera MTPR, Silva MA, Hegab B, et al. Specialist early and immediate repair of post-laparoscopic cholecystectomy bile duct injuries is associated with an improved long-term outcome. Ann Surg 2011;253(3):553–60.
56. Dominguez-Rosado I, Sanford DE, Liu J, et al. Timing of surgical repair after bile duct injury impacts postoperative complications but not anastomotic patency. Ann Surg 2016;264(3):544–53.
57. Kapoor VK. Bile duct injury repair: when? what? who? J Hepatobiliary Pancreat Surg 2007;14(5):476–9.
58. Dageforde LA, Landman MP, Feurer ID, et al. A cost-effectiveness analysis of early vs late reconstruction of iatrogenic bile duct injuries. J Am Coll Surg 2012;214(6):919–27.
59. Fidelman N, Kerlan RK Jr, LaBerge JM, et al. Accuracy of percutaneous transhepatic cholangiography in predicting the location and nature of major bile duct injuries. J Vasc Interv Radiol 2011;22(6):884–92.
60. Fasoulas K, Zavos C, Chatzimavroudis G, et al. Eleven-year experience on the endoscopic treatment of post-cholecystectomy bile leaks. Ann Gastroenterol 2011;24(3):200–5.
61. Tsalis KG, Christoforidis EC, Dimitriadis CA, et al. Management of bile duct injury during and after laparoscopic cholecystectomy. Surg Endosc 2003;17(1):31–7.
62. Rainio M, Lindström O, Udd M, et al. Endoscopic therapy of biliary injury after cholecystectomy. Dig Dis Sci 2017;63(2):474–80.
63. Shin S, Klevan A, Fernandez CA, et al. Rendezvous technique for the treatment of complete common bile duct transection after multiple hepatobiliary surgeries. J Laparoendosc Adv Surg Tech A 2014;24(10):728–30.
64. Pekolj J, Alvarez FA, Palavecino M, et al. Intraoperative management and repair of bile duct injuries sustained during 10,123 laparoscopic cholecystectomies in a high-volume referral center. J Am Coll Surg 2013;216(5):894–901.
65. Bharathy KGS, Negi SS. Postcholecystectomy bile duct injury and its sequelae: pathogenesis, classification, and management. Indian J Gastroenterol 2013; 33(3):201–15.
66. Martin D, Uldry E, Demartines N, et al. Bile duct injuries after laparoscopic cholecystectomy: 11-year experience in a tertiary center. Biosci Trends 2016;10(3): 197–201.
67. Tropea A, Pagano D, Biondi A, et al. Treatment of the iatrogenic lesion of the biliary tree secondary to laparoscopic cholecystectomy: a single center experience. Updates Surg 2016;68(2):143–8.
68. Brunicardi FC, Anderson DK, Billiar TR, et al. Schwartz's principles of surgery. 10th edition. New York: McGraw-Hill; 2015. p. 1332–4.
69. Cameron JL, Cameron AM. Current surgical therapy. 11th edition. Philadelphia: Elsevier; 2014. p. 383–91.

70. Jabłońska B. End-to-end ductal anastomosis in biliary reconstruction: indications and limitations. Can J Surg 2014;57(4):271–7.
71. Jabłońska B, Lampe P, Olakowski M, et al. Hepaticojejunostomy vs. end-to-end biliary reconstructions in the treatment of iatrogenic bile duct injuries. J Gastrointest Surg 2009;13(6):1084–93.
72. de Reuver PR, Busch ORC, Rauws EA, et al. Long-term results of a primary end-to-end anastomosis in peroperative detected bile duct injury. J Gastrointest Surg 2007;11(3):296–302.
73. Mercado M-A. Iatrogenic bile duct injury with loss of confluence. World J Gastrointest Surg 2015;7(10):254.
74. Ha T-Y, Hwang S, Song G-W, et al. Cluster hepaticojejunostomy is a useful technique enabling secure reconstruction of severely damaged hilar bile ducts. J Gastrointest Surg 2015;19(8):1537–41.
75. Moris D, Papalampros A, Vailas M, et al. The hepaticojejunostomy technique with intra-anastomotic stent in biliary diseases and its evolution throughout the years: a technical analysis. Gastroenterol Res Pract 2016;1–7.
76. Li J, Frilling A, Nadalin S, et al. Timing and risk factors of hepatectomy in the management of complications following laparoscopic cholecystectomy. J Gastrointest Surg 2011;16(4):815–20.
77. Jabłońska B. Hepatectomy for bile duct injuries: when is it necessary? World J Gastroenterol 2013;19(38):6348.

Premalignant Lesions of the Biliary Tract

Zaheer S. Kanji, MD, MSc, FRCSC[a,b,1], Flavio G. Rocha, MD[a,*]

KEYWORDS

- IPNBs • Biliary cystadenomas • Choledochal cysts • ITPNs • B-MCNs

KEY POINTS

- Premalignant cystic lesions of the biliary tree are uncommon, although the incidence is poorly characterized.
- Biliary mucinous cystic neoplasms do not communicate with the biliary tree, are more common in women of reproductive age, and are resected surgically because of a 30% risk of malignant transformation.
- Intraductal papillary mucinous neoplasms of the bile duct (IPNBs) communicate with the biliary tree and have up to an 80% risk of malignancy.
- Intraductal tubular papillary neoplasms of the bile duct are a fairly new entity resembling IPNBs, but with tubular formation and without mucin production.
- Choledochal cysts are a rare congenital cystic dilatation of the bile ducts most often associated with an anomalous pancreaticobiliary junction.

INTRODUCTION

Lesions of the biliary tract encompass a range of disorders requiring a similar approach to diagnosis with a differing strategy for management. They can be subdivided into benign versus malignant, solid versus Cystic, or inflammatory versus neoplastic. As with other diseases of the liver, biliary lesions can be classified into more than 1 category and diagnosis often requires careful attention to the presenting signs and symptoms, patient history, ethnicity, and travel history. In the United States, the most common biliary tract disorder is gallstone disease. Malignancies of the biliary tract are presumed to be secondary to chronic inflammation leading to dysplasia and finally cancer. Worldwide, pathogenesis is thought to be secondary to chronic

Disclosure: The authors have nothing to disclose.
[a] Section of General, Thoracic and Vascular Surgery, Virginia Mason Medical Center, 1100 Ninth Avenue, Seattle, WA 98101, USA; [b] Division of General Surgery, Department of Surgery, Royal Inland Hospital, University of British Columbia, 311 Columbia Street, Kamloops, British Columbia V2C 2T1, Canada
[1] Present address: 400-321 Nicola Street, Kamloops, British Columbia V2C 6G6, Canada.
* Corresponding author. Virginia Mason Medical Center, C6-GS, Buck Pavilion, 1100 Ninth Avenue, Seattle, WA 98101.
E-mail address: Flavio.Rocha@virginiamason.org

Surg Clin N Am 99 (2019) 301–314
https://doi.org/10.1016/j.suc.2018.11.007
surgical.theclinics.com

infection by various parasites, bacteria, and chronic hepatitis B and C.[1] Premalignant neoplastic lesions of the bile duct have also been described, although the incidence has been poorly characterized. These lesions include biliary mucinous cystic neoplasms (B-MCNs), intraductal papillary biliary mucinous neoplasms (IPNBs), intraductal tubular papillary neoplasms (ITPNs) of the bile duct (ITPN-B), and the better-characterized choledochal cysts (CCs). This article reviews the diagnosis and management of these premalignant biliary neoplasms.

EMBRYOLOGY AND DEVELOPMENT

The biliary tract consists of the intrahepatic and extrahepatic bile ducts and the gallbladder. Grossly, the intrahepatic bile ducts include the first-order to third-order bile ducts, which are visible in a surgical specimen. Microscopically, the bile ducts can be further subdivided into septal and interlobular ducts.[1] Unlike the intrahepatic bile ducts, the extrahepatic biliary tree is completely visible grossly and includes the common hepatic duct, which joins with the cystic duct to form the common bile duct (CBD), terminating in the second portion of the duodenum at the ampulla of Vater (AOV). On histology, the bile ducts are lined by cuboidal cells in the septal/interlobular ducts and by columnar cells in the larger intrahepatic and extrahepatic ducts. Development of the biliary tree commences in the fourth week of development.[2] The hepatic diverticulum arises from the primitive midgut and enlarges to form all the organs of the hepatopancreatobiliary system. The hepatic diverticulum is divided into cranial and caudal portions. The cranial component forms the liver and extrahepatic biliary tree, whereas the caudal component divides into a superior and inferior branch. The gallbladder and cystic duct originate from the superior caudal hepatic diverticulum, whereas the pancreas forms from the inferior. Development of these structures takes approximately 1 week and is complete by the fifth week of development. The intrahepatic biliary tree continues its formation with final completion by the 12th week of development. Microscopic bile ducts and bile canaliculi originate from hepatic cells with final ingrowth of the terminal bile ducts forming the architectural structure of the hepatic parenchyma. The common origin and parallel development of the liver and biliary tree show the close association, resemblance, and presentation of diseases from both systems, which are often difficult to differentiate from one another.

BILIARY MUCINOUS CYSTIC NEOPLASMS
Epidemiology/Presentation

Originally termed biliary cystadenomas, B-MCNs are a rare group of premalignant biliary cystic tumors often detected incidentally on cross-sectional radiologic imaging.[3] These lesions originate from hepatic parenchyma or bile duct and account for less than 1% of cystic lesions of the liver.[4] They may be found in the extrahepatic biliary tree, although more commonly are seen in the liver. B-MCNs are typically detected in young women (>90%) during the reproductive years (age 30–50 years) and rarely occur in men.[5] However, malignant degeneration of B-MCNs (cystadenocarcinomas now renamed mucinous cystic carcinomas) is equally distributed between men and women and presents a decade later, on average, than their benign counterparts.[6] B-MCNs tend to be large (>10 cm) and presentation of these lesions is often nonspecific and includes abdominal pain likely secondary to stretch of the hepatic Glissonian capsule, bloating, and rarely palpation of an abdominal mass. However, most of these lesions remain asymptomatic. Uncommonly, patients may present with fever, jaundice, or ascites, and approximately 25% of patients show increase of liver enzyme levels on laboratory analysis. Rarely, large tumors can cause obstructive jaundice secondary to compression of the extrahepatic biliary tree and/or growth within intrahepatic bile ducts[5] leading to cholangitis.[7] Compression of the inferior cava may also occur, resulting in bilateral lower leg edema. Tumor hemorrhage and rupture have also been described, although, once again, at very low frequencies.[3] However, the occurrence of symptoms does not correlate with the presence or absence of malignancy.[6]

Diagnosis

Diagnosis of B-MCNs often commences with formulating a broad differential diagnosis including inflammatory and infectious causes of biliary lesions. Although no single specific laboratory marker has been associated with B-MCNs, routine bloodwork including hepatic tumor markers such as alpha fetoprotein (AFP), carcinoembryonic antigen (CEA), and carbohydrate antigen (CA) 19-9 are commonly obtained. An increased CA 19-9 level may raise suspicion for malignant degeneration of B-MCNs, although this is nonspecific. However, AFP and CEA levels remain within normal limits in both benign and malignant disease. In cases of biliary obstruction, increased levels of cholestatic liver enzymes (alkaline phosphatase [ALP], gamma-glutamyl transferase [GGT], total bilirubin) may be observed. Similarly, radiologic imaging tends to be nonspecific in the diagnosis of B-MCNs. Typically, ultrasonography is performed to assess for more common biliary disorders, like gallstone disease. B-MCNs appear as an anechoic mass with multiple septations. Papillary projections may be seen originating from the septae or cyst wall.[5] Cross-sectional imaging such as computed tomography (CT) and MRI is complementary to ultrasonography. On CT, B-MCNs appear as hypodense lesions with nodular enhancement on intravenous contrast studies. They tend to be preferentially located in the left lobe of the liver and differ from simple hepatic cysts by the presence of papillary projections and septae. Ultrasonography is superior to CT in showing the presence of intracystic septae, whereas CT surpasses ultrasonography in predicting size and delineating anatomic relationships of the tumor to surrounding hepatic parenchyma and vasculature.[3,6] MRI is also useful for surgical planning and demonstration of anatomic relationships between cyst and surrounding hepatic parenchyma. B-MCNs are typically multilocular on MRI with thickened walls and a low T1 and high T2 intensity. Diffusion weighting of MRI may further enhance cyst characterization, although the additional utility of MRI compared with CT for B-MCNs remains unclear. In addition, magnetic resonance cholangiopancreatography (MRCP) may further assist in showing lack of biliary communication and in delineating septations, although this is not commonly performed. Studies such as endoscopic retrograde cholangiopancreatography (ERCP), similarly, are rarely performed and may be useful for biliary decompression in cases of obstructive jaundice or for obtaining tissue samples for pathologic diagnosis.

In general, routine sampling of suspected B-MCNs for preoperative pathologic confirmation should be avoided because of the risk of peritoneal/pleural seeding and low clinical utility of these findings. In cases where image-guided aspiration and core biopsy has been undertaken at the discretion of the managing clinician, cyst fluid analysis for CA 19-9 and CEA has been found to be 66% sensitive for differentiating B-MCNs from other cystic lesions of the bile duct.[3] Furthermore, cyst fluid analysis is also poor at differentiating B-MCNs from invasive biliary mucinous cystic cancers and therefore is generally avoided.

Management

Although B-MCNs are uncommon, the frequency of malignant transformation has been reported to be as high as 20% to 30%.[8] For that reason, the mainstay of

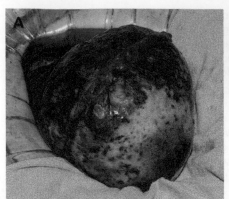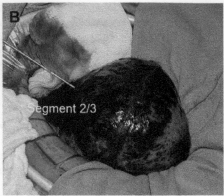

Fig. 1. (*A*) Biliary mucinous cystic neoplasm of the left lateral segment. (*B*) Transhepatic aspiration of the biliary mucinous cystic neoplasm before left lateral sectionectomy.

treatment of B-MCNs is surgical resection (**Fig. 1**). Although percutaneous aspiration/ sclerosis and ablation have been described for B-MCNs, they have been investigated in the context of single-institution studies with poor follow-up. As such, their general applicability in the clinical setting has been limited. Similarly, cyst fenestration and marsupialization have also been described, although their widespread use is limited because of the risk of cancer associated with B-MCNs. Furthermore, use of these modalities has been associated with an 80% to 90% risk of recurrence.[6] Surgical resection therefore offers the best change of cure and the only opportunity for an appropriate oncologic resection. Both open and laparoscopic approaches can be entertained, depending on the location of the lesion and the comfort level of the surgeon. Enucleation of lesions with clear gross margins is a useful strategy for central hepatic lesions in the absence of vascular involvement as a parenchymal sparing strategy, whereas more peripheral lesions can be managed with conservative hepatic resection. B-MCNs involving the extrahepatic bile ducts require resection of the biliary tree with bile duct reconstruction. In addition, liver transplant for B-MCNs has been reported, although, because of the indolent nature of both B-MCNs and mucinous cystic carcinomas, the indication for this technique remains undefined.

Pathology

As of 2010, the World Health Organization (WHO) has reclassified biliary cystic neoplasms to mirror the nomenclature for the pancreas.[9] B-MCNs are defined similar to MCNs of the pancreas pathologically by the presence of ovarian stroma expressing both estrogen and progesterone receptors.[6] Grossly, B-MCNs are multilocular and solitary, often with dense calcifications and fibrosis. Furthermore, they are lined by mucin-producing epithelium with a subsequent layer of undifferentiated mesenchymal cells. Although B-MCNs originate from the bile ducts, they are generally found to not be in communication with the biliary tree and microscopically show a well-defined capsule with a single layer of columnar or cuboidal cells that produce mucus and rarely serous fluid.[10] Immunohistochemical (IHC) analysis shows epithelial expression of both CEA and CA 19-9. In contrast, biliary mucinous cystic carcinomas are defined by a multilayer epithelium with multiple mitotic figures and loss of cellular polarity with nuclear atypia. Furthermore, IHC shows diffuse expression of CEA in the cytoplasm as opposed to solely in the epithelium with B-MCNs. In addition, the lack of ovarian stroma has been reported as a prognostic factor in patients with mucinous cystic carcinoma.

Prognosis

The prognosis of B-MCNs has not been well reported because of the rarity of the disease and the general lack of follow-up. In the largest reported series to date, the median recurrence-free survival (RFS) was 12.1 years with a 5-year RFS of 61.4%.[8] Recurrence was found to be higher in patients who underwent fenestration compared with resection in B-MCNs and was virtually universal in patients with carcinoma who did not undergo an oncologic procedure. Furthermore, the presence of margin positivity, either microscopic or gross, was independently associated with recurrence in both B-MCNs and mucinous cystic cancers. Recurrences tend to occur locally, often caused by an inadequate initial oncologic procedure, and rarely recur extrahepatically when carcinomas are present. Recurrent B-MCNs can be approached with a repeat resection and, in cases of recurrent carcinomas, salvage chemotherapy, radiation, or chemoembolization has also been described.[6] B-MCNs and their malignant counterpart tend to be indolent and, as such, overall survival (OS) is favorable, with a median OS of 8.4 years in mucinous cystic carcinomas. The 5-year OS is approximately 84%.

INTRADUCTAL PAPILLARY BILIARY MUCINOUS NEOPLASMS
Epidemiology/Presentation

Like B-MCNs, the 2010 WHO classification for cystic lesions of the bile duct have created a separate category for IPNBs recognizing their unique pathology distinct from other biliary tumors. IPNBs are a newly recognized entity also similar in nature to intraductal papillary mucinous neoplasms of the pancreas (IPMNs).[11] Like IPMNs and B-MCNs, IPNBs are mucin-secreting cystic tumors with malignant potential. The original description of IPNBs was mainly concentrated in Asia, with very few cases identified in North America, and often have been referred to as biliary papillomatosis. However, with advances in diagnostic imaging leading to surgical resection, IPNBs are being detected with increased frequency.[12] In the largest reported American series of IPNBs, the mean age of diagnosis was 67 years and, as opposed to B-MCNs, they tended to occur more commonly in men (67%).[13] However, depending on geographic location, age of diagnosis may range from 50 to 70 years, with sex preponderance favoring women in Taiwan and Japan as opposed to men in Korea and the United States.[14] The increased frequency of IPNBs in Asia is presumed to be secondary to endemic clonorchis infection and hepatolithiasis, which is thought to be at the basis of cyst pathogenesis.[15] Most cases are sporadic, with malignancy detected in 40% to 80% of resected specimens. Most IPNBs are detected incidentally by cross-sectional imaging; however, symptoms may include, most commonly, right upper quadrant pain, jaundice, and cholangitis. Cholangitis can be caused by tumor microemboli in the bile or thick mucin secretion, or can be secondary to gallstone disease, which seems to occur with increased frequency.[14] Other nonspecific findings include anemia and weight loss.

Diagnosis

The diagnosis for the cause of nonspecific abdominal findings often commences with bloodwork, including liver enzymes. The presence of IPNBs may lead to the nonspecific increase of levels of alanine transaminase, aspartate transaminase, and cholestatic enzymes such as ALP, total bilirubin, and GGT. Levels of tumor markers such as CA 19-9 and CEA can be increased secondary to obstructive jaundice or many other unrelated abdominal disorders, although an increased CEA level in the context of a known IPNB may also predict malignancy.[14] The first imaging test is often an ultrasonography scan of the abdomen performed for nonspecific biliary symptoms likely to rule out gallstone disease. This scan may show the findings of biliary dilatation and ectasia. The accuracy of ultrasonography in detecting a mass is approximately 41%, and ultrasonography is generally useful for distinguishing masses from stones.[14] CT and MRI, like B-MCNs, is complimentary to ultrasonography and may also show the findings discussed earlier. Furthermore, a cystic mass may also be detected showing an isodense or hyperenhancing pattern on CT during the late arterial phase with a hypodense pattern on venous/delayed phase. The enhancing pattern of IPNBs differs from that of other cystic lesions and biliary masses because of its suspension on a fibrovascular stalk and confinement to the biliary mucosa. In general, CT can identify a mass larger than 1 cm with a sensitivity of 50%. Like B-MCNs, lesions tend to be localized to the left lobe of the liver; however, contrary to B-MCNs, IPNBs do not show a multiloculated pattern with septations. MRI similarly shows an enhancement pattern like that observed with CT. Lesions are often hypointense on T1 phase compared with the underlying liver and hyperintense on T2 phase. The presence of mucin is not shown by ultrasonography, CT, or MRI. Cholangiography, either endoscopically or by MRI, can be useful in delineating the extent of disease, which is often underappreciated on conventional cross-sectional imaging. Furthermore, mucin hypersecretion and release from the ampulla, like IPMNs, is highly suggestive of IPNBs. This finding, in addition to diffuse biliary ductal dilatation with irregular filling defects, is pathognomonic for the presence of disease. IPNBs radiographically can be subdivided into 5 distinct subtypes[14]:

Type 1: diffuse biliary dilatation with presence of an intraductal mass (45%)
Type 2: diffuse biliary dilatation without the presence of an intraductal mass (24%)
Type 3: localized biliary dilatation with the presence of an intraductal mass (20%)
Type 4: mild biliary dilatation with intraductal casts (4%)
Type 5: focal biliary stricture with proximal ductal dilatation (7%)

Management

IPNBs are an uncommon neoplasm of the bile duct but are found in approximately 10% of cholangiocarcinomas.[16] Furthermore, 40% to 80% of lesions, as previously mentioned, harbor invasive cancer. As such, formal oncologic resection with clear margins is essential for all types of IPNBs. This is in sharp contrast with IPMNs, whereby certain branch-type lesions without worrisome or high-risk features can be serially observed. IPNBs confined to the liver are managed with hepatectomy, whereas involvement of the extrahepatic biliary tree requires bile duct resection with reconstruction. Although not well studied, percutaneous ablation, sclerosis, or cyst fenestration is not advised because of the risk of malignancy. Intraoperative frozen sections should be performed to ensure clear margins. Hilar lesions should undergo both hepatectomy and bile duct resection, although resection of the caudate lobe or vessels of the porta hepatitis should be performed selectively based on tumor involvement. In addition, although liver transplant has been described for IPNBs, patients with diffuse hepatic involvement deemed nonoperative candidates should be referred to a high-volume transplant center for further consideration.[17]

Pathology

Grossly, IPNBs show a polypoid mass that may be solitary or multifocal. Unlike B-MCNs, IPNBs have a direct communication with the dilated bile duct and may track longitudinally along the length of the involved biliary segment. Lesions may also appear as multilocular cystic masses filled with mucin.[14] Like IPMNs, the microscopic histology of IPNBs is divided into 4 categories: pancreaticobiliary, oncocytic, gastric, and intestinal subtypes (**Fig. 2**).[13] Mucin hypersecretion tends to be associated with the intestinal subtype. Furthermore, pancreaticobiliary and intestinal subtypes of IPNBs are commonly involved with high-grade dysplasia or invasive carcinoma (either tubular or colloid carcinoma). Also similar to IPMNs is the expression of mucin core-type proteins (MUCs), which differ between varying histologic subtypes. MUC1 is most commonly seen with the pancreaticobiliary subtype, whereas MUC2 is expressed on the intestinal subtype. Cystic IPNBs resemble B-MCNs histologically, but lack the characteristic ovarian stroma, which is a feature allowing differentiation between these two types of lesions.

Prognosis

Like IPMNs, invasive carcinoma associated with IPNBs is associated with improved survival compared with a pure ductal phenotype. In the largest reported series, of 39 patients, median OS was 62 months for the entire cohort and 49 months for cases with invasive cancer.[13] Five-year RFS has been described as 81% in patients having undergone a formal oncologic resection.[18] Median RFS was 82 months in patients with negative margins versus 36 months in patients with microscopic positive margins. Most recurrences occurred in the liver, although distant recurrences were also described. Factors associated with survival in addition to margin status include depth of invasion (none, <5 mm, or ≥5 mm), percentage of invasive component (0%, <10%, ≥10%), differentiation, and presence of lymphovascular invasion. On IHC, the expression of MUC1 and CEA was associated with a worse OS in benign IPNBs, whereas only MUC1 provided any prognostic information with invasive disease.

INTRADUCTAL TUBULAR PAPILLARY NEOPLASMS OF THE BILE DUCT
Epidemiology/Presentation

As was described for IPNBs, ITPNs are a fairly new entity described by the WHO classification for cystic biliary lesions, which draws similar parallels to ITPNs of the pancreas (IPTN-Ps). IPTN-Ps are a distinct entity and account for less than 1% of pancreatic lesions.[19] They are defined by the presence of intraductal growth, like IPMNs, but with tubular formation and without mucin production. They are associated with malignancy and thus management involves a formal oncologic resection, and associated invasive cancers show a more favorable prognosis then a pure ductal phenotype. Similarly, ITPNs are rare and show mostly tubular growth with some papillary elements with little to no mucin production.[20] Approximately 40% to 80% of lesions are associated with invasive carcinoma. Like IPNBs, the presentation of these lesions is nonspecific and often detected incidentally on cross-sectional imaging. Median age of diagnosis is 65 years, with a male to female preponderance of 1:2.[21] Symptoms, when present, include abdominal pain and jaundice. ITPNs are found in the biliary tree with the following frequencies: intrahepatic bile ducts (53%), perihilar bile ducts (34%), an extrahepatic bile ducts (17%). Tumors tend to be large, with a median size of 5.3 cm.

Diagnosis

Because of the recent description of ITPNs,[22] coupled with the finding that these lesions represent less than 15% of intraductal biliary neoplasms, diagnostic features, including laboratory findings and characteristic imaging findings, have not been well

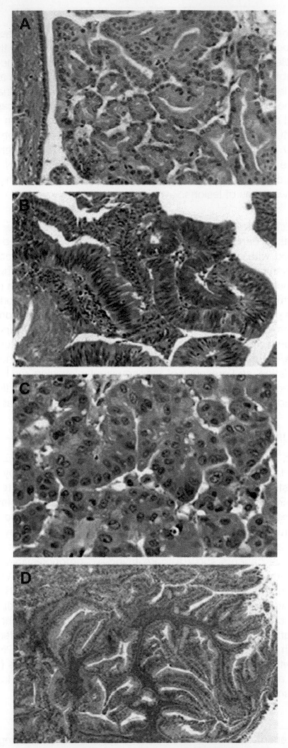

Fig. 2. Histologic subtypes of IPNBs. (*A*) Gastric-type epithelium, (*B*) intestinal-type epithelium, (*C*) oncocytic-type epithelium, (*D*) pancreatobiliary-type epithelium.

described. Often, these lesions are not discernible radiographically from IPNBs or underlying cholangiocarcinoma. In the largest published series comparing clinicopathologic and MRI features of ITPNs with IPNBs, 40% of patients with ITPNs presented with an increased serum bilirubin and liver enzyme level compared with approximately 20% with IPNBs.[23] Increased CA 19-9 level was observed in 60% of patients with ITPNs compared with 30% with IPNBs. On MRI, ITPNs showed an intraductal soft tissue mass with enhancement of the peribiliary liver and upstream biliary ductal dilatation. Lesions with cancer showed findings like those discussed earlier but with liver capsule retraction. The investigators also describe a characteristic finding of IPNBs on MRI, which included dilatations of the upstream and downstream biliary ducts and the presence of a so-called thread sign seen as curvilinear hypointense striations in the bile duct not seen with ITPNs. Unique to ITPNs are the finding of so-called cork-of-wine and 2-tone-duct signs caused by the encasement of tumor with surrounding bile.[23] The value of MRCP, ERCP, and PET scans for ITPNs has not been well characterized and thus a recommendation for or against their diagnostic utility cannot be provided.

Treatment

Because of the high frequency of associated invasive carcinoma, ITPNs should be managed with a formal oncologic resection, which includes a partial hepatectomy for intrahepatic disease. Lesions of the perihilar biliary and extrahepatic biliary tree should be managed by bile duct resection and reconstruction with or without partial hepatectomy, depending on tumor location and involvement of surrounding liver parenchyma (**Fig. 3**.). Liver transplant has been described for ITPNs; however, such patients should be referred to a formal transplant center for consideration.[12]

Pathology

ITPNs are defined by the presence of a mass-forming exophytic lesion growing from and in communication with the biliary tree. As previously described, these lesions are nonmucinous with minimal (<30%) papillary component. Microscopically, ITPNs are characterized by large, smooth nodules and tubular units with minimal or absent stroma.[20] On histology, cells are composed of columnar or cuboidal cells with occasional prominent nucleoli. Lesions associated with invasive carcinoma show a tubular formation indistinguishable from conventional cholangiocarcinoma. In up to 25% of cases, lesions show a large group of cells with smooth contours and the presence of comedonecrosis, which is unique to carcinomas arising from ITPNs. On IHC,

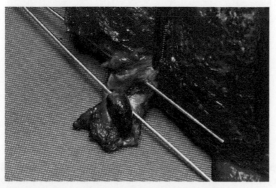

Fig. 3. Hilar cholangiocarcinoma arising in the setting of ITPN.

more than 80% of lesions express MUC1 with absence of MUC2 and MUC5A.[20] On mutational analyses of ITPNs, conventional oncogenes associated with tumorigenesis in pancreaticobiliary tumors (KRAS, GNAS, BRAF) were uninvolved. This feature, in addition to the absence of MUC2 and MUC5A, is thought to be pathognomonic of ITPNs.[21]

Prognosis

Prognostic data in ITPNs have been extrapolated from case studies and single-center case series. In general, ITPNs show indolent behavior even in the presence of invasive carcinoma. Overall 5-year survival is 90%; however, it is unclear whether the favorable prognosis is secondary to early detection or caused by the differing molecular pathways of tumorigenesis compared with other pancreaticobiliary lesions.

CHOLEDOCHAL CYSTS
Epidemiology/Presentation

Of the premalignant cystic lesions of the biliary tract, CCs are the best characterized and described in the medical literature. Despite this, CCs are a rare congenital cystic dilatation of the biliary tract, occurring at a frequency of 1 per 150,000 in the United States and 1 per 13,000 in Asia.[24] They cluster in the pediatric population and have a male to female ratio of 1:4. Although the pathogenesis of these cysts is unknown, up to 70% are associated with the presence of an anomalous pancreaticobiliary junction (APBJ). The APBJ causes the union of the pancreatic duct and CBD outside of the duodenum, forming a long common channel at least 15 mm distal to the AOV (**Fig. 4**). This long common channel predisposes to reflux of pancreatic secretions into the CBD, which is thought to contribute to the development, if not the cause, of biliary cyst formation.[25] Signs and symptoms of CCs, when present, most commonly occur in childhood or early adulthood. The classic triad of presentation of CCs is abdominal pain, jaundice, and the palpation of an abdominal mass. However, a presentation with all 3 elements of the classic triad is rare and most cases are still diagnosed incidentally on cross-sectional imaging. Adults tend to present with abdominal pain, cholangitis, or pancreatitis as opposed to the presence of an abdominal mass or jaundice. The risk of

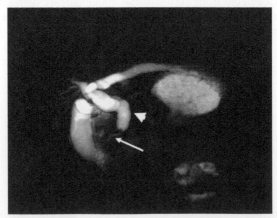

Fig. 4. Abnormal pancreatobiliary junction with choledochal cyst and gallstone. A patient with choledochal cyst. Arrow shows an abnormal pancreatobiliary junction. Arrowhead demarcates the choledochal cyst.

developing cholangiocarcinoma is 10% to 15% and the risk increases with advancing age.[26]

Diagnosis

As with other cystic lesions of the biliary tract, diagnosis often involves a combination of laboratory investigation and multiple imaging modalities. In general, laboratory abnormalities are nonspecific and rarely point toward the diagnosis of a CC. Increased liver enzyme level, including alterations in ALP and total bilirubin, may suggest some form of biliary disorder. Most commonly, the finding of a CC is made with imaging. CCs are divided into 5 distinct types:

Type 1 (80%–90%): fusiform or cystic dilatation of the extrahepatic biliary tree
   1A: cystic dilatation of the entire extrahepatic biliary tree associated with APBJ
   1B: dilatation of the distal CBD not associated with APBJ
   IC: fusiform dilatation of the entire extrahepatic biliary tree associated with APBJ
Type II (2%): true diverticulum of the extrahepatic biliary tree
Type III (1%–4%): cystic dilatation of the intraduodenal CBD at the pancreaticobiliary junction, termed choledochocele
Type IV (1%–2%): cystic dilatation of the intrahepatic and extrahepatic biliary tree
   IVA: dilatation of the extrahepatic and intrahepatic bile ducts
   IVB: multiple dilatations of the extrahepatic bile duct
Type V (<1%): isolated saccular or fusiform dilatation of the intrahepatic biliary tree with no involvement of the extrahepatic biliary tree (Caroli disease)

Typically, the first imaging modality used to diagnose suspected biliary disorder is abdominal ultrasonography. Except for type III and type V cysts, ultrasonography shows a cystic mass of the extrahepatic biliary tree.[27] The presence of intrahepatic biliary dilatation should prompt further investigation with cross-sectional imaging. CT scans have a sensitivity and specificity of greater than 90% for the detection of CCs. CT scans are useful for showing continuity of the cyst with the biliary tract and for further characterizing the remainder of the biliary tract and determining the presence of malignancy. However, the most sensitive and specific (90%–100%) noninvasive imaging modality remains MRI/MRCP, which is capable of delineating with high resolution the state of the biliary tract in relation to the CC. Although considered the most sensitive modality for imaging the biliary tract, ERCP is now used for characterizing biliary anatomy when MRI fails or for relieving biliary obstruction when present or suspected.

Treatment

Because of the increased risk of malignancy, the mainstay of management is surgical resection. For type I and IV CCs, surgical resection involves complete resection of the extrahepatic biliary tree to the level of the pancreaticobiliary junction with cholecystectomy and biliary reconstruction. In type IVA lesions, resection of the extrahepatic biliary tree is often sufficient, with resolution of the intrahepatic component in 3 to 6 months, although extensive intrahepatic disease and risk of postoperative structuring may warrant partial hepatectomy.[24] Type II lesions can be managed with diverticulectomy and primary closure because of the low risk of malignancy, and similarly small type III lesions can be managed with endoscopic sphincterotomy. Larger choledochoceles require transduodenal excision. Management of type V lesions, termed Caroli disease, depends on distribution of cystic involvement. Localized disease can be managed with partial hepatectomy; however, involvement of the entire intrahepatic biliary tree requires assessment for liver transplant.

Pathology

Pathologic findings common to all types of CCs include acute and chronic mucosa inflammation, mucosal dysplasia, and a scarcity of mucus-producing glands.[24] Irreversible changes to the liver include portal fibrosis and central venous distension, whereas parenchymal inflammation and bile duct proliferation are reversible following treatment. As previously discussed, risk of malignancy remains increased for type I and IV CCs, whereas it is negligible for types II, III, and V. This increased risk is presumed to be secondary to the presence of APBJ and thus some malignant contribution from an increased level of pancreatic enzymes. On histology, type I and IV CCs are characterized by a lack of biliary mucosa and an increase in biliary intraepithelial neoplasia with advancing age. Type II lesions resemble gallbladder tissue akin to gallbladder duplication, whereas type III CCs are lined by duodenal mucosa.

Prognosis

Outcomes following surgical resection in the absence of carcinoma remain favorable, with a 5-year OS greater than 90%. In patients with CCs associated with malignancy, the prognosis remains poor, with a median OS of 6 to 21 months.[24] Despite an adequate resection of CCs in the absence of malignancy, the risk of subsequent cancer remains increased (up to 11% 25 years after cyst excision).[28] Further analysis shows that malignancy risk increases substantially 15 years after cyst excision. Thus, continued surveillance of the biliary tree, usually with MRI, is required following bile duct excision and reconstruction.

SUMMARY

With the increasing use of cross-sectional imaging, premalignant lesions of the biliary tract are being detected with increasing frequency. Despite this, their occurrence is rare and therefore knowledge of these lesions is important because they may degenerate into cholangiocarcinoma. They are often asymptomatic or associated with nonspecific abdominal complaints such as right upper quadrant pain. Because of their risk of malignancy, patients should be referred early to a hepatobiliary surgeon for consideration of resection and managed at a center specializing in the multidisciplinary care of biliary malignancies.

REFERENCES

1. Serra S. Precursor neoplastic lesions of the biliary tract. J Clin Pathol 2014;67(10): 875–82.
2. Ando H. Embryology of the biliary tract. Dig Surg 2010;27(2):87–9.
3. Simo KA, Mckillop IH, Ahrens WA, et al. Invasive biliary mucinous cystic neoplasm: a review. HPB (Oxford) 2012;14(11):725–40.
4. Erdogan D, Kloek J, Lamers WH, et al. Mucinous cystadenomas in liver: management and origin. Dig Surg 2010;27(1):19–23.
5. Takano Y, Nagahama M, Yamamura E, et al. Prolapse into the bile duct and expansive growth is characteristic behavior of mucinous cystic neoplasm of the liver: report of two cases and review of the literature. Clin J Gastroenterol 2015; 8(3):148–55.
6. Soares KC, Arnaoutakis DJ, Kamel I, et al. Cystic neoplasms of the liver: biliary cystadenoma and cystadenocarcinoma. J Am Coll Surg 2014;218(1):119–28.
7. Pattarapuntakul T, Ovartlarnporn B, Sottisuporn J. Mucinous cystic neoplasm of the liver with extrahepatic growth presenting with ascending cholangitis

diagnosed by endoscopic ultrasound features: a case report. J Med Case Rep 2018;12(1):33.

8. Arnaoutakis DJ, Kim Y, Pulitano C, et al. Management of biliary cystic tumors: a multi-institutional analysis of a rare liver tumor. Ann Surg 2015;261(2):361–7.

9. Nakayama Y, Kato Y, Okubo S, et al. A case of mucinous cystic neoplasm of the liver: a case report. Surg Case Rep 2015;1(1):9.

10. Martel G, Alsharif J, Aubin JM, et al. The management of hepatobiliary cystade-nomas: lessons learned. HPB (Oxford) 2013;15(8):617–22.

11. Wang M, Deng BY, Wen TF, et al. An observational and comparative study on in-traductal papillary mucinous neoplasm of the biliary tract and the pancreas from a Chinese cohort. Clin Res Hepatol Gastroenterol 2016;40(2):161–8.

12. Zen Y, Jang KT, Ahn S, et al. Intraductal papillary neoplasms and mucinous cystic neoplasms of the hepatobiliary system: demographic differences between Asian and Western populations, and comparison with pancreatic counterparts. Histo-pathology 2014;65(2):164–73.

13. Rocha FG, Lee H, Katabi N, et al. Intraductal papillary neoplasm of the bile duct: a biliary equivalent to intraductal papillary mucinous neoplasm of the pancreas? Hepatology 2012;56(4):1352–60.

14. Wan XS, Xu YY, Qian JY, et al. Intraductal papillary neoplasm of the bile duct. World J Gastroenterol 2013;19(46):8595–604.

15. Ohtsuka M, Shimizu H, Kato A, et al. Intraductal papillary neoplasms of the bile duct. Int J Hepatol 2014;2014:459091.

16. Tominaga K, Kamimura K, Sakamaki A, et al. Intraductal papillary neoplasm of the bile duct: a rare liver tumor complicated by malignancy. Hepatology 2017; 66(5):1695–7.

17. Imvrios G, Papanikolaou V, Lalountas M, et al. Papillomatosis of intra- and extra-hepatic biliary tree: successful treatment with liver transplantation. Liver Transpl 2007;13(7):1045–8.

18. Lee SS, Kim MH, Lee SK, et al. Clinicopathologic review of 58 patients with biliary papillomatosis. Cancer 2004;100(4):783–93.

19. Kuscher S, Steinle H, Soleiman A, et al. Intraductal tubulopapillary neoplasm (ITPN) of the pancreas associated with an invasive component: a case report with review of the literature. World J Surg Oncol 2017;15(1):203.

20. Schlitter AM, Jang KT, Kloppel G, et al. Intraductal tubulopapillary neoplasms of the bile ducts: clinicopathologic, immunohistochemical, and molecular analysis of 20 cases. Mod Pathol 2015;28(9):1249–64.

21. Nakagawa T, Arisaka Y, Ajiki T, et al. Intraductal tubulopapillary neoplasm of the bile duct: a case report and review of the published work. Hepatol Res 2016; 46(7):713–8.

22. Park HJ, Jang KT, Heo JS, et al. A potential case of intraductal tubulopapillary neoplasms of the bile duct. Pathol Int 2010;60(9):630–5.

23. Wu CH, Yeh YC, Tsuei YC, et al. Comparative radiological pathological study of biliary intraductal tubulopapillary neoplasm and biliary intraductal papillary mucinous neoplasm. Abdom Radiol (NY) 2017;42(10):2460–9.

24. Soares KC, Arnaoutakis DJ, Kamel I, et al. Choledochal cysts: presentation, clin-ical differentiation, and management. J Am Coll Surg 2014;219(6):1167–80.

25. Gadelhak N, Shehta A, Hamed H. Diagnosis and management of choledochal cyst: 20 years of single center experience. World J Gastroenterol 2014;20(22): 7061–6.

26. Singham J, Yoshida EM, Scudamore CH. Choledochal cysts: part 1 of 3: classi-fication and pathogenesis. Can J Surg 2009;52(5):434–40.

27. Singham J, Yoshida EM, Scudamore CH. Choledochal cysts: part 2 of 3: diagnosis. Can J Surg 2009;52(6):506–11.

28. Ohashi T, Wakai T, Kubota M, et al. Risk of subsequent biliary malignancy in patients undergoing cyst excision for congenital choledochal cysts. J Gastroenterol Hepatol 2013;28(2):243–7.

Cholangiocarcinoma

Adeel S. Khan, MD, MPH[a],*, Leigh Anne Dageforde, MD, MPH[b]

KEYWORDS

- Cholangiocarcinoma (CCA) • Perihilar cholangiocarcinoma (PHCCA) • Klatskin tumor
- Intrahepatic cholangiocarcinoma (IHCCA)
- Extrahepatic cholangiocarcinoma (EHCCA)

KEY POINTS

- Cholangiocarcinoma is a rare malignancy and accounts for only 2% of all malignancies. Incidence is on the increase in the Western world.
- Cholangiocarcinoma arises from the malignant growth of the epithelial lining of the bile ducts and can be found all along the biliary tree. It can be classified into subtypes based on location: intrahepatic (arising from the intrahepatic biliary tract in the hepatic parenchyma), perihilar (at the hilum of the liver involving the biliary confluence), and distal (extrahepatic, often in the head of the pancreas).
- Despite differences in location of the cholangiocarcinoma, it is associated with a poor prognosis with surgical resection offering the best chance of cure.
- Margin status and locoregional lymph node metastases are the most important determinants of postsurgical outcomes.
- Liver transplantation is currently indicated for a select group of patients with unresectable hilar cholangiocarcinoma in absence of locoregional lymph node spread and metastatic disease in the setting of an institutional protocol involving neoadjuvant chemoradiation.

INTRODUCTION
Nature of the Problem

Cholangiocarcinomas (CCA) are rare tumors arising from the epithelium of the bile ducts (BD) and can involve any part of the biliary tract.[1] Anatomically, they can be classified as *intrahepatic* (IH), arising in the IH BDs in the hepatic parenchyma, or *extrahepatic* (EH). Extrahepatic cholangiocarcinoma (EHCCA) can further be categorized as perihilar (involving BD confluence in the liver hilum) or distal (mid or lower half of the BD, often in the head of pancreas).[1,2] Approximately 60% of CCA are perihilar; 30% arise in the mid or distal BD, and 6% to 10% are IH.[3] Historically, surgical resection has been the only potentially curable option; however, management can

[a] Section of Abdominal Transplant Surgery, Washington University St Louis, One Barnes-Jewish Hospital Plaza, Suite 6107 Queeny Tower, St Louis, MO 63110, USA; [b] Division of Transplant Surgery, Massachusetts General Hospital, 55 Fruit Street, White 511, Boston, MA 02114, USA
* Corresponding author.
E-mail address: Akhan24@wustl.edu

Surg Clin N Am 99 (2019) 315–335
https://doi.org/10.1016/j.suc.2018.12.004
0039-6109/19/© 2018 Elsevier Inc. All rights reserved.

surgical.theclinics.com

be challenging because many patients present in advanced stages with unresectable disease.[1-3] Among patients deemed resectable on initial cross-sectional imaging, approximately 30% are found to be unresectable on exploration, and many of those resected demonstrate microscopically positive margins on final pathology (R1).[3] Moreover, many patients with CCA have underlying primary sclerosing cholangitis (PSC) and/or cirrhosis, which can further complicate decision making and treatment.[1,2] In recent years, liver transplantation (LT) has emerged as a promising option in a small highly selected group of patients with unresectable perihilar cholangiocarcinoma (PHCCA) in the absence of locoregional or distant metastatic disease.

Epidemiology

CCA is a rare tumor comprising only 3% of gastrointestinal malignancies and has an annual incidence of 5000 new cases in the United States.[1-3] Worldwide, intrahepatic cholangiocarcinoma (IHCCA) is the second most common liver tumor behind hepatocellular carcinoma (HCC) and accounts for approximately 10% to 25% of all hepatobiliary malignancies.[1] CCA is far more prevalent in Asia, where in some parts the incidence is as high as 113 per 100,000.[1] In comparison, the incidence of CCA in the West is much lower at 2.1 new cases per 100,000 population; however, reports indicate a trend toward increasing rates in recent years.[4,5] CCA affects men more frequently than women with ratios of 1:1.2 to 1.5, rarely occurs before age of 40, and typically presents in the seventh decade of life.[1,2]

Risk Factors

There are several well-described risk factors for CCA.

Primary sclerosing cholangitis

PSC is an autoimmune disease resulting in inflammation and stricturing of interhepatic and/or extrahepatic BDs and is a well-established risk factor for CCA because of ongoing inflammation, epithelial proliferation, and bile stasis. The reported lifetime incidence of CCA among PSC patients is as high as 36%.[1,6]

Choledochal cysts

Patients with choledochal cysts are at a 10- to 50-fold higher risk of developing CCA (IHCCA and EHCCA).[1,2,7] The lifetime incidence of CCA in these patients ranges from 6% to 30% and is thought to be secondary to reflux of pancreatic enzymes, bile stasis, and increased concentration of intraductal bile acids in dilated ducts, which can lead to malignant transformation in the cyst epithelial cells over time.[1,7,8]

Viral hepatitis and cirrhosis

Hepatitis B virus (HBV) and C (HCV) infections and liver cirrhosis, regardless of cause, have been reported as risk factors for CCA. Sorensen and colleagues[9] followed 11,605 patients with cirrhosis over a period of 6 years and reported a 10-fold increase in risk of CCA in patients with cirrhosis. Shahib and colleagues[10] reviewed 625 cases of IHCCA in the United States and reported a significant association with HCV, whereas many studies from HBV endemic countries in Asia have implicated HBV as a risk factor for IHCCA.[1,8]

Hepatolithiasis

Hepatolithiasis is an established risk factor for IHCCA with up to 10% of patients with hepatolithiasis developing CCA in some parts of Asia.[8,11] Postulated mechanisms of malignant transformation in biliary epithelium include prolonged irritation by stones, bile stasis, and cholangitis.[1,11]

Parasitic infections
Opisthorchis viverrini and *Clonorchis sinensis* are hepatobiliary flukes that have a well-established association with CCA particularly in Southeast Asia where these infestations are common. Shin and colleagues[12] demonstrated a population-attributable risk of CCA in *C sinensis* endemic areas to be as high as 27.9% in men and 16% in women. Parasitic infections are far less common in the West and are rarely encountered as a cause of CCA.[1,2]

Other risk factors
Toxins (particularly Thorotrast exposure during the World War II), inflammatory bowel disease (both ulcerative colitis and Crohn disease), choledocholithiasis and cholangitis, diabetes and obesity, heavy alcohol use, and smoking are some of the other risk factors that have been implicated in the development of CCA.[1,2,8–10]

ANATOMY AND PATHOPHYSIOLOGY

As introduced above, CCA can develop anywhere along the BD system. The location of the CCA impacts the presentation, diagnosis, treatment options, and prognosis.

CCA is a primary biliary cancer arising from a malignant transformation cholangiocyte rather than the hepatocytes, which form the more common liver cancer HCC with malignant transformation.[13] The molecular pathogenesis of CCA involves several different signal transduction pathways. Recent data indicate some of these mutations in genetic traits may be similar between CCA and HCC.[14]

Intrahepatic Cholangiocarcinoma

Gene mutations
Regarding specific mutations and IHCCA, the KRAS mutation is one of the most frequently seen in CCA and is an oncogene shown to induce IHCCA in mouse models.[15] About 20% of IHCCA have a loss of function mutation of gene TP53, which has been shown to be oncogenic.[16] Most recently, mutations in isocitrate dehydrogenase (IDH1) and 2 (IDH2) have been appreciated in 10% to 23% of IHCCA.[17] Although mass-forming CCA is the most common IHCCA phenotype (85%), other phenotypes include periductal IHCCA that grows along the BD and intraductal-growth IHCCA.[18] The differences in these types can impact surgical management and clinical outcomes.

Staging
Until 2011, there was not a uniform TNM staging for IHCCA. After the seventh edition of American Joint Committee on Cancer (AJCC) TNM staging for IHCCA was developed. This 7th edition of AJCC TNM staging was found to be accurate and beneficial in predicting outcomes for patients undergoing resection for IHCCA.[19]

Extrahepatic Cholangiocarcinoma

Perihilar cholangiocarcinoma
Perihilar cholangiocarcinoma (PHCCA) is the most common subtype of CCA and accounts for approximately 60% of biliary tract malignancies.[20] Although considerable progress has been made in diagnosing and treating HCCA since the condition was first described by Altemeier in 1957, it still remains a challenging problem with considerable morbidity and mortality.[20]

Cause and associated gene mutations Most PHCCA cases occur spontaneously, and although chronic inflammation and bile stasis have been implicated as common risk factors, the precise cause remalns unclear. Specific genetic mutations have been linked with PHCCA and include K-ras, C-myc, p53, and Bcl-2. K-ras mutations in particular have been reported in up to 60% of patients, are more frequently seen in perihilar tumors greater than 3 cm and in patients with lymph node metastasis, and are often associated with poor survival.[21,22]

Tumor subtypes Pathologically, EHCCA can be further classified into 3 distinct subtypes: sclerosing (70%), nodular (20%), and papillary (5%–10%). Sclerosing and nodular tumors are typically firm and commonly involve the hilum. These tumors, particularly sclerosing subtype, cause circumferential thickening of the BD with radial or longitudinal tumor spread and demonstrate an early involvement of the lymphatic plexus around the BDs. These tumors are rarely confined to the BD and often demonstrate direct extension into surrounding hepatic parenchyma at the time of diagnosis. For this reason, successful resection of PHCCA almost always mandates an en bloc partial hepatectomy. Papillary tumors on the other hand are typically located in the distal BD, often have a well-defined stalk making them less likely to invade adjacent structures, and are generally associated with a favorable prognosis after resection.[21,23]

Classification and staging Classification of PHCCA involves not only differentiating it from IHCCA and distal cholangiocarcinoma (DCCA) but also stratifying tumors based on specific anatomic and prognostic factors.[20,21] In 1975, Bismuth and Corlette[24] first described their criteria for categorizing PHCCA based on the extent to which the common hepatic duct (CHD), BD confluence, and left and right ducts were involved by the tumor. The classification system and subsequent modifications by the investigators in 1992 categorized lesions into 4 subtypes and made recommendations for type and extent of surgical resection for each subtype ranging from local excision for type I lesions to hepatectomy and LT for type intravenous (IV) lesions[25] (**Table 1**). Although this classification system is useful for stratifying patients based on biliary involvement, it is limited in ability to predict resectability and survival because it does not take into consideration vascular involvement, lobar atrophy, and spread to regional lymph nodes.[20,21,23] The group at *Memorial Sloan Kettering Cancer Center (MSKCC)* attempted to expand on the Bismuth-Corlette classification by proposing a preoperative T-staging system that stratifies patients into 2 groups based on (1) extent of BDs involved by tumor, (2) portal vein involvement, and (3) presence of lobar atrophy.[26] Jarnagin and colleagues[26] demonstrated that this staging system correlated with resectability, likelihood of achieving an R0 resection, presence of metastatic disease, and median survival. Another frequently used staging system is the *AJCCTNM staging system*, which considers the size and extent of primary tumor, regional lymph node status, and distant metastasis.[27] This system is helpful in determining resectability of the tumor, but critics have questioned its ability to accurately predict survival.[21,23,28]

Table 1
Modified Bismuth-Corlette classification for hilar cholangiocarcinoma

Type	Definition
I	Stricture below the main hepatic confluence
II	Stricture confined to main hepatic confluence
IIIA	Stricture extends into main right hepatic duct
IIIB	Stricture extends into main left hepatic duct
IV	Stricture extends into right and left hepatic ducts

Distal cholangiocarcinoma

DCCA is defined as a tumor arising from the common BD below the confluence of the cystic duct and above the ampulla of Vater and constitutes approximately 20% to 40% of all diagnosed CCA. In the seventh edition of the AJCC staging manual published in 2010, for the first time distal BD tumors were classified as a separate entity and staged separately from IHCCA and PHCCA.[1,2,4,5,27] This TNM staging system considers tumor extent, lymph node spread, and presence of distant metastases and is a useful prognostic tool.

CLINICAL PRESENTATION

Table 2 summarizes the common signs and symptoms associated with CCA.

IHCCA diagnosis is often incidental. When patients do present with symptoms, they are usually symptoms such as fullness and rarely pain resulting from the size of the liver mass. Oftentimes the patients have normal liver function. Patients with EHCCA most often present with jaundice but can also have unintentional weight loss, general malaise, and occasional right upper quadrant pain.[29]

Most patients (>90%) with *EHCCA* present with symptoms of obstructive jaundice (jaundice, tea-colored urine, alcoholic stools, cholangitis, pruritis, and such). Jaundice may not be apparent if only the right- or left-sided BDs are involved, but these patients may still have other symptoms, such as vague abdominal pain, weight loss, and anorexia.[30] Patients with papillary tumors may present with intermittent episodes of obstructive jaundice due to small pieces of tumor breaking off and causing obstruction. Clinical examination may be remarkable for jaundice, possible hepatomegaly, or a palpable gallbladder if the obstruction is distal to cystic duct insertion. In addition, some patients can be diagnosed based on abnormal liver function tests, particularly alkaline phosphatase and serum bilirubin, both of which can be elevated with obstructive processes.[20,21]

DIAGNOSIS

Table 3 summarizes the commonly used diagnostic tests for IH and EHCCA.

Intrahepatic Cholangiocarcinoma

The first step in diagnosis of IHCCA includes high-quality abdominal imaging with either liver protocol triple-phase *computed tomography (CT) scan or MRI.* On CT

Table 2 Signs and symptoms of intrahepatic and extrahepatic cholangiocarcinoma		
	Signs	Symptoms
IHCCA	• Increased liver function tests • Mass found on screening ultrasound in patients with underlying liver disease • Palpable liver edge or mass in the right upper quadrant • Jaundice (rare in IHCCA)	• Malaise • Right upper-quadrant fullness • Right upper-quadrant pain • Failure to thrive/weight loss
EHCCA (PHCCA + DCCA)	• Jaundice • Elevated liver function tests and alkaline phosphatase	• Pruritus • Unintentional weight loss • Clay-colored stools • Abdominal pain

Table 3 Commonly used diagnostic tests for intrahepatic and extrahepatic cholangiocarcinoma	
	Diagnosis
IHCCA	• Imaging: CT and/or MRI • Tumor markers: CA 19-9, AFP • Imaging Guided percutaneous biopsy

EHCCA-PHCCA	• Imaging: CT and/or MRI/MRCP
	  ○ CT angiography often helpful to evaluate vessel involvement
	  ○ MRCP to evaluate BD involvement
	• Tumor markers: CA 19-9
	• ERCP with biopsy and brushings
	• FISH

EHCCA-DCCA	• Imaging: pancreas protocol CT and/or MRI/MRCP • Tumor marker: CA 19-9 • ERCP with biopsy and brushings • FISH • EUS to evaluate pancreas head for any possible mass more consistent with pancreatic adenocarcinoma

imaging, IHCCA is hypodense on noncontrasted CT and has peripheral rim enhancement in the arterial phase. There is progressive hyperattenuation on venous and delayed phases.[31,32] IHCCA on MR shows up as hypointense on T1, and hyperintense on T2-weighted images. In addition, rim hyperenhancement in the arterial phase is consistent with IHCCA.[33] Unlike the use of the Liver Reporting and Data System criteria to diagnose HCC on MRI in cirrhotic patients, imaging is not sufficient for definitive diagnosis of IHCCA, and a patient may still require a biopsy if definitive diagnosis is required. Percutaneous image-guided biopsy is usually the best approach.[31,32]

Tumor markers such as carbohydrate antigen 19-9 (CA 19-9) can be used in the setting of IHCCA but is not highly sensitive or specific for this malignancy. This tumor marker can also be elevated in benign diseases. Although elevated CA 19-9 is not always correlated with CCA, patients with unresectable CCA have significantly higher CA 19-9 levels than patients with resectable CA 19 to 9.[34] Alpha-fetoprotein (AFP) level can be elevated in HCC or mixed IHCCA/HCC tumors but is most commonly not elevated in pure CCA.[34]

Extrahepatic Cholangiocarcinoma (Perihilar Cholangiocarcinoma and Distal Cholangiocarcinoma)

Patients who are suspected of having EHCCA are subjected to *blood testing*, including complete blood count, coagulation profile, and liver function tests. Serum alkaline phosphatase and bilirubin levels are often elevated, suggestive of an obstructive pathologic condition. Tumor markers such as CA 19-9 and carcinoembryonic antigen may be falsely elevated in patients with hyperbilirubinemia, but may be relevant after biliary decompression. Moreover, 10% of the population does not express Lewis-antigen and CA 19-9 levels may be undetectable even in the setting of CCA. Tumor markers have a role for postoperative surveillance in patients who had elevated levels on initial presentation. A rising CA 19-9 level may be the first sign of recurrent disease.[20,21,23,30,34]

Traditionally, most patients presenting with painless jaundice are initially worked up with an *abdominal ultrasound*, which is a noninvasive and cost-efficient way to assess the biliary tree. Although ultrasound is sensitive for picking up biliary dilation and detecting choledocholithiasis, it is less accurate in determining site of obstruction, delineation of mass if present, and presence of metastatic disease.[28,32]

High-quality *cross-sectional imaging* is the single most important diagnostic and staging test in patients suspected of having CCA.[35] The most recent guidelines from National Comprehensive Cancer Center recommend imaging with contrast enhanced (triple or quadruple phase) CT scan or MRI /magnetic resonance cholangiopancreatography (MRCP).[23] The radiographic interpretation should focus on the location and extent of biliary involvement (staging), involvement of vascular structures (hepatic artery, portal vein, superior mesenteric vessels), and evidence of IH, locoregional (perihilar or portal lymph nodes), or distant metastatic disease.[35–37] Cross-sectional imaging for PHCCA also provides information on liver volumes, caudate involvement, and lobar atrophy; all of which are extremely valuable in planning surgical intervention. CT should be performed with IV contrast, and images should be obtained with thin 1- to 2-mm cuts in arterial pancreatic and portal venous phases of IV contrast.[21,23,35,36] MRI with MRCP has an advantage of clear delineation of extent of BD involvement and a better diagnostic specificity in diagnosing benign causes of hilar obstruction. Chryssou and colleagues[37] demonstrated MRI with MRCP to have an accuracy of approximately 80% in predicting successful resection of PHCCA. The diagnostic and staging accuracy of both modalities significantly diminishes after biliary stent placement due to decompression and imaging artifacts.[21,23]

EHCCA tend not to be fludeoxyglucose avid so *PET* has low sensitivity for diagnosing CCA or providing information on anatomic resectability. PET/CT has a specificity of about 80% for the detection of distant metastatic disease as well as lymph node metastasis, but rarely adds to information obtained from other staging modalities.[23,38]

Direct cholangiography through either *endoscopic retrograde cholangiography (ERC)* or *percutaneous transhepatic cholangiography (PTC)* offers excellent visualization of the biliary tree and can provide with a good understanding of the location and extent of stricture.[39–42] ERC and PTC also have the advantage of allowing one to obtain BD tissue for histologic examination. Because of fibrotic nature of these tumors, it is often difficult to obtain a pathologic diagnosis; endoscopic brushings and washings yield a positive result in only about 40% of EHCC patients.[20,39–42] Newer technique of fluorescent in situ hybridization (FISH) targets pericentromeric regions of chromosome 3, 7, and 17 and can significantly enhance the sensitivity of brush biopsies.[23] The finding of polysomy is diagnostic of malignancy with a sensitivity of 50% and specificity of greater than 95%.[23] However, it must be pointed out that, in the absence of suspicion for benign cause of biliary obstruction, a tissue diagnosis is not mandatory before proceeding with attempted resection or transplantation. On the other hand, pathologic confirmation is mandatory before chemotherapy or radiation, outside of an institutional transplant protocol. Use of *ERCP-guided digital cholangioscopy (Spyglass)* can further enhance the diagnostic sensitivity and specificity for CCA to 90% and 95.8%, respectively, by aiding in direct visualization of the BDs, tissue sampling, and therapeutic maneuvers.[20,21,23] *Endoscopic ultrasound (EUS)* can also provide valuable information in staging EHCC, assessing depth of tumor and relationship with adjacent vascular structures. Moreover, EUS can also allow fine needle aspiration biopsies from suspicious regional or distant lymph nodes, which can provide valuable information and can sometimes change the treatment plan.[39] Percutaneous or laparoscopic biopsy of tumors or lymph nodes is not recommended because of the high risk of disease dissemination.[43]

MANAGEMENT OPTIONS
Intrahepatic Cholangiocarcinoma

Surgical management: resection
Surgical resection is the treatment of choice for IHCCA when possible, but unfortunately, many patients present with late-stage, unresectable disease. Before surgical resection, full assessment of the extent of disease is necessary to assure complete resection of the IHCCA with sufficient functional liver remnant (FLR). Prognosis remains poor for large tumors with lymphovascular invasion, nodal disease, or multicentricity. If needed, patients can undergo pre-resection treatment to grow the remnant liver. Details on volume assessment and FLR optimization are presented under the section on PHCCA.

Surgical management: liver transplantation
LT, although a mainstay of treatment of HCC, has not been widely accepted as a treatment strategy for CCA. In very early IHCCA, there have been positive outcomes with increased survival in selected patients with small tumors. These multicenter retrospective studies were performed using liver explant pathology. The outcomes were significantly better for patients with solitary IHCCA less than 2 cm.[44,45] There is also a report of LT in 25 patients with unresectable IHCCA at University of California, Los Angeles over more than 20 years.[46] In many patients undergoing LT for IHCCA, the tumors are found incidentally postoperatively on pathology, and therefore, patients do not receive neoadjuvant chemotherapy.[47] A recent study outlines a prospective protocol for liver transplant in patients with IHCCA responsive to neoadjuvant therapy, but to date over 7 years only 6 patients have been successfully transplanted.[48]

Management of unresectable disease
Unresectable patients can receive chemotherapy, radiation therapy, placement of a hepatic artery infusion pump (HAIP), and liver-directed therapy. For patients receiving *chemotherapy* alone, combination therapy provides the best benefit. The ABC-02 trial included 410 patients treated with Gemcitabine + Cisplatin versus Gemcitabine alone in a mixed group of patients with biliary tract malignancies. Overall, addition of Cisplatin improved outcome and slowed the time of progression significantly from 5 to 8 months as well as lengthened overall survival from 8.1 to 11.7 months.[49] Recent data have shown that combining systemic chemotherapy with chemoradiation therapy improves outcomes.[50] On review of the SEER (Surveillance, Epidemiology, and End Results) database, palliative *radiotherapy* for unresectable IHCCA was associated with improved overall and cancer-free survival.[51]

Another option for patients with unresectable disease is targeted therapy using *HAIP*. After the pump is placed, the patient receives a continuous infusion of fluorodeoxyuridine in combination with systemic chemotherapy. Data from MSKCC show improved survival for patients treated with combination systemic therapy and HAIP chemotherapy.[52] The investigators describe successful downstaging in a few patients from unresectable to resectable disease, which may indicate a possible future role of intra-arterial therapy in patients with borderline resectable disease.[52]

Liver-directed therapy is an option for patients who are not surgical candidates and for patients presenting with disease too extensive for resection. Liver-directed therapy can include treatment with *radioembolization, transarterial chemoembolization, and ablation*, most commonly radiofrequency ablation (RFA). In a recent review of the National Cancer Database, patients with more advanced stage of IHCCA were less likely to receive RFA, and RFA was only associated with a survival benefit in stage I disease. Patients with more advanced disease benefited from radioembolization and radiation.[53] Radioembolization with yttrium-90 (Y-90) in unresectable IHCCA has been shown in several studies to be successful in reducing the size of unresectable IHCCA, and some patients have been able to proceed to resection following Y-90 treatment.[54,55]

Extrahepatic Perihilar Cholangiocarcinoma

Surgical management: resection
Determination of resectability Surgical resection is the best chance of long-term survival and cure in patients with PHCCA. The goals of surgical resection are to resect involved intrahepatic and extrahepatic BDs (R0 resection) along with draining portal lymph nodes. Successful resection of the biliary confluence almost always involves resection of right or left liver (depending on extent of tumor), and often the caudate lobe especially with left-sided tumors. Five-year survival rates following resection generally range from 25% to 50% with long-term survival being limited by locoregional recurrence and distant metastases.[20,21,23,26,56] Patients with positive microscopic (R1) or gross (R2) margin have a significantly worse outcome with median surgical ranging from 12 to 21 months.[23]

Resectability is determined by ability to have options for biliary reconstruction and to leave behind adequate future liver remnant (FLR). With this basic principle in mind, experts at the Americas Hepato-Pancreato-Biliary Association hilar CCA consensus meeting put forth the following criteria for categorizing a nonmetastatic PHCCA as unresectable: (1) bilateral segmental ductal extension, (2) unilateral atrophy with either contralateral segmental ductal or vascular inflow involvement, and (3) unilateral segmental ductal extension with contralateral vascular inflow involvement.[23] Despite these seemingly clear guidelines, up to 50% of patients are found unresectable at time of surgery, and of those resected, an R0 resection can only be achieved in 70% to 80% patients, indicating that there is room for improvement in preoperative workup despite the recent advances in cross-sectional imaging.[20,21,23,26]

Preoperative planning and workup Patients being considered for resection are assessed for their medical candidacy for a major hepatic resection and thorough cardiopulmonary workup performed when indicated. In addition, patients requiring right hepatectomy or extended resection for PHCCA are at risk for post-hepatectomy liver failure (PHLF) as sequelae of inadequate functional/FLR, and careful assessment of FLR quality and volume is vital before proceeding with resection. Volume optimization strategies, such a portal vein embolization (PVE), should be considered in patients with borderline or inadequate FLR.

Assessment of future liver remnant volume and quality FLR is defined as a percentage of remaining functional liver volume compared with preoperative functional liver volume (total liver volume with tumor volume subtracted). FLR volume serves as a predictor of remnant liver function, and therefore, FLR is widely used as a surrogate for risk of developing PHLF. Several 3-dimensional packages are available for use with CT and MRI for estimating liver volumes. In general, FLR $\geq$20% in otherwise healthy liver is associated with good postresection outcomes, and this cutoff has been well established as the minimum safe limit of resection.[57,58] In patients with mild steatosis, cholestasis, and early cirrhosis (Childs-Pugh A), the safe limits for FLR is in the range of 30% to 35% and increases to a minimum of 40% in patients with severe steatosis and cholestasis.[58]

In addition to the volume, it is also important to have an idea of the function of the FLR, which can be diminished in patients with hepatosteatosis, in patients with cholestasisis, and in those who have received systemic chemotherapy. Tests like indocyanine green clearance, galactose elimination test, lidocaine-monoethylglycinexylidide, test, and the ^{13}C-aminopyrine breath test are some of the available tests for functional assessment of liver before resection.[59]

Strategies for optimization of the functional liver remnant: portal vein embolization PVE is the most commonly used strategy for FLR volume optimization in PHCCA patients with inadequate or borderline FLR. It has been shown in multiple studies to be effective in inducing lobar hypertrophy with a low risk of complications (<3%).[20,23,60] Many patients with PHCCA have significant cholestasis and/or require neoadjuvant chemotherapy for locally advanced disease, and therefore, a higher FLR cutoff of 30% to 40% is used by most centers.[20] Studies have shown median FLR growth of 40% to 62% after a median of 34 to 37 days of PVE with 72% to 80% of patients able to undergo resection as originally planned.[61,62] Abulkhir and colleagues[63] reported results from a meta-analysis of 1088 patients undergoing PVE and showed a markedly lower incidence of PHLF and death compared with series reporting outcomes after major hepatectomy in patients who did not undergo PVE. All patients had FLR volume increase, and 85% went on to have liver resection after PVE with a PHLF incidence of 2.5% and a surgical mortality of 0.8%. Most of the contralateral liver hypertrophy occurs within the first 3 to 4 weeks of PVE, and rates can be slower in patients with underlying parenchymal disease and/or cirrhosis.[58] If FLR after PVE remains ≤20% or if the degree of hypertrophy is ≤5%, liver resection should be considered high risk and may be contraindicated.[64]

Preoperative biliary drainage The choice and indication of preoperative biliary drainage in patients with PHCCA remains a topic of controversy. Proponents of preoperative drainage cite studies that show major hepatic resection in the setting of jaundice, and significant biliary obstruction can impact FLR hypertrophy and contribute to PHLF and postoperative morbidity,[65–67] whereas opponents cite increased rates of cholangitis with biliary instrumentation, potential delay in therapy, and lack of studies demonstrating an impact on postoperative mortality or improvement in overall survival.[21,66,68] However, there is clear consensus that preoperative biliary drainage should be performed in PHCCA patients with cholangitis, those undergoing neoadjuvant chemotherapy, patients with hyperbilirubinemia-induced malnutrition, hepatic or renal insufficiency, and patients undergoing PVE.[23] Decompression should be prioritized for the FLR rather than biliary system within the proposed resection, because decompression of the remnant liver will aid in restoring metabolic and synthetic function in this portion and minimize potential for atrophy due to chronic biliary obstruction.[20] PTC is viewed by many to be the preferred choice of biliary decompression compared with ERC, because the former technique can allow better delineation of extent of proximal tumor spread, faster normalization of liver enzymes, and potential for decreasing cholangitis-related complications; however, modality of choice may vary from center to center depending on institutional experience with one particular technique.[20,23,67]

Surgical approach and intraoperative considerations Surgical management of PHCCA patients is considerably more challenging compared with IHCCA or DCCA, which can often be treated with hepatectomy or pancreatoduodenectomy, respectively. Patients with concerns for advanced disease on preoperative imaging should be subjected to diagnostic laparoscopy to assess for occult peritoneal metastases, which has shown to help avoid an unnecessary laparotomy incision in approximately 10% patients with peritoneal implants.[69] Definitive surgery for PHCCA required partial hepatectomy with en bloc resection of the EH BD, portal lymphadenectomy, and restoration of biliary continuity with Roux-en-Y hepaticojejunostomy. The caudate lobe is generally resected with all left-sided and most right-sided tumors because the biliary drainage of the caudate lobe is to the left duct or biliary confluence and occasionally into the right biliary system. A dilated caudate lobe duct on preoperative imaging for PHCCA indicates obstruction because of tumor and warrants removal in order to minimize the risk of biliary leak from uncontrolled caudate duct as well as to increase chances of obtaining a negative surgical margin.[20,21,23] Use of intraoperative ultrasound can confirm extent of tumor and relationship with important anatomic structures. Hilar dissection is carried out to dissect all lymph nodes and expose portal structures. Frozen section of distal BD is typically performed to rule out distal spread along BD. The portal vein and hepatic artery to the side being resected and the associated hepatic veins are typically divided extrahepatically, whereas the BD is transected sharply during parenchymal transection. There are many described techniques of parenchymal transection based on individual preference with comparable outcomes; however, the principles of maintaining low central venous pressure during resection and use of intermittent Pringle maneuver can significantly decrease blood loss during the surgery.[70]

Role of vascular resection En bloc resection of portal vein or hepatic artery may be required during hepatectomy in order to obtain a negative surgical margin. Although many centers have shown that a limited portal vein resection can be safely carried out in select patients without any significant increase in postoperative morbidity or mortality, experience with hepatic artery resection has not replicated the same success.[20,71] In select patients portal vein resection and reconstruction, with intention of obtaining a margin negative resection, is indicated for short segment vein involvement on the side of the future liver remnant. Hepatic artery involvement on the other hand is considered a contraindication to resection in most centers around the world.[20,23,71]

Adjuvant treatment Successful R0 resection provides the patient with the best chance of cure. The role of adjuvant therapy after resection in the form of either systemic chemotherapy or chemoradiation is not well defined, but there is clear evidence to suggest that it should be offered to patients with margin-positive or node-positive PHCCA. Kim and colleagues[72] demonstrated that use of adjuvant chemoradiation with capecitabine or 5-fluorouracil (5-FU) in 168 patients with resected CCA was associated with prolonged 5-year overall survival when compared with resection alone (36.5% vs 28.2%), and 5-year locoregional control was similarly increased in the chemoradiation group (58.5% vs 44.4%). Similarly, Borghero and colleagues[73] compared outcomes in 42 patients with either R1 resection or locoregional nodal involvement who received adjuvant chemoradiation with patients with negative resection margins and regional lymph nodes and demonstrated both groups to have similar 5-year overall survival (36% vs 42%, respectively).[74]

Surgical management: liver transplantation
Initial experience with LT for PHCCA included many patients with advanced disease and predictably resulted in dismal outcomes, with many centers reporting 5-year survivals of less than 30%.[73] However, in the past decade or so, LT has evolved to represent a promising option for carefully selected patients with unresectable tumors when used as part of a standardized protocol using neoadjuvant chemoradiation.[75,76] Protocol typically involves neoadjuvant treatment with chemotherapy (5-FU) and radiation (external beam radiation with or without endoluminal brachytherapy boost) for patients with

localized, nonmetastatic PHCCA without IH disease. Diagnostic laparoscopy is performed as a last step, and patients listed for LT if no metastatic and/or lymph node involvement is seen. Oral capecitabine is continued until time of LT.[75,76] The Mayo clinic group published their outcomes in 126 PHCCA patients transplanted over an 18-year period using their protocol and demonstrated a 5-year overall survival of 75% in this highly selected group. The survival in PSC patients was 80% compared with 64% for patients with de novo PHCCA.[77] Murad and colleagues[78] reviewed LT outcomes from 12 high-volume transplant centers in the United States and demonstrated a 65% recurrence-free survival after 5 years in 287 patients with PHCCA who underwent LT after neoadjuvant chemoradiation showing this form of therapy to be highly effective in this carefully selected cohort of patients. It is important to note that patients undergoing LT were highly selected, required to pass stringent inclusion criteria, and had a not insignificant risk of drop out during LT evaluation and waiting time, making it difficult to generalize the results for all patients with PHCCA. Currently, surgical resection remains the treatment of choice for resectable PHCCA patients.

Management of unresectable disease
Chemoradiation with or without intraluminal chemotherapy forms the mainstay of treatment in patients with locally advanced, unresectable tumors who are not candidates for LT with a median survival ranging from 11 months to 15 months.[23] The favored approach in patients with metastatic or locoregional recurrence is systemic chemotherapy with gemcitabine and cisplatin representing first-line chemotherapy agents.[23] Radiation for local recurrence can be associated with significant toxicity to the jejunal limb and generally is not recommended.[20,21] Photodynamic therapy and endoscopic RFA are relatively new modalities that have an evolving role in the treatment algorithm for unresectable CCA patients and may offer a survival advantage over stenting alone.[20,21,23]

Extrahepatic Distal Cholangiocarcinoma

Surgical management
Patients with DCCA are treated similar to patients with ampullary and periampullary tumors with pancreaticoduodenectomy offering the best chance of cure in patients with resectable disease. Goal of surgery should be an R0 resection with emphasis on careful assessment of BD margin with intraoperative frozen section as needed. Patients with borderline resectable disease can be considered for neoadjuvant treatment, especially when there are doubts about ability to achieve a margin-negative resection. Portal vein or superior mesenteric vein resection with reconstruction can be performed for short-segment vein involvement when the vein is clearly involved and resection would maximize chances of obtaining a negative margin. Studies have shown that long-term survival in patients undergoing R0 resection with portal vein reconstruction is similar to patients having standard resection alone.[79] Adequate lymphadenectomy at time of surgery involved removal of regional lymph nodes with pancreaticoduodenectomy specimen. The role of adjuvant therapy after margin-negative and node-negative resection is unclear with most studies not demonstrating any clear advantage with adjuvant chemoradiation or systemic chemotherapy compared with no adjuvant treatment.[80] For patients with R1 resection and/or positive lymph nodes, there is a growing body of literature that supports use of chemoradiation followed by chemotherapy or chemotherapy alone with modest improvement in disease-free and overall survival.[79,80]

Management of unresectable disease
For patients with unresectable or metastatic disease, gemcitabine and cisplatin-based palliative systemic chemotherapy is generally recommended; however, median survival in these patients is less than a year.[79]

CLINICAL OUTCOMES IN THE LITERATURE
Intrahepatic Cholangiocarcinoma

Resection

Even with resection, 5-year survival in patients with IHCCA remains low and ranges from 10% to 49%.[81,82] Tumor recurrence is common and occurs most frequently in the liver. Recurrence rates are dependent on several factors, including resection margins, IHCCA type (intraductal growth, mass forming, and periductal infiltrating), tumor size, tumor multifocality, lymphovascular invasion, neutrophil-to-lymphocyte ratio, prognostic nutritional index, elevated CA 19-9, and lymph node status[18,19,29,83–87] (**Box 1**).

Margin status mattered most in patients with node-negative disease, and R1 resection was independently related with poor survival; however, in patients with node-positive disease, margin status was not independently related to survival. In a study of 212 patients who underwent resection for mass-forming CCA, median survival was related to margin size.[19] Most IHCCA recurrences occur in the first 2 years of resection.[29,36,82]

Liver transplantation

For locally advanced IHCCA, LT has better outcomes than resection alone (5-year survival 33% vs 0% for resection), but transplant outcomes for late-stage tumors are worse than transplant for comparable HCC.[46,47] Outcomes for liver transplant for IHCCA are mixed depending on the study and stage of the tumor. Early-stage IHCCA (≤2 cm) has a better outcome following transplant that is consistent with outcomes following transplant for HCC.[44,47] One of the difficulties in comparing outcomes for patients undergoing LT for IHCCA is that many tumors are found retrospectively on explant pathology, and also that patients receive varied amounts of neoadjuvant treatment with either chemotherapy or liver-directed therapy. **Table 4** summarizes posttransplant outcomes from major studies reporting experience with LT for IHCCA.

There may be a benefit with HAIP placement in select patients ultimately leading to resection, but overall prognosis of patients with unresectable IH CCA is very poor.[52] Despite treatment with systemic chemotherapy, radiation therapy, and liver-directed therapies, median overall survival is often less than 1 year for patients with unresectable disease.[13]

Box 1
Factors associated with recurrence and worse survival after resection for intrahepatic cholangiocarcinoma

- Large tumor size >5 cm
- Tumor multifocality
- Higher TMN stage
- Lymph node metastases
- Lymphovascular invasion
- Margin status (R1 resection in node negative disease)
- Intraductal growth IHCCA type
- Elevated neutrophil-to-lymphocyte ratio
- Low prognostic nutritional index
- Perineural invasion
- Elevated CA 19-9

Table 4
Select reports of outcomes after transplantation for intrahepatic cholangiocarcinoma

Reference	Number of Patients	Recurrence Rate (%)	Median Time to Recurrence (%)	1 y Survival (%)	5 y Survival (%)
Sapisochin et al,[44] 2014					
All IHCCA	29	24.1	14.6 mo	79	45
Very Early Stage (single tumor ≤2 cm)	8	0		100	73
Late Stage	21	36.4		71	34
Hong et al,[98] 2011	25	41	Not reported	52 (2 y)	32
Lee et al,[47] 2018					
All IHCCA (included mixed IHCCA-HCC tumors)	44	36.4	Not reported	63.6	63.6
Early Stage	16	29.4		87.7	35.6
Late Stage	28	40.7		74.1	61.4
Lunsford et al,[48] 2018	6	50	7.6 mo	100	83.3

Hilar Cholangiocarcinoma

Resection

Median survival following resection is 11 to 38 months, and the 5-year survival generally ranges from 20% to 40%, with locoregional metastasis limiting long-term survival.[26,30,56,71,88–92] Results from some of the largest-volume studies on PHCCA are summarized in **Table 5**. One of the strongest determinants of survival is margin status, and patients with positive BD margins have significantly worse survival compared with patients with negative margins.[29] Five-year survival among patients with R0 resection is 27% to 45% compared with 0% to 23% for patients with R1/R2 resection.[23,26,30,46] Even after margin-negative resections, recurrence rates range from 50% to 70%.[26] Other factors associated with poor prognosis are regional lymph node metastases, high-grade tumor, tumor depth, and tumor histology (nodular sclerosing vs papillary).[20,21,28,30] Prognosis without surgery is poor, with most patients living less than a year from diagnosis.

Transplantation

A very small subset of patients with locally advanced unresectable PHCCA but without lymph node or distant metastatic disease may be eligible for LT under institutional protocol using neoadjuvant chemoradiation. Outcomes in this small group of highly selected individuals are promising with reported overall survival of 53% to

Table 5
Selected reports of outcomes after resection for perihilar cholangiocarcinoma

Series, y	N	R0 Resection (%)	5-y Survival (%)
Cho et al,[30] 2012	105	70.5	34.1
Song et al,[89] 2013	230	76.5	33
de Jong et al,[3] 2012	305	73	20
Nuzzo et al,[91] 2012	440	77	25.5
Furusawa et al,[92] 2014	144	99	35
Yu et al,[90] 2014	238	50	17

Table 6 Selected reports of postresection outcomes and poor prognostic factors for distal cholangiocarcinoma				
Reference	Number of patients	Median Survival	5-y Survival (%)	Poor Prognostic Factors
Kwon et al,[94] 2014	133		41	R2 margin Lymphovascular invasion High TNM stage
DeOliveira et al,[97] 2007	239		23	R1/R2 margin Lymph node metastases Tumor >2 cm Poorly differentiated tumors
Murakami et al,[96] 2007	43	26 mo	44	Older age Pathologic pancreatic invasion Lymph node metastases Perineural invasion R1/R2 margin TNM stage II and III
Hong et al,[46] 2009; Hong et al,[98] 2011	147	20.3 mo	18	Tumor depth >5 mm

76% and disease-free survival of 60% to 65% at 5 years after LT.[75,77,78] Posttransplant outcomes are better in PSC patients compared with those with de novo PHCCA.

Distal Cholangiocarcinoma

The median survival for patients who undergo resection for DCCA is approximately 2 years with a 5-year survival of 20% to 40% depending on extent of disease.[80,93,94] Several studies have looked at prognostic factors for patients undergoing resection for DCCA. Some of the commonly reported risk factors for cancer recurrence of poor survival are positive resection margin (R1 or R2), positive lymph nodes, tumor size >2 cm, and poorly differentiated tumors, perineural invasion, lymphovascular invasion, pancreatic invasion, and depth of tumor invasion.[80,93–98] Murakami and colleagues[96] looked at their experience with resection margins and lymph node involvement in resection specimens in 43 patients and reported significantly worse 5-year survival in patients with positive margins compared with negative margins (8% vs 60%) and in patients with involved lymph nodes compared with patients without lymph node involvement (18% vs 40%). **Table 6** summarizes outcomes and poor prognostic factors after resection for DCCA in several large studies. Median survival in patients with unresectable DCCA is poor with most patients living less than a year after diagnosis.[80]

SUMMARY

CCA is the most common primary biliary malignancy and can arise in the IH or EH biliary system. The prognosis is generally quite poor because many patients present at an advanced stage where surgery is not an option. However, among patients with resectable disease, surgery with negative margins offers the best chance of cure. Margin status and locoregional lymph node metastases are the most important determinants of postsurgical outcomes with increased risk of recurrence in patients with positive BD margins or lymph node metastasis. A very small group of patients with unresectable hilar CCA without spread to regional lymph nodes or distant sites might benefit from LT when carried out under an institutional protocol involving neo-adjuvant chemoradiation therapy.

REFERENCES

1. Tyson GL, El-Serag HB. Risk factors for cholangiocarcinoma. Eur J Gastroenterol Hepatol 2011;54:173–84.
2. Welzel TM, Graubard BI, El-Serag HB, et al. Risk factors for intrahepatic and extrahepatic cholangiocarcinoma in the Unites States: a population-based case-control study. Clin Gastroenterol Hepatol 2007;5:1221–8.
3. de Jong MC, Marques H, Clary BM, et al. The impact of portal vein resection on outcomes for hilar cholangiocarcinoma. A Multi-institutional analysis of 305 cases. Cancer 2012;118:4737–47.
4. Yang JD, Kim B, Sanderson SO, et al. Biliary tract cancers in Olmsted County, Minnesota, 1976-2008. Am J Gastroenterol 2012;107(8):1256–62.
5. Saha SK, Zhu AX, Fuchs CS, et al. Forty-year trends in cholangiocarcinoma incidence in the U.S.: intrahepatic disease on the rise. Oncologist 2016;21(5):594–9.
6. LaRusso NF, Shneider BL, Black D, et al. Primary sclerosing cholangitis: summary of a workshop. Hepatol 2006;44:746–64.
7. Soreide K, Korner H, Havnen J, et al. Bile duct cysts in adults. Br J Surg 2004;91:1538–48.
8. Blechacz BR, Gores GJ. Cholangiocarcinoma. Clin Liver Dis 2008;12:131–50.
9. Sorensen HT, Friis S, Olsen JH, et al. Risk of liver and other types of cancer in patients with cirrhosis: a nationwide cohort study in Denmark. Hepatol 1998;28:921–5.
10. Shahib YH, El-Serag HB, Davila JA, et al. Risk factors of intrahepatic cholangiocarcinoma in the Unites States: a case-control study. Gastroenterology 2005;128:620–6.
11. Kubo S, Kinoshita H, Hirohashi K, et al. Hepatolithiasis associated with cholangiocarcinoma. World J Surg 1995;19:637–41.
12. Shin HR, Oh JK, Lim MK, et al. Descriptive epidemiology of cholangiocarcinoma and clonorchiasis in Korea. J Korean Med Sci 2010;25:1011–6.
13. Bridgewater J, Galle PR, Khan SA, et al. Guidelines for the diagnosis and management of intrahepatic cholangiocarcinoma. J Hepatol 2014;60(6):1268–89.
14. Palmer WC, Patel T. Are common factors involved in the pathogenesis of primary liver cancers? A meta-analysis of risk factors for intrahepatic cholangiocarcinoma [review]. J Hepatol 2012;57(1):69–76 [Erratum in: J Hepatol 2012;57(5):1160].
15. O'Dell MR, Huang JL, Whitney-Miller CL, et al. Kras(G12D) and p53 mutation cause primary intrahepatic cholangiocarcinoma. Cancer Res 2012;72(6):1557–67.
16. Farazi PA, Zeisberg M, Glickman J, et al. Chronic bile duct injury associated with fibrotic matrix microenvironment provokes cholangiocarcinoma in p53-deficient mice. Cancer Res 2006;66(13):6622–7.
17. Borger DR, Tanabe KK, Fan KC, et al. Frequent mutation of isocitrate dehydrogenase (IDH)1 and IDH2 in cholangiocarcinoma identified through broad-based tumor genotyping. Oncologist 2012;17(1):72–9.
18. Bagante F, Weiss M, Alexandrescu S, et al. Long-term outcomes of patients with intraductal growth sub-type of intrahepatic cholangiocarcinoma. HPB (Oxford) 2018;20(12):1189–97.

19. Farges O, Fuks D, Boleslawski E, et al. Influence of surgical margins on outcome in patients with intrahepatic cholangiocarcinoma: a multicenter study by the AFC-IHCC-2009 study group. Ann Surg 2011;254(5):824–9 [discussion: 830].

20. Lidsky ME, Jarnagin WR. Surgical management of hilar cholangiocarcinoma at Memorial Sloan Kettering Cancer Center. Ann Gastroenterol Surg 2018;2:304–12.

21. Poruk KE, Pawlik TM, Weiss MJ. Perioperative management of hilar cholangiocarcinoma. J Gastrointest Surg 2015;19(10):1889–99.

22. Isa T, Tomita S, Nakachi A, et al. Analysis of microsatellite instability, K-ras gene mutation and p53 protein overexpression in intrahepatic cholangiocarcinoma. Hepatogastroenterology 2002;49(45):604–8.

23. Mansour JC, Aloia TA, Crane CH, et al. Hilar cholangiocarcinoma: expert consensus statement. HPB (Oxford) 2015;17:691–9.

24. Bismuth H, Corlette MB. Intrahepatic cholangioenteric anastomosis in carcinoma of the hilus of liver. Surg Gynecol Obstet 1975;140:170–8.

25. Bismuth H, Nakache R, Diamond T. Management strategies in resection for hilar cholangiocarcinoma. Ann Surg 1992;215(1):31–8.

26. Jarnagin WR, Fong Y, DeMatteo RP, et al. Staging, resectability, and outcome in 225 patients with hilar cholangiocarcinoma. Ann Surg 2001;234:507–17.

27. Edge SB, Compton CC. The American Joint Committee on Cancer: the 7th edition of AJCC cancer staging annual and the future of TNM. Ann Surg Oncol 2010; 17(6):1471–4.

28. de Jong MC, Hong SM, Augustine MM, et al. Hilar cholangiocarcinoma: tumor depth as a predictor of outcome. Arch Surg 2011;146(6):697–703.

29. Endo I, Gonen M, Yopp AC, et al. Intrahepatic cholangiocarcinoma: rising frequency, improved survival, and determinants of outcome after resection. Ann Surg 2008;248(1):84–96.

30. Cho MS, Kim SH, Park SW. Surgical outcomes and predicting factors of curative resection in patients with hilar cholangiocarcinoma: 10 year single-institution experience. J Gastrointest Surg 2012;16(9):1672–9.

31. Valls C, Gumà A, Puig I, et al. Intrahepatic peripheral cholangiocarcinoma: CT evaluation. Abdom Imaging 2000;25(5):490–6.

32. Choi BL, Lee JM, Han JK. Imaging of intrahepatic and hilar cholangiocarcinoma. Abdom Imaging 2004;29(5):548–57.

33. Ni T, Shang XS, Wang WT, et al. Different MR features for differentiation of intrahepatic mass-forming cholangiocarcinoma from hepatocellular carcinoma according to tumor size. Br J Radiol 2018;91(1088):20180017.

34. Patel AH, Harnois DM, Klee GG, et al. The utility of CA 19-9 in the diagnoses of cholangiocarcinoma in patients without primary sclerosing cholangitis. Am J Gastroenterol 2000;95(1):204–7.

35. Aloia TA, Charnasangavej C, Faria S, et al. High-resolution computed tomography accurately predicts resectability in hilar cholangiocarcinoma. Am J Surg 2007;193:702–6.

36. Chen HW, Lai EC, Pan AZ, et al. Preoperative assessment and staging of hilar cholangiocarcinoma with 16 multidetector-row computed tomograpy cholangiography and angiography. Hepatogastroenterology 2009;56(91–92):578–83.

37. Chryssou E, Guthrie JA, Ward J, et al. Hilar cholangiocarcinoma: MR correlation with surgical and histological findings. Clin Radiol 2010;65(10):781–8.

38. Breitenstein S, Apesteugi C, Clavien PA. Positron emission tomography (PET) for cholangiocarcinoma. HPB (Oxford) 2008;10:120–1.

39. Tamada K, Ushio J, Sugano K. Endoscopic diagnosis of extrahepatic bile duct carcinoma: advances and current limitations. World J Clin Oncol 2011;10(2): 203–16.

40. De Bellis M, Sherman S, Fogel EL, et al. Tissue sampleing at ERCP in suspected malignant biliary strictures (Part 1). Gastrointest Endosc 2002;56:552–61.

41. Silva MA, Tekin K, Aytekin F, et al. Surgery for hilar cholangiocarcinoma: a 10 year experience of a tertiary referral center in the UK. Eur J Surg Oncol 2005;31(5): 633–9.

42. Park MS, Kim TK, Kim KW, et al. Differentiation of extrahepatic bile duct cholangiocarcinoma from benign stricture: findings at MRCP versus ERCP. Radiology 2004;233(1):234–40.

43. Heimbach KM, Sanchez W, Rosen CM, et al. Trans-peritoneal fine needle aspiration biopsy of hilar cholangiocarcinoma is associated with disease dissemination. HPB (Oxford) 2011;13:356–60.

44. Sapisochin G, Rodríguez de Lope C, Gastaca M, et al. "Very early" intrahepatic cholangiocarcinoma in cirrhotic patients: should liver transplantation be reconsidered in these patients? Am J Transplant 2014;14(3):660–7.

45. Sapisochin G, de Lope CR, Gastaca M, et al. Intrahepatic cholangiocarcinoma or mixed hepatocellular-cholangiocarcinoma in patients undergoing liver transplantation: a Spanish matched cohort multicenter study. Ann Surg 2014;259(5): 944–52.

46. Hong JC, Jones CM, Duffy JP, et al. Comparative analysis of resection and liver transplantation for intrahepatic and hilar cholangiocarcinoma: a 24-year experience in a single center. Arch Surg 2011;146(6):683–9.

47. Lee DD, Croome KP, Musto KR, et al. Liver transplantation for intrahepatic cholangiocarcinoma. Liver Transpl 2018;24(5):634–44.

48. Lunsford KE, Javle M, Heyne K, et al. Methodist–MD Anderson Joint Cholangiocarcinoma Collaborative Committee (MMAJCCC). Liver transplantation for locally advanced intrahepatic cholangiocarcinoma treated with neoadjuvant therapy: a prospective case-series. Lancet Gastroenterol Hepatol 2018;3(5):337–48 [Erratum in: Lancet Gastroenterol Hepatol 2018;3(6):e3].

49. Valle J, Wasan H, Palmer DH, et al. ABC-02 Trial Investigators. Cisplatin plus gemcitabine versus gemcitabine for biliary tract cancer. N Engl J Med 2010; 362(14):1273–81.

50. Verma V, Kusi Appiah A, Lautenschlaeger T, et al. Chemoradiotherapy versus chemotherapy alone for unresected intrahepatic cholangiocarcinoma: practice patterns and outcomes from the national cancer database. J Gastrointest Oncol 2018;9(3):527–35.

51. Shao F, Qi W, Meng FT, et al. Role of palliative radiotherapy in unresectable intrahepatic cholangiocarcinoma: population-based analysis with propensity score matching. Cancer Manag Res 2018;10:1497–506.

52. Konstantinidis IT, Groot Koerkamp B, Do RK, et al. Unresectable intrahepatic cholangiocarcinoma: Systemic plus hepatic arterial infusion chemotherapy is associated with longer survival in comparison with systemic chemotherapy alone. Cancer 2016;122(5):758–65.

53. Kolarich AR, Shah JL, George TJ Jr, et al. Non-surgical management of patients with intrahepatic cholangiocarcinoma in the United States, 2004-2015: an NCDB analysis. J Gastrointest Oncol 2018;9(3):536–45.

54. Rayar M, Sulpice L, Edeline J, et al. Intra-arterial yttrium-90 radioembolization combined with systemic chemotherapy is a promising method for downstaging

unresectable huge intrahepatic cholangiocarcinoma to surgical treatment. Ann Surg Oncol 2015;22(9):3102–8.

55. Shaker TM, Chung C, Varma MK, et al. Is there a role for Ytrrium-90 in the treatment of unresectable and metastatic intrahepatic cholangiocarcinoma? Am J Surg 2018;215(3):467–70.

56. Kobayashi A, Miwa S, Nakata T, et al. Disease recurrence patterns after R0 resection of hilar cholangiocarcinoma. Br J Surg 2010;97:56–64.

57. Abdalla EK, Adam R, Bilchik AJ, et al. Improving resectability of hepatic colorectal metastases: expert consensus statement. Ann Surg Oncol 2006;13: 1271–80.

58. Khan AS, Garcia-Aroz S, Ansari MA, et al. Assessment and optimization of liver volume before major hepatic resection: current guidelines and a narrative review. Int J Surg 2018;52:74–81.

59. Gazzaniga GM, Cappato S, Belli FE, et al. Assessment of hepatic reserve for the indication of hepatic resection: how I do it. J Hepatobiliary Pancreat Surg 2005; 12:27–30.

60. Abdalla E. Portal vein embolization (prior to major hepatectomy) effects on regeneration, resectability and outcome. J Surg Oncol 2010;102:960–7.

61. Worni M, Shah KN, Clary BM. Colorectal cancer with potentially resectable hepatic metastases: optimizing treatment. Curr Oncol Rep 2014;16:407.

62. Shindoh J, Vauthey JN, Zimmitti G. Analysis of the efficacy of portal vein embolization for patients with extensive liver malignancy and very low future liver remnant volume, including a comparison with the associating liver partition with portal vein ligation for stated hepatectomy approach. J Am Coll Surg 2013;217: 126–33.

63. Abulkhir A, Limongelli P, Healey AJ, et al. Preoperative portal vein embolization for major liver resection: a meta-analysis. Ann Surg 2008;247:49–57.

64. Ribero D, Abdalla EK, Madoff DC, et al. Portal vein embolization before major hepatectomy and its effect on regeneration, resectability and outcome. Br J Surg 2007;94:1386–94.

65. Nimura Y. Preoperative biliary drainage before resection for cholangiocarcinoma (Pro). HPB (Oxford) 2008;10:130–3.

66. Iacono C, Ruzzenente A, Campagnaro T, et al. Role of preoperative biliary drainage in jaundiced patients who are candidates for pancreatoduodenectomy or hepatic resection: highlights and drawbacks. Ann Surg 2013;257:191–204.

67. Kennedy TJ, Yopp A, Qin Y, et al. Role of preoperative biliary drainage of liver remnant prior to extended liver resection for hilar cholangiocarcinoma. HPB (Oxford) 2009;11:445–51.

68. Laurent A, Taylor C, Cherqui D. Cholangiocarcinoma: preoperative biliary drainage (Con). HPB (Oxford) 2008;10:126–9.

69. Bird N, Elmasry M, Jones R, et al. Role of staging laparoscopy in the stratification of patients with perihilar cholangiocarcinoma. Br J Surg 2017;104:418–25.

70. Melendez JA, Arslan V, Fischer ME, et al. Perioperative outcomes of major hepatic resections under low central venous pressure anesthesia: blood loss, blood transfusion and the risk of postoperatiec renal dysfunction. J Am Coll Surg 1998;187:620–5.

71. Abbas S, Sandroussi C. Systematic review and meta-analysis of the role of vascular resection in the treatment of hilar cholangiocarcinoma. HPB (Oxford) 2013;15:492–503.

72. Kim TH, Han SS, Park SJ, et al. Role of adjuvant chemoradiotherapy for resected extrahepatic biliary tract cancer. Int J Radiat Oncol Biol Phys 2011l;81:e853–9.

73. Borghero Y, Crane CH, Szklaruk J, et al. Extrahepatic bile duct adenocarcinoma: patients at high risk for local recurrence treated with surgery and adjuvant chemoradiation have an equivalent overall survival to patients with standard-risk treated with surgery alone. Ann Surg Oncol 2008;15:3147–56.

74. Shimoda M, Farmer DG, Colquhoun SD, et al. Liver transplantation for cholangiocellular carcinoma: analysis of a single center experience and review of literature. Liver Transpl 2001;7(12):1023–33.

75. Heimbach JK, Haddock MG, Alberts SR, et al. Transplantation for hilar cholangiocarcinoma. Liver Transpl 2004;10(suppl.2):65–8.

76. Rea DJ, Heimbach JM, Rosen CB, et al. Liver transplantation with neoadjuvant chemoradiation is more effective trhan resection for hilar cholangiocarcinoma. Ann Surg 2005;242:451–8.

77. Rosen CB, Heimbach JK, Gores GJ. Liver transplantation for cholangiocarcinoma. Transpl Int 2010;23(7):692–7.

78. Murad SW, Kim WR, Harnoid DM, et al. Efficacy of neoadjuvant chemoradiation followed by liver transplantation, for perihilar cholangiocarcinoma at 12 US centers. Gastroenterology 2012;143:88–98.e3.

79. Chua TC, Saxena A. Extended pancreaticoduodenectomy with vascular resection for pancreatic cancer: a systematic review. J Gastrointest Surg 2010;14(9): 1442–52.

80. Dickson PV, Behrman SW. Distal cholangiocarcinoma. Surg Clin North Am 2014; 94:325–42.

81. de Jong MC, Nathan H, Sotiropoulos GC, et al. Intrahepatic cholangiocarcinoma: an international multi-institutional analysis of prognostic factors and lymph node assessment. J Clin Oncol 2011;29(23):3140–5.

82. Conci S, Ruzzenente A, Viganò L, et al. Patterns of distribution of hepatic nodules (single, satellites or multifocal) in intrahepatic cholangiocarcinoma: prognostic impact after surgery. Ann Surg Oncol 2018;25(12):3719–27.

83. Farges O, Fuks D, Le Treut YP, et al. AJCC 7th edition of TNM staging accurately discriminates outcomes of patients with resectable intrahepatic cholangiocarcinoma: by the AFC-IHCC-2009 study group. Cancer 2011;117(10):2170–7.

84. Buettner S, Spolverato G, Kimbrough CW, et al. The impact of neutrophil-to-lymphocyte ratio and platelet-to-lymphocyte ratio among patients with intrahepatic cholangiocarcinoma. Surgery 2018;164(3):411–8.

85. Hyder O, Hatzaras I, Sotiropoulos GC, et al. Recurrence after operative management of intrahepatic cholangiocarcinoma. Surgery 2013;153(6):811–8.

86. Choi SB, Kim KS, Choi JY, et al. The prognosis and survival outcome of intrahepatic cholangiocarcinoma following surgical resection: association of lymph node metastasis and lymph node dissection with survival. Ann Surg Oncol 2009; 16(11):3048–56.

87. Ribero D, Pinna AD, Guglielmi A, et al, Italian Intrahepatic Cholangiocarcinoma Study Group. Surgical Approach for Long-term Survival of Patients With Intrahepatic Cholangiocarcinoma: A Multi-institutional Analysis of 434 Patients. Arch Surg 2012;147(12):1107–13.

88. Lee SG, Song GW, Hwang S, et al. Surgical treatment of hilar cholangiocarcinoma in the new era: the Asan experience. J Hepatobiliary Pancreat Sci 2010;17: 476–89.

89. Song SC, Choi DW, Kow AWC, et al. Surgical outcomes f 230 resected hilar cholangiocarcinoma in a single center. ANZ J Surg 2013;83:268–74.

90. Yu W, Shao, Gu Z, et al. Effect evaluation of vascular resection for patients with hilar cholangiocarcinoma: original data and meta-analysis. Hepatogastroenterology 2014;61(130):307–13.
91. Nuzzo G, Giuliante F, Ardito F, et al. Improvement in perioperative and long-term outcome after surgical treatment of hilar cholangiocarcinoma: results of an Italian multicenter analysis of 440 patients. Arch Surg 2012;147(1):26–34.
92. Furusawa N, Kobayashi A, Yokoyama T, et al. Surgical treatment of 144 cases of hilar cholangiocarcinoma without liver-related mortality. World J Surg 2014;38(5): 1164–76.
93. Distal bile duct. In: Edge SB, Byrd DR, editors. AJCC cancer staging manual. 7th edition. New York: Springer; 2010. p. 227–33.
94. Kwon HJ, Kim SG, Chun JM, et al. Prognostic factors in patients with middle and distal bile duct cancers. World J Gastroenterol 2014;20(21):6658–65.
95. Lim KH, Oh DY, Chie EK, et al. Adjuvant concurrent chemoradiation therapy (CCRT) alone versus CCRT followed by adjuvant chemotherapy: which is better in patients with radically resected extrahepatic biliary tract cancer? A nonrandomized single center study. BMC Cancer 2009;9:345.
96. Murakami Y, Uemura K, Hayashidani Y, et al. Prognostic significance of lymph node metastasis and surgical margin status for distal chaolangiocarcinoma. J Surg Oncol 2007;95(3):207–12.
97. DeOliveira ML, Cunningam SC, Camreon JL, et al. Cholangiocarcinoma: thirty-one year experience with 564 patients at a single institution. Ann Surg 2007; 245(5):755–62.
98. Hong SM, Pawlik TM, Cho HJ, et al. Depth of tumor invasion better predicts prognosis than the current American Joint Committee on Cancer T classification for distal bile duct carcinoma. Surgery 2009;146(2):250–7.

Gallbladder Cancer

Diagnosis, Surgical Management, and Adjuvant Therapies

Laura Hickman, MD, Carlo Contreras, MD*

KEYWORDS

- Gallbladder cancer • Incidental gallbladder cancer • Gallbladder polyps
- Radical cholecystectomy • Staging laparoscopy • Adjuvant chemoradiotherapy

KEY POINTS

- Gallbladder cancer (GBC) has a poor prognosis, but R0 resection is potentially curative. Presenting symptoms may be misdiagnosed as biliary colic or chronic cholecystitis. Risk factors include advanced age, female sex, gallbladder polyps greater than 1 cm, and cholelithiasis.
- Patients with GBC diagnosed after cholecystectomy for suspected benign disease represent more than half of new cases. Incidentally discovered GBCs have improved survival, because they are often diagnosed at an earlier stage.
- Preoperative imaging should include computed tomography (CT), with MRI or PET-CT reserved for special cases. Biopsy is only indicated if the tumor is unresectable to provide prognostic information and tissue diagnosis for chemotherapy. GBC found at the time of operation should undergo intraoperative lymph node sampling and delayed definitive resection.
- For incidental gallbladder cancer (IGBC) after laparoscopic cholecystectomy, observation is recommended for pT1a; other tumors pT1b or greater necessitate more extensive resection.
- At the time of radical cholecystectomy, confirm cancer diagnosis by frozen section (for non-IGBC); an adequate operation includes staging laparoscopy, R0 en bloc resection, and locoregional lymph node clearance.

INTRODUCTION

Gallbladder cancer (GBC) is a relatively rare occurrence with a poor prognosis (overall 5-year survival is 50% for stage I cancers and 3% for stage IV cancers[1]). Surgical resection is the only potentially curative therapy, but success is variable and

Disclosure: The authors have nothing to disclose.
Division of Surgical Oncology, Department of Surgery, University of Alabama at Birmingham, Birmingham, AL, USA
* Corresponding author. BDB 612 1808 7th Avenue South, Brimingham, AL 35294.
E-mail address: ccontreras@uabmc.edu

Surg Clin N Am 99 (2019) 337–355
https://doi.org/10.1016/j.suc.2018.12.008
0039-6109/19/© 2018 Elsevier Inc. All rights reserved.

surgical.theclinics.com

dependent on stage, tumor biology, and completeness of resection. From a multi-center US study including patients undergoing resection with curative intent, median survival is around 25 months.[2] More than half of GBCs are diagnosed on pathologic examination after cholecystectomy for cholecystitis or cholelithiasis.[3] Approximately 1 in 250 laparoscopic cholecystectomies will yield a pathologic diagnosis of incidental gallbladder cancer (IGBC)[4,5] For the remainder of GBC diagnosed preoperatively, the presenting symptoms are commonly jaundice or weight loss. IGBCs are often diagnosed at an earlier stage, thus have improved survival over non-IGBC.[6]

EPIDEMIOLOGY

The growing popularity of laparoscopic cholecystectomies has led to an increase in incidence of GBC. Although GBC is a rare cause of malignancy in the Western hemisphere, it continues to be a significant source of mortality in Japan, India, and Chile, among other countries.[7] In the United States, there are more than 1000 new cases GBC each year with an average age of 71 at diagnosis.[8] Seventy percent of GBCs are in women, with a 2.41:1 ratio to men. Sixty-four percent of GBC is diagnosed in Caucasians, 17% in Hispanics, 9% in African Americans, and 2% in Asian/Pacific Islanders.[9] GBC disproportionately affects Hispanics, Alaskan natives, and Native Americans in the United States.[10,11] In more than 15,000 GBC cases in the Surveillance, Epidemiology, and End Results (SEER) database, improved survival was seen in women, Asian/Pacific Islanders, and patients who underwent curative resection and/or chemotherapy.[12]

GBC is an aggressive disease with common local invasion, early and widespread nodal metastases, and frequent distant metastases. Presenting symptoms are often misdiagnosed as biliary colic or chronic cholecystitis, further delaying diagnosis. As such, a large proportion of cases is diagnosed at advanced stage; unfortunately, longitudinal database studies show this proportion has increased since 2001 to roughly 40% of all cases.[12] Compared with hilar cholangiocarcinoma, GBC has worse survival and shorter time to recurrence.[13]

ANATOMY

The gallbladder (GB) is adherent to portions of segments IV and V of the liver, and it can be divided into 2 distinct surfaces. The hepatic surface lacks a peritoneal lining, which contributes to relatively common tumor extension into the liver parenchyma; the peritoneal surface is covered by visceral peritoneum (**Fig. 1**). The GB most commonly receives its blood supply from the right hepatic artery via the cystic artery, and venous drainage is via the liver bed or cystic vein typically into the right portal system. The cystic duct joins the common hepatic duct to create the common bile duct (CBD) before emptying into the duodenum.

The wall of the GB is different from most other hollow viscous organs because it lacks a submucosal layer. The wall of the GB consists of the mucosa, lamina propria, a muscular layer, perimuscular connective tissue, and serosa (or visceral peritoneum). The latest edition of the American Joint Committee on Cancer (AJCC) guidelines (8th edition; 2017) accounts for the difference in tumor biology observed when tumors present on the peritoneal side of the GB compared with the hepatic side.[14]

STAGING

The 8th edition the AJCC staging system was implemented January 1, 2018. The T category describes the depth of tumor penetration within the GB wall. T1a lesions

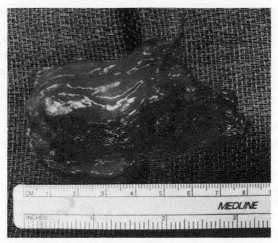

Fig. 1. The peritoneal surface of the GB is covered in serosa (visceral peritoneum), seen on the top half of the specimen.

invade the lamina propria, and the T1b lesion invades the muscular layer. The 8th edition the T2 classification now differentiates between the peritoneal and hepatic surfaces (T2a and T2b, respectively). T3 tumors perforate the GB serosa or penetrate into the liver or one other adjacent organ. T4 tumors are defined as those that invade the main portal vein, hepatic artery, or tumors that invade 2 or more extrahepatic organs. The updated N-category is defined by the number of metastatic lymph nodes (LN; N1 = 1–3 LN metastases, N2 = 4 or more LN metastases), instead of their anatomic position.[1] In the absence of LN metastasis, T1 tumors are stage I; T2a tumors are stage IIA; T2b tumors are stage IIB; and T3 tumors are stage IIIA. T3N1 disease is defined as stage IIIB. Stage IV tumors include all T4 lesions (stage IVA), all N2 disease (stage IVB), and all metastatic disease (stage IVB).

RISK FACTORS

The most significant risk factors for development of GBC are female sex,[8] advanced age,[8] cholelithiasis or other benign GB pathology[15] (approximately 0.7% of laparoscopic cholecystectomies are found to have IGBC[5]), chronic infection with *Salmonella* species or *Helicobacter pylori*,[11] anomalous pancreatobiliary duct junction,[11] porcelain GB,[11] GB polyps,[16] and obesity.[17] Secondary risk factors for development of GBC include family history of cholelithiasis,[11] chronic cholecystitis,[11] high parity,[11] tobacco consumption,[11] chemical exposure (benzene),[11] high carbohydrate intake,[10] and chronic diarrhea.[10] A familial link in GBC is unclear, because population-based studies from Utah and Sweden are discordant.[18,19]

In patients undergoing laparoscopic cholecystectomy for presumed benign disease, risk factors for finding IGBC include female sex,[4] older age,[4] jaundice,[4] acute cholecystitis,[4] dilated bile ducts,[20] or GB wall thickening.[20]

Gallbladder Polyps

GB polyps are seen in up to 12% of cholecystectomy specimens and 5% to 7% of biliary ultrasound studies, but only 0.6% of polyps are malignant.[16,21] Most GB polyps are cholesterol or fibromyoglandular lesions with no malignant potential,[22] unlike true papillary neoplasms (adenomas). In patients with polyps, the likelihood of malignancy increases in polyps greater than 1 cm, age greater than 50, cholelithiasis, solitary sessile polyps, and primary sclerosing cholangitis.[16]

Although there is conflicting evidence about the threshold for intervention on a GB polyp, it is largely accepted that polyps less than 1 cm are often benign and polyps greater than 2 cm are often neoplastic. The Americas Hepato-Pancreato-Biliary Association (AHPBA) suggests that any polyp greater than 1 cm or with a vascular pedicle should be removed secondary to increased incidence of cancer (45%–65% likelihood).[7,16] The term intracholecystic papillary-tubular neoplasm (ICPN) was established to describe any preinvasive adenomatous polypoid or papillary neoplasms of the GB greater than 1 cm; diagnosis of this lesion should prompt more extensive pathologic sectioning of the cholecystectomy specimen because ICPN can be a marker for unappreciated carcinoma.[22]

Historically, "porcelain" or calcification of the GB wall has been associated with GB carcinoma in up to 61% of patients, often prompting cholecystectomy on this indication alone. More recent series have clarified this risk, noting that discontiguous, rather than diffuse, calcification of the entire GB wall is associated with carcinoma, but at a much lower frequency, approximately 2% to 7%.[23,24] Consequently, active surveillance is appropriate in asymptomatic patients without other features suspicious for malignancy or patients with significant comorbidities.[24]

DIAGNOSIS
Pathology

A recent consensus statement from the AHPBA[7] recommends a minimum of 3 representative samples and the cystic duct margin should be microscopically examined in a normal-appearing GB specimen. Any specimen with suspicion of polyp on preoperative imaging, abnormal gross appearance, or dysplasia should be completely sampled. Other high-risk disorders should prompt complete sampling: choledochal cysts, anomalous union of the pancreatobiliary ducts, primary sclerosing cholangitis, and hyalinizing cholecystitis. In the event neoplasia is identified, it is also important to identify involvement of Rokitansky-Aschoff sinuses, multifocal lesions, involvement of hepatic versus peritoneal surface, and the cystic duct margin.[7] The most common cancer of the GB is adenocarcinoma,[22] although neuroendocrine tumors,[25] small cell tumors,[26] primary non-Hodgkin lymphoma,[27] and metastases have been reported (**Fig. 2**).

Symptoms

Presenting symptoms of GBC mimic that of biliary colic and thus can be difficult to differentiate from benign disease. As with other biliary tract cancers, weight loss and jaundice are often associated with more advanced disease. Jaundice is a relative contraindication to resection, because these patients only have a mean disease-free survival of 6 months, even after R0 resection.[28] A retrospective review of almost 400 patients found patients with obstructive jaundice were more likely to have metastatic (48% vs 37%) and unresectable disease (25% vs 10%).[29] Another study found the overall survival (OS) after curative resection of the jaundiced cohort was 14 months versus 32 months in the nonjaundiced cohort.[30] Poor long-term survival was associated with gastric outlet obstruction, obstructive jaundice, nodal involvement, extension into adjacent organs, and higher TNM stage.[29]

Imaging

On imaging, GBC can present as a mass adjacent to the GB, GB polyps, or wall thickening. Uniform wall thickening is indicative of benign disease, such as cholecystitis or

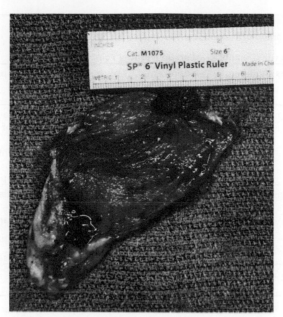

Fig. 2. Melanoma polyp on GB mucosa (immediately underneath the ruler).

adenomyomatosis.[16] Findings that favor GBC include discontinuity or irregular mucosal thickening, irregular serosal thickening, or loss of differentiation between the 3 layers.[31]

A GB mass discovered on pathology or routine ultrasound should undergo contrast-enhanced abdominal computed tomography (CT) of the chest, abdomen, and pelvis[7,9] (**Table 1**). The advantages of CT over ultrasound alone are the potential to identify portal lymphadenopathy, peritoneal implants, or vascular invasion; CT is the most accurate modality to determine resectability with a sensitivity of 99% and specificity of 76%.[32] The role of gadolinium-enhanced MRI is primarily in examination of the biliary ducts or liver parenchyma.

The presence of nodal disease, especially in the porta hepatis, left gastric and aortocaval basins, is important to identify to avoid laparotomy in unresectable cases and for prognostic purposes. A meta-analysis found the sensitivity of PET with fludeoxyglucose F18-CT for detecting primary tumors was 93% and the specificity was 80%.[33] However, PET-CT has only 56% sensitivity for detecting occult metastases.[34] In patients with potentially resectable GBC on conventional CT, the addition of PET-CT changed the management of 23% of patients.[35] The 2018 National Comprehensive Cancer Network (NCCN) guidelines recommend PET-CT when findings on conventional studies are equivocal, because the use of PET-CT has not been established in preoperative planning.[9] PET-CT may be most applicable for IGBC (which are often diagnosed at more advanced stages), because identification of occult nodal metastases may avoid subsequent laparotomy.[36]

Duodenal involvement is a risk factor for unresectability, although not a contraindication to attempted resection. Symptoms of gastric outlet obstruction, mural thickening on CT, mucosal irregularity on CT, and infiltration of tumor into duodenal mucosa on endoscopy are each associated with unresectability at the time of operation.[37]

Table 1
Guidelines for workup of known or suspected gallbladder cancer

Circumstances of GBC Diagnosis	Workup and Key Points[9]
Preoperative mass identified	• Contrasted CT of chest, abdomen, and pelvis • Liver function tests and tumor markers • Consider SL
Incidental finding at surgery	• Frozen section of GB if suspicious for cancer • Intraoperative staging with resection of any suspicious LNs and cystic duct node • Definitive surgery should be delayed until full imaging and pathologic workup is complete • Contrasted CT of chest, abdomen, and pelvis
Incidental findings on pathology	• Observation recommended for T1a patients with R0 resection • Contrasted CT/MRI of chest, abdomen, and pelvis for T1b or greater • Consider SL for T1b or greater • Consider neoadjuvant therapy in N1 disease
Unresectable (on SL or imaging)	• Biopsy if tissue not available • Genetic testing

Data from Benson AB III, D'Angelica MI, Abbot DE, et al. NCCN Clinical Practice Guidelines in Oncology: Hepatobiliary Cancers. Version 5.2018. 2018.

There is no role for preoperative biopsy of a primary tumor that appears resectable on imaging. However, if workup reveals any feature suspicious for unresectability (ie, intrahepatic tumors, extension into vascular structures, lymphadenopathy outside the hepatoduodenal ligament, or peritoneal implants), preoperative biopsy should be performed. In addition to providing prognostic information, biopsy can also facilitate genetic testing to guide chemotherapy.[9]

MANAGEMENT OPTIONS
Previously Diagnosed Gallbladder Cancer

Patients with suspicion for cancer diagnosis will likely not have a tissue biopsy before laparotomy. In this case, it is imperative to send multiple core-needle biopsy specimens for frozen section to confirm cancer before radical resection.[7] Although imaging is helpful in differentiating benign masses, mass-forming xanthogranulomatous cholecystitis can be mistaken for GBC.[38]

Staging laparoscopy (SL) is an important adjunct to identify peritoneal implants and nodal disease outside of the hepatoduodenal ligament in patients with proven or suspected GBC. GBC tends to undergo early nodal spread to the cystic duct node and choledochal nodes. Spread outside of the hepatoduodenal ligament (including celiac, retropancreatic, and aortocaval nodes) generally represents metastatic disease and precludes resection. These nodes should be assessed early during laparoscopy or laparotomy.[28] SL in this setting is encouraged in both NCCN guidelines and the 2014 AHPBA consensus statement for GBC.[7,9] In a prospective study by Agarwal and colleagues,[39] 409 patients with GBC underwent SL with a single umbilical port; 95 patients (23.2%) were found to have either surface liver metastases or peritoneal implants and avoided laparotomy. Three hundred fourteen patients underwent subsequent laparotomy, with an additional 75 patients found to have unresectable disease (most with nonhepatoduodenal LNs or local tumor extension). In other words, SL identified 56% (95 of 170) of unresectable patients before laparotomy. Laparoscopic ultrasound (to identify local extension) and aortocaval LN frozen sections can further increase accuracy of identifying unresectable disease before laparotomy.[39] This study also highlights the importance of aortocaval and celiac LN sampling before resection, because 28% (47 of 170) of unresectable patients presented with nonhepatoduodenal nodal involvement *without* signs of surface metastases.[39]

There have been no randomized controlled trials to compare laparoscopic versus open radical cholecystectomy for GBC, but there are a multitude of single-institution series showing the safety and feasibility of a laparoscopic approach. A meta-analysis of more than 1200 patients found laparoscopic resection was associated with less blood loss, a shorter hospital stay, equivalent recurrence rate, and improved survival rate.[40] Laparoscopic radical cholecystectomy should be reserved for high-volume, specialized centers.

Incidentally Diagnosed Gallbladder Cancer

The safety and convenience of laparoscopic surgery have led to an increase in referrals for minimally invasive cholecystectomy, although it has allowed for controversy in the treatment of GBC. The popularity of laparoscopic cholecystectomies has led to an increase in incidentally diagnosed cancers, which account for approximately 0.7% of all specimens.[41] In fact, more than half of GBCs are now diagnosed at the time of cholecystectomy or on surgical pathology report.[41–43]

Incidental diagnosis of GBC has led to earlier discovery of cancers, and thus, improved oncologic outcomes.[44,45] A multicenter US retrospective study[6] identified 445 patients with GBC, 60% of whom who were diagnosed incidentally. Eighty-five percent of the cohort underwent attempted resection, and 72% had a completed resection. The patients with non-IGBC were more likely to have distant disease upon exploration (36% vs 21%, P<.001), a higher incidence of R1 or R2 resections, T3 or T4 disease (70% vs 40%, P<.001), poorly differentiated tumors (50% vs 31%, P = .001), and positive LNs (60% vs 43%, P = .009). Half of the patients who underwent curative resection received adjuvant therapy (no difference between groups), but recurrence was more prevalent in non-IGBC (50% vs 35%, P = .04). Poor survival prognostic factors on multivariate analysis included non-IGBC (hazard ratio 2.18, 95% confidence interval [CI] 1.16–4.09, P = .15), advanced T stage, and lymphovascular invasion. Median OS for non-IGBC was significantly worse compared with IGBC (17 vs 32 months, P = .001, excluding 30-day mortalities and R2 resections).[6] A single-center series of 107 patients[43] found an overall 5-year survival of 15%, with a 33% OS for patient with IGBC. Non-IGBC was also associated with a worse median OS of 8 versus 21 months.[43]

Initial operation

Most IGBC are diagnosed on pathologic review. However, if cancer is diagnosed by frozen section at the time of initial operation, the surgeon should carefully inspect the peritoneal cavity for signs of distant spread and consider biopsy of any suspicious LNs before closure. It is paramount to handle the GB with care and use a laparoscopic specimen retrieval bag for extraction, because worse outcomes are observed with any bile spillage.[44] An R1 resection at the initial operation has outcomes comparable to stage IV GBC, necessitating that a formal resection attempt be performed by a hepatobiliary specialist.[46] Current guidelines for IGBC recommend re-resection for T1b, T2, and T3 tumors, unless distant spread on preoperative imaging or poor functional status[7,9] (Table 2).

Table 2 Surgical principles in the treatment of gallbladder cancer	
Surgical Principle	**Key Points[9]**
Staging laparoscopy	• Highest yield in non-IGBC, T3 or greater, unfavorable tumor biology, or positive margins after cholecystectomy
Initial exploration	• Metastases to celiac axis or aortocaval nodes makes further resection futile
Hepatic resection	• Standard resection is segments IVB and V, although additional segments may be indicated for R0 resection
Lymphadenectomy	• Must include all nodes in porta hepatis, and preferably 6 or more nodes for complete staging
Bile duct resection	• Routine resection is not recommended, but may be necessary for R0 resection in advanced stages
Port-site resection	• Routine resection is not recommended, because port-site disease is a marker for disseminated intra-abdominal spread
Extent of resection	• T1a tumors: simple cholecystectomy • T1b and greater: radical cholecystectomy (hepatic resection + portal lymphadectomy + cholecystectomy) • Surgical morbidity nears 50% and perioperative mortality is approximately 5%[28]

Data from Benson AB III, D'Angelica MI, Abbot DE, et al. NCCN Clinical Practice Guidelines in Oncology: Hepatobiliary Cancers. Version 5.2018. 2018.

The status of the cystic duct node on initial operation is predictive of additional positive nodes in the porta hepatis. However, if the subsequent radical cholecystectomy shows no evidence of residual disease, the disease-free survival of these patients is similar to N0 rather than N1.[47]

Subsequent operation

Staging laparoscopy It is important to identify patients with unresectable or metastatic disease, given the morbidity of a laparotomy and limited role for palliative resection in advanced disease. Some investigators have advocated for SL in IGBC; Butte and colleagues[48] found that of 46 patients who underwent diagnostic laparoscopy, 2 were found to have unresectable disease at the time of laparoscopy and an additional 8 were found to have unresectable disease at the time of laparotomy. The study demonstrated a diagnostic yield for 20%, but given the minimal risk associated with laparoscopy, the investigators advocate for routine diagnostic laparoscopy in this population. Risk factors associated with disseminated disease include advanced T stage, positive margin after initial cholecystectomy, and high tumor grade.[48]

Extent of resection Reoperation for IGBC should achieve R0 resection and locoregional LN clearance; the type of hepatic resection has been proven to be less important than simply achieving R0 resection.[49] Studies have shown equivalent survival rates for patients undergoing hepatic wedge resection versus formal segmentectomy (IVb and V) or hemihepatectomy.[3,28,50,51] In addition, major hepatic resections are associated with worse perioperative morbidity without survival benefit.[42,44] However, there are times when an R0 resection necessitates a formal hepatectomy (because of right portal vein invasion, for example).

For early-stage tumors (T1b or T2), patients should undergo radical cholecystectomy with en bloc resection of adjacent liver parenchyma and hepatoduodenal lymphadenectomy. Resection of the CBD with Roux-en-Y hepaticojejunostomy is not routinely recommended, because it increases morbidity without any survival benefit. However, extrahepatic bile duct resection is necessary if the patient has a positive cystic duct margin on intraoperative frozen section or direct extension.[28] CBD involvement is a marker for decreased survival, even after R0 resection.[52] D'Angelica and colleagues[28] found a 5-year survival of 21% for patients with CBD involvement compared with 49% for patients without CBD involvement.

For later-stage tumors (T3 or T4), the extent of resection is debated in the literature. For patients with tumor extension into the gastrointestinal tract but without signs of distant nodal involvement, radical en bloc resections have been reported.[28] These operations have shown increased morbidity and mortality without any disease-free survival or OS benefit outside of small case series. The most important predictors of long-term survival are tumor biology and stage, rather than the extent of resection.[7,28]

Lymphadenectomy Lymphadenectomy is standard for T1b tumors or greater.[9] LN evaluation is essential in radial resection and confers a survival benefit compared with radial resection without lymphadenectomy.[53] The presence of hepatoduodenal nodal disease is not a contraindication to resection, but patients may benefit from neoadjuvant chemotherapy.[9] A portal lymphadenectomy for GBC includes the porta hepatis, gastrohepatic ligament, and retroduodenal space. Tumor-related para-aortic and celiac lymphadenopathy is generally considered metastatic. In a study by Shirai and colleagues,[54] patients with pathologic negative nodes had a median 5-year survival of 80% compared with 43% in node-positive patients.[54] Apart from positivity, the LN ratio has also been shown to predict survival after surgery.[55] This calculation takes into account the tumor biology (positive LNs) and the extent of lymphadenectomy (total LN count in specimen).

It has been proposed adequate staging requires 6 LNs from the hepatoduodenal ligament (supplemented with LNs from more distant sites if needed).[55-57] However, a recent study examining 2800 patients from National Cancer Database (NCDB) found that only half of the patients had any LN retrieved and only 12% had 6 or more nodes.[37]

Port-site metastases A systematic review[58] of 27 studies found the rate of port-site metastasis in the 1990s to be significantly higher than the modern era (2000–2014) (10.3% compared with 18.6%). However, the extraction port still carries a higher risk of disease than nonextraction sites.[58] When comparing patients who tested positive and negative for port-site metastases, metastasis decreased survival from 42 to 17 months in a study of 113 patients.[59] However, there was no difference in disease-free survival or OS when patients were adjusted for T and N staging; instead, port-site metastases are a marker of more advanced disease and worse prognosis.[60] A multicenter study of 449 patients found that port-site excision was not associated with improved OS and carries the same risk of recurrence. Empiric port-site excision is not recommended, because it does not change prognosis but carries a 15% risk of ventral hernia.[3,9]

Residual disease The probability of finding residual disease upon re-resection after IGBC diagnosis is dependent on tumor biology. For early-stage tumors (T1), the incidence of residual disease at any location was 37.5%.[61] For higher-stage tumors (T2 or T3), the incidence approached 70% to 80%.[3,51,61] Risk factors for residual disease include T3 tumors, perineural invasion, and lymphovascular invasion. Even after R0 resection, residual disease is associated with a 5-year disease-specific survival of only 19% compared with 74% of patients with no disease on re-resection.[62] Patients with IGBC who underwent re-resection had a significant survival benefit (41% 5-year

OS) compared with IGBC without re-resection (15% 5-year OS).[3] Studies looking specifically at IGBC with T1b tumors found an improved 5-year OS with re-resection (87.5% vs 61.3%), but no difference in T1a tumors.[63,64] This also held true for patients with residual disease or later stage (T2 or T3) tumors.[65] Any patient with incidentally diagnosed T1b, T2, or T3 disease limited to the GB should undergo re-resection.

Tumor location The location of tumor within the GB has surgical and prognostic implications. Shindoh and colleagues[66] published a series of 437 patients from 4 international centers who underwent curative resection for GBC. For T2 tumors, those on the hepatic surface of the GB (as opposed to the peritoneal side) had higher rates of vascular invasion (51% vs 19%, $P<.01$), neural invasion (33% vs 8%, $P<.01$), and nodal metastases (40% vs 17%, $P<.01$). For T2 tumors only, intrahepatic recurrence rate after liver resection was significantly higher for hepatic-sided tumors than peritoneal-sided tumors (23% vs 3%, $P = .003$), as was distant nodal recurrence after regional lymphadenectomy (16% vs 3%, $P = .019$). The investigators state that resection alone may be sufficient for peritoneal-sided T2 tumors, but adjuvant therapy is needed in hepatic-sided T2 tumors. Five-year survival was 42.6% for hepatic-sided T2 tumors compared with 64.7% for peritoneal-sided T2 tumors.[66] Lee and colleagues[67] also advocate that liver resection may not be necessary to T2 tumors on the peritoneal surface, because they did not find a significant difference in 5-year OS.

Surgical timing and approach There is conflicting literature regarding the timing of re-resection for IGBC. Ethun and colleagues[41] found optimal timing for reoperation is 4 to 8 weeks in a multi-institutional study of 207 patients, because there was a significant increase in OS compared with shorter or longer intervals after initial cholecystectomy (<4 weeks: 17.4 months, 4–8 weeks: 40.4 months, greater than 8 weeks: 22.4 months, $P = .03$). In contrast, Ausania and colleagues[68] demonstrated an optimal delay of 3 months after cholecystectomy in a cohort of 46 patients. The investigators thought this time allowed patients with biological unfavorable cancer to declare themselves and avoid an operation without changing survival outcomes for those that eventually undergo resection.

Laparoscopic radical cholecystectomy has been described in the literature, and 2 studies have compared laparoscopic (a combined total of 43 laparoscopic cases) and open approaches. Both studies found no difference in recurrence rates, but lower blood loss and shorter hospital stay for laparoscopy.[69,70] It has been suggested that perioperative blood transfusions are associated with shorter OS and recurrence-free survival on multivariate analysis; judicious use of blood in this population may be warranted.[71]

Role of Neoadjuvant and Adjuvant Therapy

An analysis of the NCDB found no increase in the proportion of GBC patients who received adjuvant therapy for GBC over time, despite findings that both chemotherapy and chemoradiotherapy (CRT) improve OS in patients with T2 tumors or greater. Currently, less than one-third of patients receive adjuvant therapy.[72]

Neoadjuvant chemoradiotherapy in resectable gallbladder cancer

A retrospective cohort of 74 patients with locally advanced or node-positive GBC was treated with neoadjuvant gemcitabine or gemcitabine + platinum regimens and then reevaluated for resection.[73] Thirty percent of patients (n = 22) were eligible for surgical attempt, with 14% undergoing R0 resection (n = 10). However, the difference in survival between the persistently unresectable subset and the eventually resectable group was marked (OS 11 months vs 51 months, $P = .003$).[73] This finding suggests that patients who are initially unresectable but who respond to chemotherapy should be reevaluated by a surgeon.

Adjuvant chemotherapy in resected gallbladder cancer

The latest NCCN guidelines recommend consideration of chemotherapy or CRT after resection of GBC.[9] However, the data are limited, and no regimen has emerged as superior in this cohort (no high-quality randomized controlled trials). There are numerous single-center studies, but several large studies offer valuable insight. Decisions for adjuvant therapy should take into account individual risks and benefits.

Horgan and colleagues[74] published a meta-analysis of 6712 patients from 1960 to 2010 for patients with either GBC or bile duct cancer undergoing resection. There was a modest, nonsignificant survival benefit overall, with a greater benefit in those with either node-positive disease or R1 resection.[74] Similarly, Ma and colleagues[75] published a meta-analysis that revealed adjuvant therapy was associated with improved survival among patients with R1 resections, positive LNs, and combined stages II/III.[75] Using SEER data, Wang and colleagues[76] found that adjuvant CRT provides a survival benefit in patients with at least T3 or N1 disease.

Mantripragada and colleagues[77] published an analysis of 4775 resected GC patients identified from the NCBD. They propensity matched 4708 patients to compare patients who underwent resection alone versus resection + adjuvant therapy. Interestingly, adjuvant therapy did not confer a survival benefit except in patients with T3 or node-positive disease who received CRT within 3 months of surgery. In that small subset, adjuvant CRT increased median survival by 3 months at 5 years postoperatively.[77] A similar NCDB study[78] supports adjuvant chemotherapy in node-positive disease to have an average OS of 20 months postresection compared with 8.6 months in patients not receiving chemotherapy. Despite this, only 22% of node-positive postresection patients are currently receiving chemotherapy.[78]

Finally, Ghidini and colleagues[79] analyzed a total of 22,499 patients (3967 that underwent resection) including Western and Asiatic cohorts. They compared any adjuvant treatment to surgery only and found a 4.3-month (95% CI 0.88–7.79, $P = .014$) increase in survival with adjuvant treatment.

Adjuvant chemoradiotherapy in resected gallbladder cancer

After R0 resection, there have been some data that suggest a survival benefit with the use of adjuvant radiotherapy.[77,80] A cohort of 78 patients with stage T2-4 resectable GC was propensity matched to determine the effect of adjuvant CRT on OS after curative resection.[81] The adjuvant CRT group was treated with treated with external beam radiation + either monotherapy (capecitabine) or dual-agent chemotherapy (oxaliplatin-based). The group that received adjuvant CRT had a significantly longer OS (27 vs 13 months, $P = .004$) and disease-free survival (23 vs 7 months, $P = .004$).[79]

Kim[82] advocates that patients with pT2 disease or R1 resection for GC are at highest risk for locoregional recurrence and thus would benefit the most from adjuvant CRT before progression.[82] An NCDB analysis of node-positive patients revealed the best OS with R0 resection combined with adjuvant CRT.[83]

Chemotherapy in unresectable gallbladder cancer

The phase 3 trial ABC-02 by Valle and colleagues[84] supports the use of gemcitabine/cisplatin compared with gemcitabine alone for advanced or metastatic biliary tract cancers, not exclusively GB carcinoma. The OS difference for the groups was statistically significant (11.7 vs 8.1 months, $P<.001$), although both dismal compared with survival after resection.[84] However, gemcitabine/cisplatin offered measurable efficacy in 80% of patients. Population-based studies since the original publication in 2010 have identified risk factors that predict worse survival: male gender, elevated initial CA 19-9 level, metastases, poor performance status, and measurable disease by RECIST (Response Evaluation Criteria In Solid Tumors) criteria.[85] However, either regimen offers better OS compared with best supportive care in metastatic GC (35.6 vs 13 weeks).[86]

Chemoradiotherapy in unresectable gallbladder cancer

Chemotherapy is the traditional therapy for unresectable GBC (level 1 evidence for use of gemcitabine/cisplatin in NCCN guidelines, version 2.2018[9]), and no RCTs have been conducted to examine the role of locoregional therapy (ie, radiation therapy) for unresectable cancer.[87] In fact, most recurrences after resection are locoregional (85%–90%), with locoregional recurrence being the primary cause of tumor-related mortality.[88]

An analysis of the NCDB from 2004 to 2013 for unresected but nonmetastatic GBC compared outcomes for patients receiving chemotherapy alone (CT) with CRT.[87] In the cohort of 1199 patients, 872 (73%) underwent CT and 327 (27%) underwent CRT. OS analysis revealed a statistically significant difference of 7.8 months (95% CI 7.5–8.5) in the CT group compared with 12.9 months (95% CI 11.0–14.7) in CRT group.[87] These data support the need for a prospective study to examine the role of CRT in unresected, nonmetastatic GC.

Targeted therapeutic agents in gallbladder cancer

The advanced stage of diagnosis and limited adjuvant chemotherapeutic options have paved the way for targeted therapeutics using next-generation sequencing. **Table 3** presents some of the common mutations in GBC and corresponding potential clinical targets.[89,90] Erlotinib has shown some clinical benefit as a monotherapy[91] and in combination with bevacizumab,[92] but showed no significant benefit in a small series of patients treated with sorafenib + erlotinib.[93] A phase 3 trial showed no survival benefit with gemcitabine, oxaliplatin, + erlotinib compared with gemcitabine + oxaliplatin alone, although the erlotinib group had improved progression-free survival and tumor shrinkage.[94] A small cohort of GBC patients received *HER2/neu*-directed therapy with

Table 3
Targetable genetic mutations in gallbladder cancer

Targetable Mutations	Prevalence (%)	Potential Therapeutics
EGFR	4–13	Afatinib, Erlotinib, Cetuximab
HER2/neu amplification	10–16	Trastuzumab, Lapatinib, Pertuzumab
TP53	4–47	Bevacizumab
ERBB3	0–12	Seribantumab, Pertuzumab, Trastuzumab
PTEN PIK3CA	0–4 6–14	mTOR inhibitors (everolimus)
KRAS	4–13	Trametinib, Selumetinib
AR1D1A	15	mTOR inhibitor (everolimus), anti-PD-L1 (Pembrolizumab) for tumors with microsatellite instability
CDKN2A/B loss	6–19	Palbociclib

Data from Jain A, Javle M. Molecular profiling of biliary tract cancer: a target rich disease. J Gastrointest Oncol 2016;7(5):797–803; and Sicklick JK, Fanta PT, Shimabukuro K, et al. Genomics of gallbladder cancer: the case for biomarker-driven clinical trial design. Cancer Metastasis Rev 2016;35(2):263–75.

more than half showing some degree of response.[95] One-third of patients receiving cetuximab, gemcitabine, + oxaliplatin went on to curative resection after tumor response.[96]

Palliative Therapy

Similar to other biliary cancers, the mainstay of palliative treatment in GBC is maintenance of adequate biliary drainage, nutrition, and local compressive symptoms. Biliary drainage can be achieved via percutaneous catheter placement or endoscopic biliary stents and is ideally performed before initiation chemotherapy.[9] Biliary tumors often cause duodenal or gastric outlet compression, necessitating distal feeding access or gastrojejunal bypass to maintain adequate nutrition. Patients with stage IV GBC enrolled in ABC-02 derived a modest survival benefit from gemcitabine/cisplatin.[84]

SURVIVAL IN GALLBLADDER CANCER

Tumor stage is the most important factor for predicting patient survival (Table 4).[57,97] Unfortunately, most patients are diagnosed at later stages and will develop lethal metastases even after aggressive surgical therapy. Current staging systems used variables at the time of diagnosis or surgery to predict long-term survival. Buettner and colleagues[2] propose a prediction tool for patients undergoing curative resection based on conditional survival (CS); this takes into account that if a patient is alive 2 years after surgery, then they are significantly more likely to be alive 5 years after surgery than their stage based on variables at diagnosis would predict.[2] They found the 5-year OS for all tumors to be 31.6%, with a positive surgical margin, larger tumor, higher tumor grade, and LN metastases. Not surprising, they found that CS increases as time from surgery increases, with the most significant discrepancy between OS and CS in patients with the worst initial prognosis (ie, T3/4 tumors, positive nodes).[2] For example, for a patient who is 5 years postoperative from resection of a T3/T4 tumor, the predicted OS at 8 years is only 9.7% compared with CS of 75.2%.[2] Wang and colleagues[76] used SEER data to create a Web-based tool to predict survival after surgery or surgery + CRT in GBC (found at http://skynet.ohsu.edu/nomograms).

There are no data to support frequency or duration of follow-up imaging for GBC, but NCCN recommends imaging every 6 months for 2 years and then annually up to 5 years.[9]

Table 4
Five-year survival for GBC by American Joint Committee on Cancer T-classification and stage

	5 Year OS[97] (%)		5-Year OS[57] (%)
T1a	85.9	Stage I	62.5
T1b		Stage IIA	50.2
T2	56.1	Stage IIB	
T3	19.2	Stage IIIA	25.7
T4	14.1	Stage IIIB	22.1
		Stage IVA	15.7
		Stage IVB	6.7

Data from Miyakawa S, Ishihara S, Horiguchi A, et al. Biliary tract cancer treatment: 5,584 results from the Biliary Tract Cancer Statistics Registry from 1998 to 2004 in Japan. J Hepatobiliary Pancreat Surg 2009;16(1):1–7.[97]

REFERENCES

1. American Joint Committee on Cancer. AJCC cancer staging handbook: from the AJCC cancer staging manual. 7th edition. New York: Springer; 2010.
2. Buettner S, Margonis GA, Kim Y, et al. Changing odds of survival over time among patients undergoing surgical resection of gallbladder carcinoma. Ann Surg Oncol 2016;23(13):4401–9.
3. Fuks D, Regimbeau JM, Le Treut YP, et al. Incidental gallbladder cancer by the AFC-GBC-2009 Study Group. World J Surg 2011;35(8):1887–97.
4. Muszynska C, Lundgren L, Lindell G, et al. Predictors of incidental gallbladder cancer in patients undergoing cholecystectomy for benign gallbladder disease: Results from a population-based gallstone surgery registry. Surgery 2017;162(2): 256–63.
5. Choi KS, Choi SB, Park P, et al. Clinical characteristics of incidental or unsuspected gallbladder cancers diagnosed during or after cholecystectomy: a systematic review and meta-analysis. World J Gastroenterol 2015;21(4):1315–23.
6. Ethun CG, Le N, Lopez-Aguiar AG, et al. Pathologic and prognostic implications of incidental versus nonincidental gallbladder cancer: a 10-Institution Study from the United States Extrahepatic Biliary Malignancy Consortium. Am Surg 2017; 83(7):679–86.
7. Aloia TA, Jarufe N, Javle M, et al. Gallbladder cancer: expert consensus statement. HPB (Oxford) 2015;17(8):681–90.
8. Lau CSM, Zywot A, Mahendraraj K, et al. Gallbladder carcinoma in the United States: a population based clinical outcomes study involving 22,343 patients from the surveillance, epidemiology, and end result database (1973-2013). HPB Surg 2017;2017:1532835.
9. Benson AB III, D'Angelica MI, Abbot DE, et al. NCCN Clinical Practice Guidelines in Oncology: Hepatobiliary Cancers. Version 5.2018 2018. Available at: https://www.nccn.org/professionals/physician_gls/pdf/hepatobiliary_blocks.pdf. Accessed October 2, 2018.
10. Zatonski WA, Lowenfels AB, Boyle P, et al. Epidemiologic aspects of gallbladder cancer: a case-control study of the SEARCH Program of the International Agency for Research on Cancer. J Natl Cancer Inst 1997;89(15):1132–8.
11. Sharma A, Sharma KL, Gupta A, et al. Gallbladder cancer epidemiology, pathogenesis and molecular genetics: recent update. World J Gastroenterol 2017; 23(22):3978–98.
12. Rahman R, Simoes EJ, Schmaltz C, et al. Trend analysis and survival of primary gallbladder cancer in the United States: a 1973-2009 population-based study. Cancer Med 2017;6(4):874–80.
13. Jarnagin WR, Ruo L, Little SA, et al. Patterns of initial disease recurrence after resection of gallbladder carcinoma and hilar cholangiocarcinoma: implications for adjuvant therapeutic strategies. Cancer 2003;98(8):1689–700.
14. American Joint Committee on Cancer. AJCC cancer staging manual. 8th edition. New York: Springer Internltional Publishing; 2017.
15. Shrikhande SV, Barreto SG, Singh S, et al. Cholelithiasis in gallbladder cancer: coincidence, cofactor, or cause! Eur J Surg Oncol 2010;36(6):514–9.
16. Elmasry M, Lindop D, Dunne DF, et al. The risk of malignancy in ultrasound detected gallbladder polyps: a systematic review. Int J Surg 2016;33(Pt A):28–35.
17. Campbell PT, Newton CC, Kitahara CM, et al. Body size indicators and risk of gallbladder cancer: pooled analysis of individual-level data from 19 prospective cohort studies. Cancer Epidemiol Biomarkers Prev 2017;26(4):597–606.

18. Samadder NJ, Smith KR, Wong J, et al. Familial risk of biliary tract cancers: a population-based study in Utah. Dig Dis Sci 2016;61(12):3627–32.
19. Hemminki K, Li X. Familial liver and gall bladder cancer: a nationwide epidemiological study from Sweden. Gut 2003;52(4):592–6.
20. Koshenkov VP, Koru-Sengul T, Franceschi D, et al. Predictors of incidental gallbladder cancer in patients undergoing cholecystectomy for benign gallbladder disease. J Surg Oncol 2013;107(2):118–23.
21. Sandrasegaran K, Menias CO. Imaging and screening of cancer of the gallbladder and bile ducts. Radiol Clin North Am 2017;55(6):1211–22.
22. Adsay V, Jang KT, Roa JC, et al. Intracholecystic papillary-tubular neoplasms (ICPN) of the gallbladder (neoplastic polyps, adenomas, and papillary neoplasms that are ≥1.0 cm): clinicopathologic and immunohistochemical analysis of 123 cases. Am J Surg Pathol 2012;36(9):1279–301.
23. Stephen AE, Berger DL. Carcinoma in the porcelain gallbladder: a relationship revisited. Surgery 2001;129(6):699–703.
24. DesJardins, Haley, et al. Porcelain Gallbladder: Is Observation a Safe Option in Select Populations? JACS 2018;226(6).1064–9.
25. Okada H, Uchida Y, Matsuzaki N, et al. A case of neuroendocrine carcinoma in the hepatic hilar lymph nodes concomitant with an adenocarcinoma of the gallbladder. World J Surg Oncol 2016;14(1):284.
26. Adachi T, Haraguchi M, Irie J, et al. Gallbladder small cell carcinoma: a case report and literature review. Surg Case Rep 2016;2(1):71.
27. Ayub A, Rehmani S, Al-Ayoubi AM, et al. Primary non-hodgkin's lymphoma of the gallbladder: a population-based analysis. Anticancer Res 2017;37(5):2581–6.
28. D'Angelica M, Dalal KM, DeMatteo RP, et al. Analysis of the extent of resection for adenocarcinoma of the gallbladder. Ann Surg Oncol 2009;16(4):806–16.
29. Mishra PK, Saluja SS, Prithiviraj N, et al. Predictors of curative resection and long term survival of gallbladder cancer - A retrospective analysis. Am J Surg 2017; 214(2):278–86.
30. Tran TB, Norton JA, Ethun CG, et al. Gallbladder cancer presenting with jaundice: uniformly fatal or still potentially curable? J Gastrointest Surg 2017;21(8): 1245–53.
31. Kim SW, Kim HC, Yang DM, et al. Gallbladder carcinoma: causes of misdiagnosis at CT. Clin Radiol 2016;71(1):e96–109.
32. Li B, Xu XX, Du Y, et al. Computed tomography for assessing resectability of gallbladder carcinoma: a systematic review and meta-analysis. Clin Imaging 2013; 37(2):327–33.
33. Annunziata S, Pizzuto DA, Caldarella C, et al. Diagnostic accuracy of fluorine-18-fluorodeoxyglucose positron emission tomography in gallbladder cancer: a meta-analysis. World J Gastroenterol 2015;21(40):11481–8.
34. Rodriguez-Fernandez A, Gomez-Rio M, Medina-Benitez A, et al. Application of modern imaging methods in diagnosis of gallbladder cancer. J Surg Oncol 2006;93(8):650–64.
35. Corvera CU, Blumgart LH, Akhurst T, et al. 18F-fluorodeoxyglucose positron emission tomography influences management decisions in patients with biliary cancer. J Am Coll Surg 2008;206(1):57–65.
36. Butte JM, Redondo F, Waugh E, et al. The role of PET-CT in patients with incidental gallbladder cancer. HPB (Oxford) 2009;11(7):585–91.
37. Kalayarasan R, Javed A, Puri AS, et al. A prospective analysis of the preoperative assessment of duodenal involvement in gallbladder cancer. HPB (Oxford) 2013; 15(3):203–9.

38. Agarwal AK, Kalayarasan R, Javed A, et al. Mass-forming xanthogranulomatous cholecystitis masquerading as gallbladder cancer. J Gastrointest Surg 2013; 17(7):1257–64.
39. Agarwal AK, Kalayarasan R, Javed A, et al. The role of staging laparoscopy in primary gall bladder cancer–an analysis of 409 patients: a prospective study to evaluate the role of staging laparoscopy in the management of gallbladder cancer. Ann Surg. 2013;258(2):318–23.
40. Zhao X, Li XY, Ji W. Laparoscopic versus open treatment of gallbladder cancer: A systematic review and meta-analysis. J Minim Access Surg 2018;14(3):185–91.
41. Ethun CG, Postlewait LM, Le N, et al. Association of optimal time interval to re-resection for incidental gallbladder cancer with overall survival: a multi-institution analysis from the US extrahepatic biliary malignancy consortium. JAMA Surg 2017;152(2):143–9.
42. Duffy A, Capanu M, Abou-Alfa GK, et al. Gallbladder cancer (GBC): 10-year experience at Memorial Sloan-Kettering Cancer Centre (MSKCC). J Surg Oncol 2008;98(7):485–9.
43. Shih SP, Schulick RD, Cameron JL, et al. Gallbladder cancer: the role of laparoscopy and radical resection. Ann Surg 2007;245(6):893–901.
44. Hueman MT, Vollmer CM Jr, Pawlik TM. Evolving treatment strategies for gallbladder cancer. Ann Surg Oncol 2009;16(8):2101–15.
45. Jensen EH, Abraham A, Habermann EB, et al. A critical analysis of the surgical management of early-stage gallbladder cancer in the United States. J Gastrointest Surg 2009;13(4):722–7.
46. Butte JM, Kingham TP, Gonen M, et al. Residual disease predicts outcomes after definitive resection for incidental gallbladder cancer. J Am Coll Surg 2014;219(3): 416–29.
47. Vega EA, Vinuela E, Yamashita S, et al. Extended lymphadenectomy is required for incidental gallbladder cancer independent of cystic duct lymph node status. J Gastrointest Surg 2018;22(1):43–51.
48. Butte JM, Gonen M, Allen PJ, et al. The role of laparoscopic staging in patients with incidental gallbladder cancer. HPB (Oxford) 2011;13(7):463–72.
49. Cavallaro A, Piccolo G, Di Vita M, et al. Managing the incidentally detected gallbladder cancer: algorithms and controversies. Int J Surg 2014;12(Suppl 2). S108–s119.
50. Araida T, Higuchi R, Hamano M, et al. Hepatic resection in 485 R0 pT2 and pT3 cases of advanced carcinoma of the gallbladder: results of a Japanese Society of Biliary Surgery survey–a multicenter study. J Hepatobiliary Pancreat Surg 2009; 16(2):204–15.
51. Butte JM, Waugh E, Meneses M, et al. Incidental gallbladder cancer: analysis of surgical findings and survival. J Surg Oncol 2010;102(6):620–5.
52. Nishio H, Ebata T, Yokoyama Y, et al. Gallbladder cancer involving the extrahepatic bile duct is worthy of resection. Ann Surg 2011;253(5):953–60.
53. Jensen EH, Abraham A, Jarosek S, et al. Lymph node evaluation is associated with improved survival after surgery for early stage gallbladder cancer. Surgery 2009;146(4):706–11 [discussion: 711–3].
54. Shirai Y, Wakai T, Sakata J, et al. Regional lymphadenectomy for gallbladder cancer: rational extent, technical details, and patient outcomes. World J Gastroenterol 2012;18(22):2775–83.
55. Negi SS, Singh A, Chaudhary A. Lymph nodal involvement as prognostic factor in gallbladder cancer: location, count or ratio? J Gastrointest Surg 2011;15(6): 1017–25.

56. Ito H, Ito K, D'Angelica M, et al. Accurate staging for gallbladder cancer: impli-cations for surgical therapy and pathological assessment. Ann Surg 2011; 254(2):320–5.

57. Lee AJ, Chiang Y-J, Lee JE, et al. Validation of American Joint Committee on Can-cer eighth staging system for gallbladder cancer and its lymphadenectomy guidelines. J Surg Res 2018;230:148–54.

58. Berger-Richardson D, Chesney TR, Englesakis M, et al. Trends in port-site metas-tasis after laparoscopic resection of incidental gallbladder cancer: a systematic review. Surgery 2017;161(3):618–27.

59. Shoup M, Fong Y. Surgical indications and extent of resection in gallbladder can-cer. Surg Oncol Clin N Am 2002;11(4):985–94.

60. Maker AV, Butte JM, Oxenberg J, et al. Is port site resection necessary in the sur-gical management of gallbladder cancer? Ann Surg Oncol 2012;19(2):409–17.

61. Pawlik TM, Gleisner AL, Vigano L, et al. Incidence of finding residual disease for incidental gallbladder carcinoma: implications for re-resection. J Gastrointest Surg 2007;11(11):1478–86 [discussion: 1486–7].

62. Vinuela E, Vega EA, Yamashita S, et al. Incidental gallbladder cancer: residual cancer discovered at oncologic extended resection determines outcome: a report from high- and low-incidence countries. Ann Surg Oncol 2017;24(8): 2334–43.

63. Abramson MA, Pandharipande P, Ruan D, et al. Radical resection for T1b gall-bladder cancer: a decision analysis. HPB (Oxford) 2009;11(8):656–63.

64. Hari DM, Howard JH, Leung AM, et al. A 21-year analysis of stage I gallbladder carcinoma: is cholecystectomy alone adequate? HPB (Oxford) 2013;15(1):40–8.

65. Dixon E, Vollmer CM Jr, Sahajpal A, et al. An aggressive surgical approach leads to improved survival in patients with gallbladder cancer: a 12-year study at a North American Center. Ann Surg 2005;241(3):385–94.

66. Shindoh J, de Aretxabala X, Aloia TA, et al. Tumor location is a strong predictor of tumor progression and survival in T2 gallbladder cancer: an international multi-center study. Ann Surg 2015;261(4):733–9.

67. Lee W, Jeong CY, Jang JY, et al. Do hepatic-sided tumors require more extensive resection than peritoneal-sided tumors in patients with T2 gallbladder cancer? Results of a retrospective multicenter study. Surgery 2017;162(3):515–24.

68. Ausania F, Tsirlis T, White SA, et al. Incidental pT2-T3 gallbladder cancer after a cholecystectomy: outcome of staging at 3 months prior to a radical resection. HPB (Oxford) 2013;15(8):633–7.

69. Agarwal AK, Javed A, Kalayarasan R, et al. Minimally invasive versus the conven-tional open surgical approach of a radical cholecystectomy for gallbladder can-cer: a retrospective comparative study. HPB (Oxford) 2015;17(6):536–41.

70. Itano O, Oshima G, Minagawa T, et al. Novel strategy for laparoscopic treatment of pT2 gallbladder carcinoma. Surg Endosc 2015;29(12):3600–7.

71. Lopez-Aguiar AG, Ethun CG, McInnis MR, et al. Association of perioperative transfusion with survival and recurrence after resection of gallbladder cancer: A 10-institution study from the US Extrahepatic Biliary Malignancy Consortium. J Surg Oncol 2018;117(8):1638–47.

72. Mitin T, Enestvedt CK, Jemal A, et al. Limited use of adjuvant therapy in patients with resected gallbladder cancer despite a strong association with survival. J Natl Cancer Inst 2017;109(7):1–9.

73. Creasy JM, Goldman DA, Dudeja V, et al. Systemic chemotherapy combined with resection for locally advanced gallbladder carcinoma: surgical and survival out-comes. J Am Coll Surg 2017;224(5):906–16.

74. Horgan AM, Amir E, Walter T, et al. Adjuvant therapy in the treatment of biliary tract cancer: a systematic review and meta-analysis. J Clin Oncol 2012;30(16): 1934–40.

75. Ma N, Cheng H, Qin B, et al. Adjuvant therapy in the treatment of gallbladder cancer: a meta-analysis. BMC Cancer 2015;15:615.

76. Wang SJ, Lemieux A, Kalpathy-Cramer J, et al. Nomogram for predicting the benefit of adjuvant chemoradiotherapy for resected gallbladder cancer. J Clin Oncol 2011;29(35):4627–32.

77. Mantripragada KC, Hamid F, Shafqat H, et al. Adjuvant therapy for resected gallbladder cancer: analysis of the national cancer data base. J Natl Cancer Inst 2017;109(2) [pii:djw202].

78. Bergquist JR, Shah HN, Habermann EB, et al. Adjuvant systemic therapy after resection of node positive gallbladder cancer: Time for a well-designed trial? (Results of a US-national retrospective cohort study). Int J Surg 2018;52:171–9.

79. Ghidini M, Tomasello G, Botticelli A, et al. Adjuvant chemotherapy for resected biliary tract cancers: a systematic review and meta-analysis. HPB (Oxford) 2017;19(9):741–8.

80. Hoehn RS, Wima K, Ertel AE, et al. Adjuvant therapy for gallbladder cancer: an analysis of the national cancer data base. J Gastrointest Surg 2015;19(10): 1794–801.

81. Gu B, Qian L, Yu H, et al. Concurrent chemoradiotherapy in curatively resected gallbladder carcinoma: a propensity score-matched analysis. Int J Radiat Oncol Biol Phys 2018;100(1):138–45.

82. Kim TG. Patterns of initial failure after resection for gallbladder cancer: implications for adjuvant radiotherapy. Radiat Oncol J 2017;35(4):359–67.

83. Tran Cao HS, Zhang Q, Sada YH, et al. The role of surgery and adjuvant therapy in lymph node-positive cancers of the gallbladder and intrahepatic bile ducts. Cancer Cytopathol 2018;124(1):74–83.

84. Valle J, Wasan H, Palmer DH, et al. Cisplatin plus gemcitabine versus gemcitabine for biliary tract cancer. N Engl J Med 2010;362(14):1273–81.

85. Kim BJ, Hyung J, Yoo C, et al. Prognostic factors in patients with advanced biliary tract cancer treated with first-line gemcitabine plus cisplatin: retrospective analysis of 740 patients. Cancer Chemother Pharmacol 2017;80(1):209–15.

86. Singh SK, Talwar R, Kannan N, et al. Chemotherapy compared with best supportive care for metastatic/unresectable gallbladder cancer: a non-randomized prospective cohort study. Indian J Surg Oncol 2016;7(1):25–31.

87. Verma V, Surkar SM, Brooks ED, et al. Chemoradiotherapy versus chemotherapy alone for unresected nonmetastatic gallbladder cancer: National practice patterns and outcomes. J Natl Compr Cancer Netw 2018;16(1):59–65.

88. Macdonald OK, Crane CH. Palliative and postoperative radiotherapy in biliary tract cancer. Surg Oncol Clin N Am 2002;11(4):941–54.

89. Jain A, Javle M. Molecular profiling of biliary tract cancer: a target rich disease. J Gastrointest Oncol 2016;7(5):797–803.

90. Sicklick JK, Fanta PT, Shimabukuro K, et al. Genomics of gallbladder cancer: the case for biomarker-driven clinical trial design. Cancer Metastasis Rev 2016;35(2): 263–75.

91. Philip PA, Mahoney MR, Allmer C, et al. Phase II study of erlotinib in patients with advanced biliary cancer. J Clin Oncol 2006;24(19):3069–74.

92. Lubner SJ, Mahoney MR, Kolesar JL, et al. Report of a multicenter phase II trial testing a combination of biweekly bevacizumab and daily erlotinib in patients with

unresectable biliary cancer: a phase II Consortium study. J Clin Oncol 2010; 28(21):3491–7.

93. El-Khoueiry AB, Rankin C, Siegel AB, et al. S0941: a phase 2 SWOG study of sorafenib and erlotinib in patients with advanced gallbladder carcinoma or cholangiocarcinoma. Br J Cancer 2014;110(4):882–7.

94. Kim ST, Jang KT, Lee SJ, et al. Tumour shrinkage at 6 weeks predicts favorable clinical outcomes in a phase III study of gemcitabine and oxaliplatin with or without erlotinib for advanced biliary tract cancer. BMC Cancer 2015;15:530.

95. Javle M, Churi C, Kang HC, et al. HER2/neu-directed therapy for biliary tract cancer. J Hematol Oncol 2015;8:58.

96. Gruenberger B, Schueller J, Heubrandtner U, et al. Cetuximab, gemcitabine, and oxaliplatin in patients with unresectable advanced or metastatic biliary tract cancer: a phase 2 study. Lancet Oncol 2010;11(12):1142–8.

97. Miyakawa S, Ishihara S, Horiguchi A, et al. Biliary tract cancer treatment: 5,584 results from the Biliary Tract Cancer Statistics Registry from 1998 to 2004 in Japan. J Hepatobiliary Pancreat Surg 2009;16(1):1–7.

Ampullary Cancer

Rui Zheng-Pywell, MD, Sushanth Reddy, MD*

KEYWORDS

- Ampullary cancer • Pancreaticoduodenectomy • Biliary obstruction

KEY POINTS

- There are 2 distinct subtypes of ampullary cancers: pancreaticobiliary and intestinal. Pancreaticobiliary tumors are more aggressive.
- Because these tumors present earlier, most patients can undergo curative resection. Fit patients should be considered for pancreaticoduodenectomy.
- There is a survival benefit from adjuvant chemotherapy. The role of radiation therapy remains controversial for ampullary cancers.
- Patients with ampullary adenomas or those who cannot tolerate a formal pancreaticoduodenectomy should be considered for an endoscopic or surgical ampullectomy.

INTRODUCTION: NATURE OF THE PROBLEM

A majority of periampullary cancers (PACs) are pancreatic adenocarcinomas. Ampullary cancers are rare: they comprise 0.2% of all gastrointestinal cancers and 16% to 28% of all PACs.[1–3] These tumors have a slight male preponderance and patients tend to be in their seventh decade of life. Data from the United States Surveillance, Epidemiology, and End Results Program demonstrate an overall incidence of 0.49 cases per 100,000 individuals. The incidence of PACs has been steadily rising, however, over the past 4 decades.[4] Patients with these cancers do have better overall survival than those with pancreatic or distal bile duct cancers.[5]

RELEVANT ANATOMY/PATHOPHYSIOLOGY

The ampulla of Vater is formed by the union of the pancreatic duct with the common bile duct. Eponymously named for the German anatomist Abraham Vater, the ampulla is often confused with the sphincter of Oddi. The sphincter is actually a group of circular muscle fibers surrounding the submucosal portion of the ducts proximal to the duodenal papilla at the site of entry of the ampulla itself.[6] Anatomically, the ampulla is the landmark between the foregut and the hindgut.

The authors have nothing to disclose.
Department of Surgery, University of Alabama at Birmingham, 1808 7th Avenue South, BDB 607 Birmingham, AL 35233-3411, USA
* Corresponding author.
E-mail address: sreddy@uabmc.edu

Surg Clin N Am 99 (2019) 357–367
https://doi.org/10.1016/j.suc.2018.12.001
0039-6109/19/© 2018 Elsevier Inc. All rights reserved.

The epithelial lining of the ampulla and the immediately surrounding tissues is complex. The surrounding duodenum is made up of intestinal (IT) epithelium with goblet cells whereas the actual duodenal papilla contains goblet cells in a foveolar-like epithelium. Both the distal bile duct and the pancreatic duct have columnar, mucus-secreting cells.[7] Adenocarcinomas can develop from any one of these epithelial linings. The behavior of each cancer differs greatly. Conceptually the distinction of these 4 epithelia seems straightforward. In practice, most tumors of the periampullary region grow to involve not only the ampulla but also the pancreas, distal bile duct, and duodenum. These different cancers often can be distinguished from one another only histologically on the final resected specimen by an experienced group of pathologists.[3]

CLINICAL PRESENTATION/EXAMINATION

Patients with ampullary cancer present in a manner similar to those with pancreatic head adenocarcinomas and distal bile duct cholangiocarcinomas. Most patients' primary complaint is jaundice. Please see **Table 1** for details.

DIAGNOSTIC PROCEDURES

The differential diagnosis of a patient with jaundice is large and outside the scope of this review. Nonetheless, practitioners should focus on determining whether jaundice is related to obstruction. Obstructive jaundice is classically defined by elevation in the direct (or conjugated bilirubin) and intrahepatic and extrahepatic biliary ductal dilation. Different diagnostic modalities are discussed in **Table 2**.

AVAILABLE PROCEDURES

Patients with periampullary malignancies should be evaluated in a high-volume center with a multidisciplinary discussion prior to initiating treatment. At the authors' institution, upfront chemotherapy is preferred for pancreatic cancers. This approach is supported for patients with pancreatic cancer but not as well defined for those with ampullary cancers. Other centers advocate for a surgery-first approach to these diseases.

Most patients have undergone some imaging prior to referral. If patients have evidence of metastatic disease, they should have endoscopic biliary decompression, biopsy for tissue diagnosis, consultation for palliative chemotherapy, and discussions regarding end-of-life issues.

For those patients with localized disease, the authors advocate the procedural paradigm shown in **Fig. 1**. If an upfront chemotherapy approach is used, individualized centers should establish criteria for high-risk cancers. Several studies have attempted to clarify high-risk features for pancreatic cancer, with limited reproducibility. Such definitions have yet to be established for ampullary cancer. The authors have defined high-risk ampullary cancers as primary tumors larger than 3 cm on cross-sectional

Table 1	
Common clinical presentations and examination findings	
Clinical Presentation	**Examination**
Biliary obstruction (80%)	Painless jaundice Acholic stool
Diarrhea	Steatorrhea
Gastrointestinal bleed (33%)	Melena (can be exacerbated by antiplatelet/anticoagulant use)

Table 2
Diagnostic tests with associated advantages and disadvantages

Test	Advantages	Disadvantages
CT of abdomen with and without contrast	• Fast, relatively inexpensive • Details arterial and venous involvement • Easy to see aberrant arterial anatomy • Can see liver metastases	• Nephrotoxic and limited utility in patients with renal dysfunction • Often is the second CT scan these patients undergo • Additional radiation exposure
MRI of abdomen with contrast	• No radiation exposure • No contrast-related renal injury • Helpful for smaller liver lesions	• No standardization of technique • Expensive and time consuming • Difficult for larger or claustrophobic patients, those with pacemakers
ERCP	• Can be diagnostic and therapeutic	• Invasive • Biliary stenting associated with increased infection risk after surgery • Biliary brushings with limited utility in diagnosis
Endoscopic ultrasound	• Reliably obtain tissue diagnosis • Helps delineate anatomic origin	• Invasive • Very operator dependent • Postprocedure pancreatitis

imaging, periampullary lymph nodes larger than 2 cm, or serum carbohydrate antigen 19-9 (CA 19-9) level greater than 200 ng/ml after biliary decompression. The decision to operate is determined by proximity of the tumor to local vessels, absence of metastatic disease to solid organs, and patient fitness to undergo a pancreatoduodenectomy (PD). Compared with pancreatic cancers, ampullary cancers are less likely to involve the splenomesenteric venous confluence, the superior mesenteric artery (SMA), or hepatic arterial branches of the celiac axis. Ampullary cancers, therefore, are more likely to be categorized as resectable. Involvement of these structures should classify these tumors as either locally advanced or borderline resectable. Patients with vascular involvement should proceed through an upfront chemotherapy pathway. These anatomic features are best delineated on high-quality, thin-cut CT scans with and without intravenous contrast (eg, pancreatic protocol CT scan).

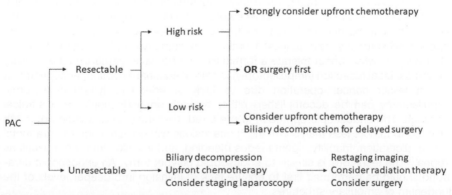

Fig. 1. Management algorithm for PAC.

PROCEDURE TECHNIQUE

The operation of choice for ampullary cancer is a PD. Given the high morbidity and mortality from this operation, most patients should be seen at a tertiary referral center. Prior to surgery a high-quality CT scan is advised to delineate anatomy—paying extra attention to aberrant hepatic arterial vasculature. An aberrant right hepatic artery or an aberrant left hepatic artery originating from the SMA or the left gastric artery, respectively, is present in 15% to 20% of patients. A PD begins with a thorough abdominal exploration for metastatic disease. The exact steps differ from surgeon to surgeon; however, the fundamental moves remain the same. Typically, the duodenum is mobilized out of the retroperitoneum with a wide Kocher or Cattell-Braasch maneuver. Using this approach, the tumor's relationship to the SMA is established. Next, the superior mesenteric vein (SMV) is identified. Some surgeons widely open the lesser sac to trace the right gastroepiploic vein's confluence into the SMV. Others dissect the transverse mesocolon off the pancreatic head to identify the SMV in a groove in this location. The right gastroepiploic vein must be ligated and divided. This exposes the inferior border of the pancreas and is necessary to safely create a tunnel behind the neck of the pancreas. The hepatoduodenal ligament is dissected to identify the hepatic arteries and the common bile duct. Care should be exercised with circumferential control of the bile duct to avoid injuring the portal vein or (if present) an aberrant right hepatic artery. The gastroduodenal artery should be identified, test clamped, ligated, and divided. By dividing the common bile duct and the gastroduodenal artery, the portal vein can be easily identified. If the gall bladder is present, it can be removed at this point. The tunnel behind the neck of the pancreas can be completed. Surgeons differ on their approach to the pylorus. No data support a pylorus-preserving operation or a classic PD. Nonetheless, after division of the stomach or duodenum, the neck of the pancreas is well exposed. The pancreas is then divided, thereby exposing the splenomesenteric venous confluence. The uncinate attachments to the SMA are ligated and divided with special attention to the inferior pancreaticoduodenal artery. After widely opening the ligament of Treitz, the proximal jejunum divided with a stapler. The jejunal mesentery can be ligated and divided completing the resection. Some surgeons divide the jejunum and its mesentery prior to completing the uncinate dissection. The specimen is then passed off and processed with special attention to specialized margins (**Fig. 2**). Reconstruction typically follows a "reverse question mark approach" where the jejunum is delivered with a retrocolic approach to the pancreatic neck and bile duct. Several different approaches have been advocated for the pancreatic anastomosis to the jejunum or stomach—none has proved consistently superior to another. The biliary reconstruction typically is straightforward: a single layer of hand-sewn absorbable sutures. The duodenojejunostomy or gastro-jejunostomy can be accomplished in either a hand-sewn or stapled fashion. Most experienced surgeons leave at least 1 drain at the completion of reconstruction.

For patients who cannot tolerate a formal PD or who have premalignant ampullary adenomas, local resection (ampullectomy) is also a reasonable option, accepting that it is a lesser cancer operation due to lack of adequate lymphadenectomy. Ampullectomy can be accomplished either through an endoscopic or a surgical approach. The endoscopic approach is preferred. Generally, endoscopic approach is limited to tumors less than 5 cm and those lesions without evidence of intraductal growth, ulceration, friability, spontaneous bleeding, and invasion into the muscularis propria.[8] The technique is similar to endoscopic polypectomy. An endoscopic ultrasound should be performed first to ensure lack of invasion into deeper levels of the duodenum or ampullary structures.

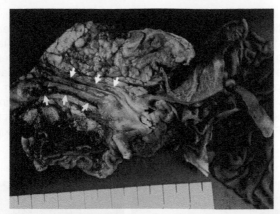

Fig. 2. This is an en bloc pancreaticoduodenectomy specimen from a patient with ampullary cancer. The black arrow is pointing at ampullary cancer. The white arrows designate the pancreatic duct. The yellow arrows designate the common bile duct.

Surgical ampullectomy is safe and associated with low recurrence.[9] In surgery, the duodenum is mobilized out of the retroperitoneum. Stay sutures are placed prior to a longitudinal duodenotomy. The ampulla is typically in the distal portion of the second part of the duodenum. Identification of the ampulla prior to opening the duodenum can allow for a smaller duodenotomy. If the gallbladder has not been previously removed, the cystic duct can facilitate ampullary identification: After completing a cholecystectomy, the cystic duct ostia is cannulated with a small Fogarty catheter that is advanced distally into the duodenum. The catheter's balloon is palpated after insufflation while gently pulling back on the Fogarty. If this technique is used, the surgeon should take great care to avoid damaging the common bile duct. If the cystic duct

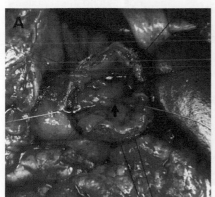
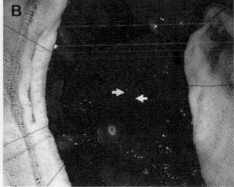

Fig. 3. Surgical ampullectomy (*A*) The ampullary adenoma (*black arrow*) with a metallic probe is entering the ampulla of Vater following a longitudinal enterotomy along the second portion of the duodenum. (*B*) After removal of the ampullary mass, the pancreatic (*white arrow*) and common bile (*yellow arrow*) ducts are exposed. Numerous stay sutures were placed around the ampulla prior to resection to facilitate exposure. The pancreatic and bile ducts will be approximated to the surrounding duodenal mucosa with absorbable sutures.

opening is small, a catheter may not be inserted safely. Furthermore, in patients with obstructive jaundice, this technique should not be attempted because the catheter will not pass through the ampulla safely. In jaundiced patients, the ampullary mass is typically large enough to palpate, or the biliary stent (if placed preoperatively) can be manually identified to find the ampulla. Several stay sutures are placed around the ampulla. This facilitates lifting the duodenal mucosa much like in an endoscopic approach. In **Fig. 3**A, a probe has been inserted into the ampulla going into the common bile duct. The ampulla is excised with cautery exposing the pancreatic and common bile ducts (**Fig. 3**B). These 2 structures should then be approximated with fine

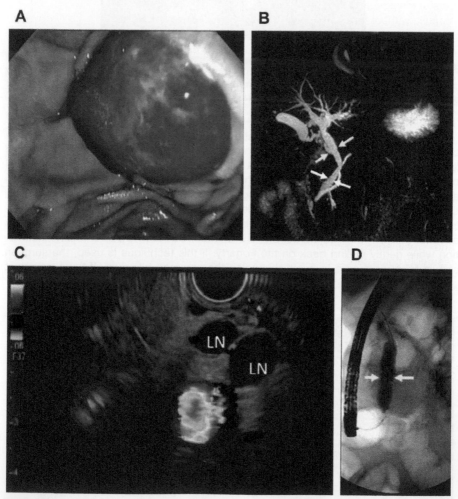

Fig. 4. Diagnosis of ampullary cancer. ERCP, endoscopic retrograde cholangiopancreatography. (*A*) Endoscopic view of an ampullary cancer causing biliary obstruction. (*B*) Magnetic resonance cholangiopancreatography images of the tumor demonstrating both dilation of the pancreatic duct (*white arrows*) and the common bile duct (*yellow arrows*). (*C*) Using endoscopic ultrasound, 2 malignant-appearing lymph nodes (LN) are identified. Note the lack of color flow in the nodes in comparison to the surrounding vasculature. (*D*) ERCP images of the common bile duct (*yellow arrows*) demonstrating marked biliary ductal dilation.

absorbable sutures to the surrounding duodenal mucosa. In addition, these ducts should be sutured together to close the septum between the 2 structures. The duodenum is then closed transversely in a Heineke-Mikulicz manner. If an extended duodenotomy was used, the surgeon should consider a Finney pyloroplasty or a Jaboulay duodenogastrostomy. Many surgeons buttress the closure with a portion of omentum or the round ligament. Again, the surgical field is widely drained.

DIAGNOSIS

Patients with ampullary cancer typically present with obstructive jaundice. Unlike cancers of the pancreas and common bile duct, most of these lesions are localized to the ampulla without invasion into the surrounding vasculature. These lesions are typically small and are difficult to see on cross-sectional imaging. Their presence is suspected based on dilation of the common bile and pancreatic (less common) ducts (**Fig. 4**). In centers with a surgical first approach to PAC, a tissue diagnosis is not necessary provided the patient is fit to undergo a PD and has resectable disease without metastases on reliable cross-sectional imaging. At centers where a chemotherapy-first approach is used for pancreatic cancers, patients typically have a biopsy through an endoscopic ultrasound. Many patients undergo endoscopic retrograde cholangiopancreatography (ERCP) prior to surgical consultation.

MANAGEMENT OPTIONS
Clinical Outcomes in the Literature

Several different histopathologic classifications of ampullary cancers have been published (**Box 1**[10]). Predominantly, 2 distinct subtypes are used: pancreatobiliary (PB) and IT.[11] PB ampullary cancers histologically consist of simple or branching glands and small solids nest of cells and have desmoplastic stroma. IT-type cancers resemble colon cancer and are composed of tubular to elongated glands.[12] In addition to their microscopic differences, these 2 subtypes differ greatly clinically. PB cancers

---

Box 1
PAC Histopathology

Histopathology of PACs

Carcinoma in situ

Adenocarcinoma
   Adenocarcinoma, IT type

Clear cell adenocarcinoma

Mucinous adenocarcinoma

Signet ring cell adenocarcinoma

Adenosquamous carcinoma

Small cell carcinoma

Undifferentiated
   Spindle cell type
   Giant cell type

Papillary carcinoma
   Invasive
   Noninvasive

Table 3
TNM staging of periampullary cancer

T stage

Tx	Primary tumor not assessed
T0	No evidence of primary tumor
Tis	Carcinoma in situ
T1	Tumor limited to ampulla of Vater or sphincter of Oddi or has perisphincteric invasion (beyond the sphincter of Oddi and/or into the duodenal submucosa)
T1a	Tumor limited to ampulla of Vater or sphincter of Oddi
T1b	Perisphincteric tumor invasion (beyond the sphincter of Oddi and/or into the duodenal submucosa)
T2	Tumor invades the muscularis propria of duodenum
T3	Tumor either invades the pancreas directly up to 0.5 cm, extends beyond 0.5 cm into pancreas, or extends into peripancreatic tissue/periduodenal tissue/duodenal serosa without involvement of the celiac axis or SMV
T3a	Tumor directly invades pancreas (≤0.5 cm)
T3b	Tumor extends >0.5 cm into pancreas or extends into peripancreatic tissue/periduodenal tissue/ duodenal serosa without involvement of the celiac axis SMA
T4	Tumor (of any size) with involvement of celiac axis, SMA, and/or common hepatic artery

N stage

Nx	Regional lymph nodes cannot be assessed
N0	No regional lymph node metastasis
N1	Metastasis to 1–3 regional lymph nodes
N2	Metastasis to >4 regional lymph nodes

M stage

M0	No distant metastasis
M1	Distant metastasis

Table 4
Summary of adjuvant therapies approaches for ampullary cancers

Author, Year	N	Therapy	Survival	P Value
Bhatia et al,[19] 2006	N = 29	50.4-Gy XRT, 5FU	3.4 y	.01
	N = 96	Surgery alone	1.6 y	
Sikora et al,[20] 2005	N = 49	50.4-Gy XRT, 5FU	34.6 mo	.3
	N = 55	Surgery alone	29.5 mo	
Zhou et al,[21] 2009	N = 50	50.4-Gy XRT, varied chemotherapy	33.4 mo	.969
	N = 61	Surgery alone	36.2 mo	
Lee et al,[22] 2000	N = 13	48.6-Gy XRT, 5FU	81%[a]	.132
	N = 26	Surgery alone	47%[a]	
Takada et al,[23] 2002	N = 24	MMF + 5FU	28.1%[b]	NS
	N = 24	Surgery alone	34.3%[b]	
Neoptolemos et al,[24] 2012	N = 99	Gem	70.8 mo	<.05 (gem vs surgery)
	N = 99	5FU	57.8 mo	
	N = 99	Surgery alone	40.6 mo	

Abbreviations: FU, fluorouracil; gem, gemcitabine; MMF, mycophenolate mofetil; NS, not significant; XRT, radiotherapy.
[a] Three-year survival.
[b] Five-year survival.

Box 2
Pitfalls in management

• Pay careful attention to any aberrant arteries.

• Wide mobilization of the duodenum helps with closure.

• Be prepared to convert to formal resection if ampullectomy is technically difficult or cancer is present.

• PD is the preferred approach for all patients with ampullary cancer.

---

are much more likely to have lymph nodes metastases, advanced T stage, and perineural invasion compared with IT cancers.[11,13] For staging, see **Table 3** Finally, PB cancers are associated with far worse survival than IT-type cancers (5-year survival rate 5%–36% vs 50%–100%).[14–18] No studies to date have demonstrated a difference in approach for the 2 histopathologic subtypes.

Because ampullary cancer is rare, clinical trials focused on this disease are unlikely to be performed. The data on ampullary cancers are either extracted from other larger trials focusing on pancreaticobiliary malignancies with subset analyses or through retrospective institutional reviews of ampullary cancer patients. A summary of known adjuvant therapies for ampullary cancers is shown in **Table 4**. In general, adjuvant chemotherapy may play a role in treating ampullary cancers whereas adjuvant radiation therapy has less support. Studies focusing on preoperative chemotherapy and radiation therapy have not been published. Series describing upfront therapy focus on PAC as a whole and contain small numbers of ampullary cancer patients.

SUMMARY

Although rare, ampullary cancers are the second most common PAC after pancreatic adenocarcinoma. Surgery is the mainstay of treatment. For adenomas, endoscopic or local surgical therapy is the preferred treatment. In patients with ampullary cancer, PD is essential to achieving cure. These are technically demanding operations; patients should likely be sent to a referral center. Originally believed a single entity, new histologic evidence suggests that ampullary cancer subtypes behave differently. There are no consensus guidelines regarding chemotherapy or radiotherapy options for patients with ampullary cancer. Although survival with this disease is far better than with pancreatic cancer or cholangiocarcinoma, most patients still succumb to their disease. See **Box 2** for pitfalls in management.

REFERENCES

1. He J, Ahuja N, Makary MA, et al. 2564 resected periampullary adenocarcinomas at a single institution: trends over three decades. HPB (Oxford) 2014;16(1): 83–90.
2. Hatzaras I, George N, Muscarella P, et al. Predictors of survival in periampullary cancers following pancreaticoduodenectomy. Ann Surg Oncol 2010;17(4):991–7.
3. Pomianowska E, Grzyb K, Westgaard A, et al. Reclassification of tumour origin in resected periampullary adenocarcinomas reveals underestimation of distal bile duct cancer. Eur J Surg Oncol 2012;38(11):1043–50.
4. Albores-Saavedra J, Schwartz AM, Batich K, et al. Cancers of the ampulla of vater: demographics, morphology, and survival based on 5,625 cases from the SEER program. J Surg Oncol 2009;100(7):598–605.

5. Jean M, Dua K. Tumors of the ampulla of Vater. Curr Gastroenterol Rep 2003;5(2): 171–5.

6. Kirk J. Observations on the histology of the choledocho-duodenal junction and papilla duodeni, with particular reference to the ampulla of Vater and sphincter of Oddi. J Anat 1944;78(Pt 4):118–120.3.

7. Adsay V, Ohike N, Tajiri T, et al. Ampullary region carcinomas: definition and site specific classification with delineation of four clinicopathologically and prognostically distinct subsets in an analysis of 249 cases. Am J Surg Pathol 2012; 36(11):1592–608.

8. De Palma GD, Forestieri P. Role of endoscopy in the bariatric surgery of patients. World J Gastroenterol 2014;20(24):7777–84.

9. Schneider L, Contin P, Fritz S, et al. Surgical ampullectomy: an underestimated operation in the era of endoscopy. HPB (Oxford) 2016;18(1):65–71.

10. AJCC. AJCC cancer staging manual. In: Amin MB, Edge S, Greene F, et al, editors. Continuing to build a bridge from a "population-based" to a more "personalized" approach. 8th edition. Switzerland: Springer International Publishing; 2018. Available at: https://www.springer.com/us/book/9783319406176#aboutBook.

11. Kimura W, Futakawa N, Yamagata S, et al. Different clinicopathologic findings in two histologic types of carcinoma of papilla of Vater. Jpn J Cancer Res 1994; 85(2):161–6.

12. Perysinakis I, Margaris I, Kouraklis G. Ampullary cancer–a separate clinical entity? Histopathology 2014;64(6):759–68.

13. Kim WS, Choi DW, Choi SH, et al. Clinical significance of pathologic subtype in curatively resected ampulla of vater cancer. J Surg Oncol 2012;105(3):266–72.

14. Carter JT, Grenert JP, Rubenstein L, et al. Tumors of the ampulla of vater: histopathologic classification and predictors of survival. J Am Coll Surg 2008; 207(2):210–8.

15. Roh YH, Kim YH, Lee HW, et al. The clinicopathologic and immunohistochemical characteristics of ampulla of Vater carcinoma: the intestinal type is associated with a better prognosis. Hepatogastroenterology 2007;54(78):1641–4.

16. Ruemmele P, Dietmaier W, Terracciano L, et al. Histopathologic features and microsatellite instability of cancers of the papilla of vater and their precursor lesions. Am J Surg Pathol 2009;33(5):691–704.

17. Westgaard A, Schjolberg AR, Cvancarova M, et al. Differentiation markers in pancreatic head adenocarcinomas: MUC1 and MUC4 expression indicates poor prognosis in pancreatobiliary differentiated tumours. Histopathology 2009; 54(3):337–47.

18. Westgaard A, Tafjord S, Farstad IN, et al. Resectable adenocarcinomas in the pancreatic head: the retroperitoneal resection margin is an independent prognostic factor. BMC Cancer 2008;8:5.

19. Bhatia S, Miller RC, Haddock MG, et al. Adjuvant therapy for ampullary carcinomas: the Mayo Clinic experience. Int J Radiat Oncol Biol Phys 2006;66(2): 514–9.

20. Sikora SS, Balachandran P, Dimri K, et al. Adjuvant chemo-radiotherapy in ampullary cancers. Eur J Surg Oncol 2005;31(2):158–63.

21. Zhou J, Hsu CC, Winter JM, et al. Adjuvant chemoradiation versus surgery alone for adenocarcinoma of the ampulla of Vater. Radiother Oncol 2009;92(2):244–8.

22. Lee JH, Whittington R, Williams NN, et al. Outcome of pancreaticoduodenectomy and impact of adjuvant therapy for ampullary carcinomas. Int J Radiat Oncol Biol Phys 2000;47(4):945–53.

23. Takada T, Amano H, Yasuda H, et al. Is postoperative adjuvant chemotherapy useful for gallbladder carcinoma? A phase III multicenter prospective randomized controlled trial in patients with resected pancreaticobiliary carcinoma. Cancer 2002;95(8):1685–95.
24. Neoptolemos JP, Moore MJ, Cox TF, et al. Effect of adjuvant chemotherapy with fluorouracil plus folinic acid or gemcitabine vs observation on survival in patients with resected periampullary adenocarcinoma: the ESPAC-3 periampullary cancer randomized trial. JAMA 2012;308(2):147–56.

Endoscopic Management of Biliary Disorders
Diagnosis and Therapy

Rajesh Krishnamoorthi, MD, Andrew Ross, MD*

KEYWORDS

- Biliary disorders • Endoscopic ultrasound • ERCP • EUS • Ampullary adenoma
- Altered anatomy ERCP • Endoscopic retrograde cholangiopancreatography

KEY POINTS

- Since its introduction into clinical practice, endoscopic retrograde cholangiopancreatography has evolved from a diagnostic and therapeutic tool to a predominantly therapeutic tool.
- There is a limited role for diagnostic endoscopic retrograde cholangiopancreatography in current practice with widespread availability of magnetic resonance cholangiopancreatography and endoscopic ultrasound examination.
- The availability of specialized stents like lumen-apposing metal stents has improved the success rates of transmural biliary drainage.
- The novel cautery-tip delivery system available with lumen-apposing metal stent has helped to shorten the time of complex procedures.
- At the present time, endoscopic retrograde cholangiopancreatography remains the standard of care for patients requiring biliary decompression.

INTRODUCTION

Endoscopic cannulation of ampulla of Vater was first described by McCune and colleagues[1] in 1968; they reported a cannulation rate of 25% in a series of 50 patients. Since then, dedicated duodenoscopes have been developed and endoscopic retrograde cholangiopancreatography (ERCP) has assumed a major role in management of biliary disease. Owing to the introduction of less invasive imaging technologies such as magnetic resonance cholangiopancreatography (MRCP) and endoscopic ultrasound (EUS) examination, ERCP has evolved from a diagnostic to predominantly therapeutic modality. A recent study reported a greater than 75% decrease in the rate of diagnostic ERCPs between 1998 and 2013 using the Nationwide Inpatient

Dr Krishnamoorthi has nothing to disclose. Dr Ross receives funding from Boston Scientific.
Digestive Diseases Institute, Virginia Mason Medical Center, Seattle, WA 98101, USA
* Corresponding author.
E-mail address: Andrew.Ross@virginiamason.org

Surg Clin N Am 99 (2019) 369–386
https://doi.org/10.1016/j.suc.2018.12.002
0039-6109/19/© 2018 Elsevier Inc. All rights reserved.
surgical.theclinics.com

Sample dataset.[2] In current practice, diagnostic ERCP is rarely performed. Compared with ERCP, EUS is a newer endoscopic modality that has evolved from a tool for diagnostic imaging and tissue acquisition to one with an array of therapeutic capabilities that can complement ERCP in obtaining biliary access and drainage. This article reviews the diagnostic and therapeutic applications of ERCP and EUS in the management of biliary diseases.

DIAGNOSTIC ENDOSCOPIC RETROGRADE CHOLANGIOPANCREATOGRAPHY

The decrease in diagnostic ERCP parallels the widespread availability of MRCP and EUS. MRCP can accurately define ductal anatomy and diagnose several biliary diseases including choledocholithiasis, choledochal cysts, and biliary tumors.[3–5] EUS has a high sensitivity and specificity for choledocholithiasis and helps to obtain a tissue diagnosis in malignant biliary strictures.[6]

Indeterminate Biliary Strictures

In patients with indeterminate biliary strictures (with equivocal imaging and histologic characteristics), an ERCP with cholangioscopy might help to establish the underlying diagnosis.[7] Cholangioscopy enables direct visualization of the biliary epithelium and targeted biopsies. This can be performed by advancing (1) a cholangioscope though the working channel of duodenoscope or (2) a small-caliber forward viewing scope directly into the bile duct (direct peroral cholangioscopy).[8] The modern digital single operator cholangioscopy system (SpyGlass DS, Boston Scientific, Natick, MA) is a single-use, disposable cholangioscope that offers high-resolution imaging. It can be advanced into the bile duct over a guide wire and enables tissue acquisition using a dedicated biopsy forceps (Spy-Bite, Boston Scientific; **Fig. 1**). Cholangioscopes also have therapeutic role in management of large bile duct stones. Specialized catheters with an electrohydraulic lithotripsy or laser tip can be advanced through the cholangioscope to fragment large stones (**Fig. 2**).

A novel low-profile probe has been recently developed that can be used to perform optical coherence tomography of the biliary tract. It can generate cross-sectional images of bile duct (up to 6 cm in 90 seconds) and help to differentiate between inflammatory and malignant strictures. A recent in vivo study on the safety and efficacy of direct cannulation with the low-profile probe during ERCP and optical coherence tomography for indeterminate biliary strictures has reported promising results.[9]

Primary sclerosing cholangitis (PSC) is an autoimmune disease that results in fibrosis of the biliary tree. MRCP has largely replaced ERCP-aided cholangiography in making a diagnosis of PSC. However, when the clinical suspicion of PSC is high but MRCP is normal or equivocal, ERCP can be helpful. In addition to obtaining a cholangiogram, ERCP enables tissue sampling (with brush or forceps) and treatment of dominant strictures, if necessary (with balloon dilation). The brushing sample from biliary strictures can be analyzed using fluorescent in situ hybridization to diagnose cholangiocarcinoma when the cytology examination is equivocal.[10]

Sphincter of Oddi Dysfunction

The updated Rome IV classification has renamed sphincter of Oddi dysfunction (SOD) with new terminology.[11] Patients with sphincter stenosis or obstruction (formerly SOD type I) have elevated liver tests during pain attacks and dilated bile duct on imaging.

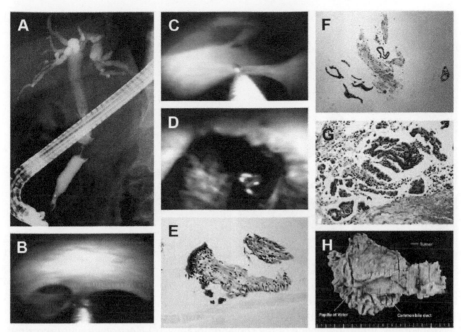

Fig. 1. (*A*) A case of distal cholangiocarcinoma. Endoscopic retrograde cholangiography demonstrated a distal bile duct stricture. (*B*) Cholangioscopic-guided mapping biopsy was performed from the B4 confluence, (*C*) the confluence of the anterior and posterior segmental ducts, (*D*) and the main lesion. (*E*) Histopathologic examination of the biopsy specimens revealed that the B4 confluence and (*F*) the confluence of the anterior and posterior segmental ducts had nonneoplastic mucosa and that (*G*) the main lesion had adenocarcinoma. (*H*) Mapping of the resected specimen. (From Ogawa et al., Usefulness of cholangioscopic-guided mapping biopsy using SpyGlass DS for preoperative evaluation of extrahepatic cholangiocarcinoma: a pilot study, CC BY-NC-ND 4.0 Endosc Int Open 2018;06(02):E199–E204. DOI: 10.1055/s-0043-117949 © Georg Thieme Verlag KG 2017, with permission.)

Patients with functional biliary sphincter disorder (formerly SOD type II) have either elevated liver tests or dilated bile duct (not both). SOD type III (normal liver tests and bile duct) has been reclassified as functional pain.

Biliary pressure at the SOD can be assessed by ERCP-aided manometry. It has a role in management of biliary sphincter disorder (formerly SOD type II), because elevated pressure predicts response to endoscopic sphincterotomy. Manometry is not indicated in SOD type I, because these patients uniformly respond to sphincterotomy. Current practice guidelines recommend against diagnostic or therapeutic ERCP in patients with functional abdominal pain (SOD III),[12] because a recent prospective, randomized trial showed no symptomatic benefit with sphincterotomy in patients with SOD III disease when compared with a sham procedure.[13]

THERAPEUTIC ENDOSCOPIC RETROGRADE CHOLANGIOPANCREATOGRAPHY
Bile Duct Stones

Most common bile duct (CBD) stones can be removed using an extraction balloon and/or basket after performing a biliary sphincterotomy. The success rate for complete removal of CBD stones that are less than 1.5 cm is extremely high, particularly when ERCP is performed by an experienced endoscopist.[8] CBD stones that are greater

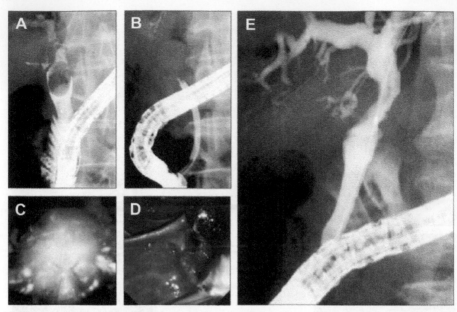

Fig. 2. (*A*) Cholangiography showing a large stone at the confluence of the bile duct. (*B*) Electrohydraulic lithotripsy image of the cholangiography. (*C*) Electrohydraulic lithotripsy image of the cholangioscope. (*D*) After the fragmentation of the bile duct stone, the stone removal is performed using a standard technique. (*E*) Complete stone clearance was achieved. (*From* Kamiyama R, Ogura T, Okuda A, et al. Electrohydraulic lithotripsy for difficult bile duct stones under endoscopic retrograde cholangiopancreatography and peroral transluminal cholangioscopy guidance. Gut Liver 2018;12(4):457; with permission.)

than 1.5 cm might need additional techniques like mechanical, laser, or electrohydraulic lithotripsy for successful removal. Combined sphincterotomy with sphincteroplasty (with large dilation balloons) can help to avoid lithotripsy even in large stones.[14] The extraction of CBD stones with sphincteroplasty alone (without sphincterotomy) is associated with a higher risk of post-ERCP pancreatitis; thus,[15] this approach is reserved for removal of small stones in patients with a high risk of bleeding.[8]

In patients with failed or incomplete extraction of large CBD stones, plastic stents can be placed to bypass the stones and drain bile. Interval ERCP after a few months of stent placement improves the success rate of complete stone removal.[16] Fully covered self-expanding metal stents (fcSEMS) also have a role in management of complex CBD stones.[17,18] Although plastic stents cause mechanical friction and fragment stones to aid stone removal, the mechanism by which fcSEMS help stone removal is unclear.[19]

Bile Leak

Bile leak is most commonly seen after cholecystectomy. Other etiologies include liver transplantation, hepatectomy, trauma, liver biopsy, and percutaneous transhepatic cholangiography.[20] Most bile leaks are maintained by the high pressure gradient across the biliary sphincter. This gradient can be reduced by biliary sphincterotomy alone, the placement of a plastic biliary stent alone, or both. All 3 approaches are equally effective in the treatment of bile leak.[21] Biliary sphincterotomy with plastic stent placement for 4 to 6 weeks is the most common approach in current practice.[22]

In addition to plastic stents, fcSEMS have a role in treatment of bile leak. It can be effective in refractory leaks (defined as a persistent leak after combined biliary sphincterotomy and plastic stent placement) and high-grade leaks (defined as extravasation of contrast with no filling of the intrahepatic ducts).[23,24] A fcSEMS may be superior to plastic stents in posthepatectomy bile leaks, because they are usually complex leaks and require bridging stents.[25] One drawback of fcSEMS is that they require a dilated biliary tree for placement and therefore may not be an appropriate treatment option for some patients.

Acute Cholecystitis

In patients with acute cholecystitis who are deemed high risk for cholecystectomy, endoscopic drainage of the gallbladder (GB) is an alternative to percutaneous cholecystostomy. There are 2 endoscopic options: (1) ERCP-aided transpapillary GB stenting (TGS) and (2) EUS-guided transmural GB drainage. Transmural GB drainage is discussed elsewhere in this article.

A systematic review and metaanalysis estimated the technical and clinical success of TGS in acute cholecystitis as 96% and 88%, respectively.[26] Double pigtail plastic stents are commonly used for TGS with one pigtail in the GB and other in the duodenum. Before stent placement, the cystic duct is cannulated with a guidewire, which is then advanced and coiled into the GB (**Fig. 3**). A recent study described TGS with a

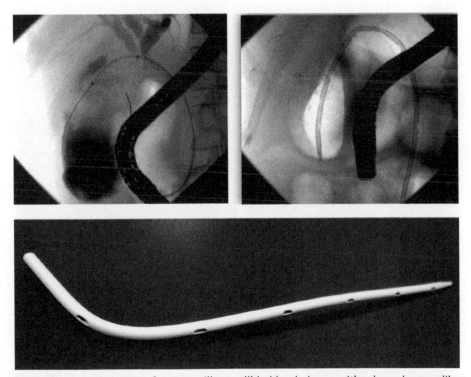

Fig. 3. Fluoroscopic image of transpapillary gallbladder drainage with a long, large-caliber fenestrated plastic stent (Johlin stent). (*From* Ogawa et al., Usefulness of cholangioscopic-guided mapping biopsy using SpyGlass DS for preoperative evaluation of extrahepatic cholangiocarcinoma: a pilot study, CC BY-NC-ND 4.0 Endosc Int Open 2018;06(02):E199–E204. DOI: 10.1055/s-0043-117949. © Georg Thieme Verlag KG 2017, with permission.)

novel long large caliber fenestrated plastic stent (Johlin stent, Wilson-Cook Medical Inc., Winston-Salem, NC).[27]

Benign Biliary Strictures

There are several etiologies for benign biliary strictures (BBS) including postcholecystectomy stricture, PSC, IgG4 cholangiopathy, chronic pancreatitis, and anastomotic stricture after liver transplantation. Endoscopic treatment of most BBS involves ERCP with balloon dilation and placement of 1 or more stents followed by interval stent exchanges.

Because plastic stents are easily removable and relatively inexpensive, they are the treatment of choice for BBS in most institutions (**Fig. 4**). However, the need for multiple ERCPs at short intervals for stent exchange is a potential drawback of plastic stents. Also, the placement of side-by-side plastic stents in tight strictures and strictures located at the hepatic bifurcation can be challenging.[28]

A fcSEMS is an alternative to plastic stents in management of BBS. These stents can be left in place for a longer duration and can theoretically be removed without difficulty. Two recent randomized clinical trials comparing fcSEMS versus multiple plastic stents for the treatment of BBS reported similar success rates.[29,30] Although the success rates were similar, fewer ERCPs were needed with fcSEMS. As noted, the placement of a fcSEMS for the treatment of BBS may be limited by the caliber of the biliary tree upstream from the stenosis.

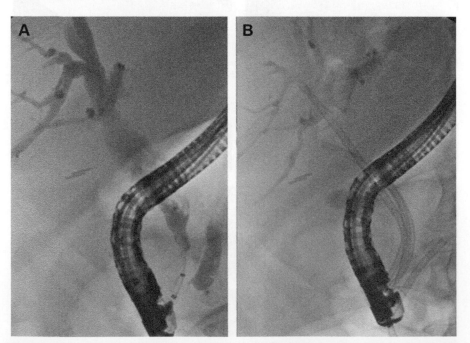

Fig. 4. Multiple plastic stents in the biliary duct. (*A*) Endoscopic retrograde cholangiopancreatography images showing distal common bile duct stricture from chronic pancreatitis. (*B*) Multiple plastic stents in the common bile duct along with a plastic stent in the pancreatic duct. (*From* Perri V, Familiari P, Tringali A, et al. Plastic biliary stents for benign biliary diseases. Gastrointest Endosc Clin N Am 2011;21(3):417; with permission.)

Malignant Biliary Stricture

Preoperative biliary drainage

In current practice, preoperative biliary drainage (PBD) is not routinely performed in jaundiced patients with a resectable periampullary or pancreatic malignancy.[31] Common indications for PBD are symptomatic jaundice (intractable pruritus, dehydration), acute cholangitis, and the need for neoadjuvant chemotherapy.

The choice of stent for PBD (plastic stent vs SEMS) should be individualized for each patient. Plastic stents are relatively inexpensive compared with SEMS. SEMS have a 3-fold larger diameter than a 10F plastic stent and thus remain patent for a longer duration with a lesser need for reintervention. Two recent studies comparing plastic stents versus SEMS for PBD reported conflicting results on stent-related complications.[32,33] Tol and colleagues[32] reported lower complication rate with fcSEMS compared with plastic stents (6% vs 31%), whereas Song and colleagues[33] reported no difference (14% vs 16.3%). Both studies reported no difference in surgery-related complications.

In patients with upfront resectable disease who require drainage, plastic stents may be considered over SEMS because they are less expensive. In patients who need neoadjuvant chemotherapy, SEMS should be preferred over plastic stents given the need for adequate and durable biliary drainage until the surgery.

Palliative biliary drainage

Practice guidelines from American Society for Gastrointestinal Endoscopy and European Society of Gastrointestinal Endoscopy recommend the use of SEMS for palliative biliary drainage in pancreas cancer, when the life expectancy is 6 months or more.[28,34] A recent cost-effectiveness study found the initial placement of SEMS to be more cost effective than plastic stents for pancreatic cancer–related biliary stricture.[35] However, it should be noted that a recent systematic review and metaanalysis reported no survival difference between plastic stents and SEMS when used for malignant obstruction.[36]

Tumor ingrowth can cause biliary obstruction in uncovered SEMS, necessitating reintervention. The fcSEMS were developed in an effort to prevent tumor ingrowth. However, studies comparing the duration of stent patency between fcSEMS and uncovered SEMS have reported conflicting results.[37] Although fcSEMS help to prevent tumor ingrowth, stent migration is a drawback. Partially covered metal stents were developed in an effort to strike a balance of lower tumor ingrowth and lesser stent migration. However, there are limited data to support the superiority of the partially covered metal stents to uncovered or fully covered stent.

Side-by-side plastic stents are an alternate option to SEMS for the management of malignant obstruction. Lawrence and Romagnuolo[38] reported promising results with this approach, with more than one-half of the study patients having clinically patent stents at 221 days. Given the cost difference between plastic stents and SEMS, this finding might be relevant in resource-limited settings.

Hilar strictures

The endoscopic management of malignant hilar strictures is more complex as compared with distal biliary strictures.[19] Several factors determine unilateral versus bilateral stenting, including candidacy for surgical resection, associated liver atrophy, and tumor burden. Plastic stents and SEMS can be used for palliation of hilar strictures. Whereas SEMS stay patent for a longer duration, reintervention through existing SEMS can be extremely challenging. When SEMS are used for bilateral drainage, they can be placed in a stent-in-stent (Y configuration) or side-by-side configuration (**Fig. 5**). Decisions on stent placement for hilar strictures can be complex and should

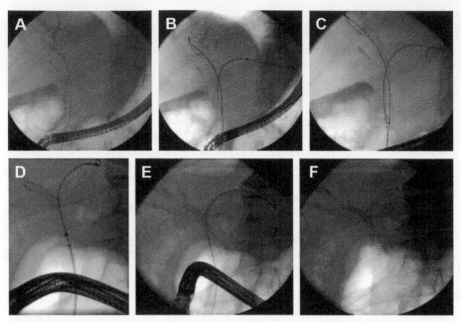

Fig. 5. (A) An 0.035 guidewire placed bilaterally. (B) Bilateral delivery systems placed over the guidewire. (C) Hilar stents placed side by side. (D) Endoscopic retrograde cholangiopancreatography image showing the right stent in the right hepatic duct and a delivery system over a guide wire passing through the interstices of the stent. (E) Delivery system over the guidewire. (F) Bilateral stents deployed by a stent-in-stent Y-shaped configuration. (From Law R, Baron TH. Bilateral metal stents for hilar biliary obstruction using a 6Fr delivery system: outcomes following bilateral and side-by-side stent deployment. Dig Dis and Sci 2013;58(9):2669; with permission.)

always been done in a multidisciplinary manner when surgical resection is being considered.

In patients with hilar cholangiocarcinoma who are not surgical candidates, photodynamic therapy or radiofrequency ablation can be delivered endoscopically for palliation.[39,40]

Endoscopic Retrograde Cholangiopancreatography in Altered Anatomy

Roux-en-Y gastric bypass

A standard sideviewer scope cannot be used to perform ERCP in patients with Roux-en-Y gastric bypass anatomy because the gastric pouch is disconnected from the rest of the stomach and duodenum. There are several approaches to performing ERCP in patients with a Roux-en-Y gastric bypass anatomy and each has its unique advantages and disadvantages. When available, enteroscopy-assisted ERCP is the least invasive approach for the management of biliary diseases, and specifically for CBD stones. In this approach, a forward viewing scope (pediatric colonoscope or balloon-assisted enteroscope) is advanced from gastric pouch into the Roux limb up to the jejunojejunostomy. At this point, the pancreatobiliary limb is identified and the scope is advanced upstream to identify the major papilla in the second part of the duodenum. Biliary cannulation with forward viewing scopes can be challenging and the success rate varies based on the experience of the endoscopy center.[8,41] Balloon-assisted enteroscopy (BAE) using a double (Fujinon, Wayne, NJ) or single balloon (Olympus, Center Valley, PA) enteroscope is often required in patients with a long Roux limb. These endoscopes are longer than a pediatric colonoscope and require the use of dedicated, long cannulation devices and wires.

Laparoscopy-assisted ERCP is an alternate approach when BAE is not available or when BAE-ERCP fails. This approach provides direct access into the excluded stomach through a gastrostomy and a standard sideviewer scope can be used to perform ERCP. Although this approach is technically less challenging than BAE-ERCP, it requires coordination between multiple specialties, which comes with added costs and inconvenience.

More recently, a novel approach has been developed, which involves the placement of a lumen-apposing metal stent (LAMS) from the gastric pouch into the excluded stomach using EUS guidance, followed by advancement of a standard duodenoscope through the LAMS to perform ERCP (**Fig. 6**). Patients consenting for this procedure need to understand the off-label use of LAMS and the risk of persistent gastrogastric fistula (after the removal of the LAMS), which can lead to weight gain. The reported success rate of this hybrid approach is promising.[42] However, further prospective studies comparing the adverse events (short term and long term) of this technique with BAE-ERCP and laparoscopy-assisted ERCP are needed.

Pancreatoduodenectomy

In most patients who have undergone pancreatoduodenectomy (Whipple surgery), ERCP can be performed using a therapeutic upper scope or colonoscope. Rarely, BAE might be needed. A common indication for ERCP in these patients is biliary obstruction secondary to anastomotic stricture at the hepaticojejunostomy. Most of these strictures respond well to balloon dilation and stent placement. In patients with biliary obstruction secondary to afferent limb syndrome, double pigtail plastic stents can placed across the jejunal strictures to accomplish biliary drainage.[43]

Ampullary Adenoma

Ampullary adenoma is a precancerous lesion involving the major papilla and surrounding duodenal mucosa. It is being increasingly detected due to widespread use of upper gastrointestinal endoscopy.[44] Endoscopic ampullectomy is a minimally invasive alternative to pancreatoduodenectomy. Intraductal adenoma growth of greater than 1 cm (into the CBD or pancreatic duct) limits the ability of endoscopic resection to achieve complete eradication.

Ampullectomy is similar to polypectomy in the rest of the gastrointestinal tract except that it is performed using a sideviewing duodenoscope (**Fig. 7**). The routine placement of a prophylactic pancreatic duct stent to prevent post-ERCP pancreatitis is recommended after an ampullectomy. Surveillance endoscopy after ampullectomy is determined based on adenoma size, resection technique, and histology of the resected specimen. Small residual intraductal adenoma can be endoscopically treated using radiofrequency ablation or other ablative modalities (Argon Plasma Coagulation, photodynamic therapy, and thermal probes).[45]

In patients with small well-differentiated T1 ampullary cancers (<6 mm) who are considered high-risk surgical candidates, ampullectomy might be a reasonable option because the risk of nodal metastasis is low (<4%).[46] Pancreaticoduodenectomy is the preferred management for larger and invasive tumors, as long as the patient is a

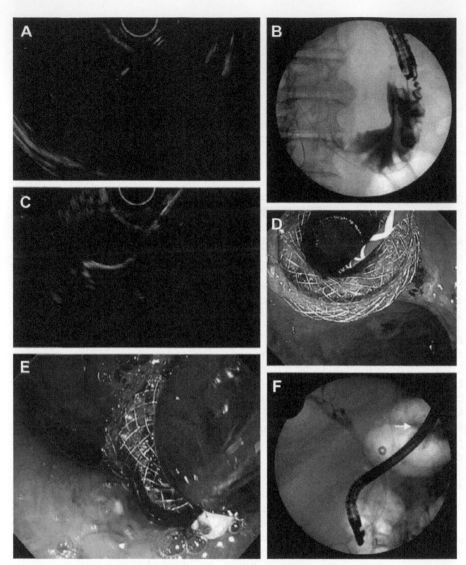

Fig. 6. (*A*) Endosonographic image of the excluded stomach accessed with an endoscopic ultrasound (EUS) needle from the remnant gastric pouch. (*B*) Fluoroscopic image showing a wire coiled within the lumen of the excluded stomach after being advanced through the EUS needle. (*C*) Endosonographic image of the distal flange of the lumen-apposing metallic stent (LAMS) after being deployed into the excluded stomach. (*D*) Endoscopic image of the proximal flange of the LAMS after being deployed into the proximal afferent jejunal limb. (*E*) Endoscopic image showing the lumen of the LAMS dilated with a 15-mm dilating balloon. (*F*) Fluoroscopic image showing a duodenoscope through the LAMS (*arrow*) with successful placement of a self-expanding metal stent in the bile duct. (*From* Bukhari M, Kowalski T, Nieto J, et al. An international, multicenter, comparative trial of EUS-guided gastrogastrostomy-assisted ERCP versus enteroscopy-assisted ERCP in patients with Roux-en-Y gastric bypass anatomy. Gastrointest Endosc 2018;88(3):488; with permission.)

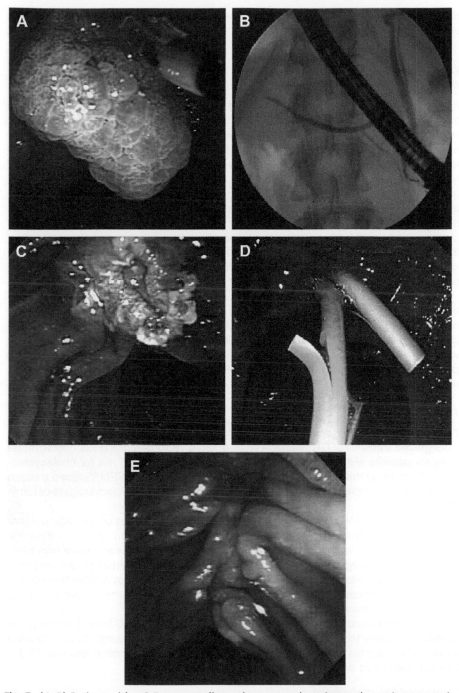

Fig. 7. (*A–D*) Patient with a 2.5-cm ampullary adenoma undergoing endoscopic retrograde cholangiopancreatography and ampullectomy. (*E*) The same patient 8 weeks after papillectomy. (*From* Irani S, Arai A, Ayub K, et al. Papillectomy for ampullary neoplasm: results of a single referral center over a 10-year period. Gastrointest Endosc 2009;70(5):926; with permission.)

reasonable surgical candidate; ampullectomy does not accomplish removal of the regional lymph nodes.

ENDOSCOPIC ULTRASOUND EXAMINATION
Diagnostic Endoscopic Ultrasound Examination

EUS examination has high sensitivity and specificity for diagnosing cholelithiasis and choledocholithiasis.[6,8] A recent systematic review and metaanalysis reported that for the same pretest probability of choledocholithiasis, EUS examination has a higher posttest probability when the result is positive and a lower posttest probability when the result is negative when compared with MRCP.[47]

In patients with high clinical suspicion of choledocholithiasis but nondiagnostic imaging (abdominal ultrasound examination and MRCP), EUS examination is the ideal next step. EUS examination is specifically helpful in patients with suspected CBD stones, who cannot undergo MRCP because of large body habitus or claustrophobia. If a CBD stone is identified on EUS examination, an ERCP can be performed during the same procedure. If no stones are seen, an unnecessary ERCP and the associated complications can be avoided.

In patients with obstructive jaundice with or without imaging evidence of ampullary tumor or biliary stricture, EUS examination enables direct visualization of the biliary obstruction and tissue acquisition using fine needle aspiration and biopsy. In the case of malignancy, EUS examination aids in cancer staging by assessing for vascular and lymph node involvement in addition to hepatic spread. ERCP is usually performed during the same endoscopy procedure when biliary decompression is required.

Therapeutic Endoscopic Ultrasound

Transmural gallbladder drainage

EUS-guided transmural GB drainage is an alternative to percutaneous cholecystostomy for patients with acute cholecystitis who are deemed high risk for cholecystectomy. Transmural drainage of GB is usually performed using fcSEMS placed through the duodenal (cholecytoduodenostomy) or gastric wall (cholecystogastrostomy; **Fig. 8**).

For the purpose of GB drainage, LAMS has several advantages over plastic or other fcSEMS (without the lumen-apposing feature). The apposition of GB wall to the duodenal or gastric wall decreases the risk of bile leak peritonitis and stent migration. LAMS also has a larger diameter that aids prompt drainage of thick sludge and pus. The cautery tip available in the novel LAMS delivery system (Hot AXIOS-Boston Scientific) can significantly shorten the endoscopy procedure time by removing the need for dilating the tract.

A recent systematic review and metaanalysis on use of LAMS for GB drainage reported impressive technical and clinical success rates of 93.8% and 92.5%, respectively.[48] It is important to note, however, that the overall complication rate was 18.3% with an associated perforation rate of 6.7%.

Transmural biliary drainage

The role of EUS in providing biliary access for ERCP through a rendezvous approach (after failed cannulation) is well-established. With recent advances in EUS and stent technology, direct transmural biliary drainage using covered metal stents is becoming more common.

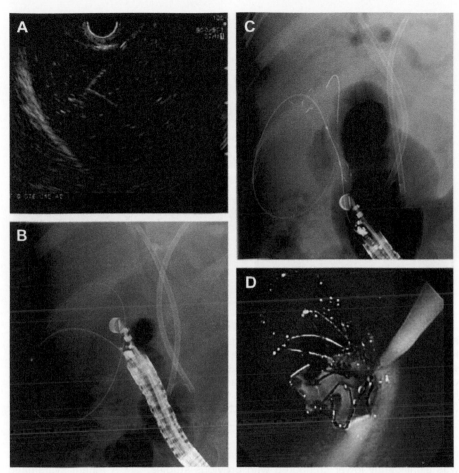

Fig. 8. (*A*) Endoscopic ultrasound image showing Needle tip in the gallbladder (GB), (*B*) Guidewire coiled in the GB under fluoroscopic guidance. (*C*) A self-expanding metal stent proximal flange deployed in the GB. (*D*) Distal flange of the covered self-expanding metal stent opened in the gastric lumen. (*From* Choi JH, Park DH, Lee SS, et al. Can endoscopic ultrasound help to drain the gallbladder? Gastrointestinal Intervention 2013;2(1):32; with permission.)

Over the last decade, EUS-guided transmural biliary drainage emerged as a rescue option after failed ERCP, before consideration of percutaneous transhepatic biliary drainage.[49] Two common approaches for EUS-guided transmural biliary drainage are (1) choledochoduodenostomy, accessing the main bile duct through the duodenal wall, and (2) hepaticogastrostomy, accessing the intrahepatic ducts though the stomach wall (**Figs. 9** and **10**). Hepaticogastrostomy can be especially useful in patients with postsurgical altered anatomy.

Over the last few years, studies have explored the role for EUS-guided transmural biliary drainage as primary method of biliary decompression (instead of ERCP).[49,50] Two recent randomized control trials comparing EUS-guided transmural biliary drainage versus ERCP for primary treatment of malignant biliary obstruction reported similar success rates and adverse events.[49,50] The rate of adverse

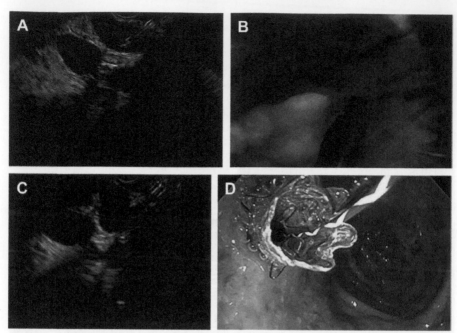

Fig. 9. Steps of endoscopic ultrasound-guided biliary drainage. After puncturing the extra-hepatic bile duct using a 19-gauge needle (*A*), a guidewire is inserted into the intrahepatic system (*B*). The transmural tract is balloon dilated (*C*), followed by insertion of a fully covered metal stent (*D*). (*From* Bang JY, Navaneethan U, Hasan M, et al. Stent placement by EUS or ERCP for primary biliary decompression in pancreatic cancer: a randomized trial (with videos). Gastrointest Endosc 2018;88(1):12; with permission.)

events with EUS-guided transmural biliary drainage reported in these studies was significantly lower compared with previous studies.[51,52] A recent systematic review and metaanalysis on safety of EUS-guided cholechoduodenostomy reported an adverse event rate of 17.7%.[53] It must be noted that the 2 recent randomized control trials were from tertiary referral centers with extensive expertise in EUS and ERCP and their results might not be generalizable at the current time.[49,50]

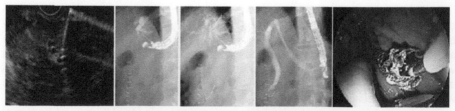

Fig. 10. Endoscopic ultrasound and fluoroscopic images showing the deployment of a long partially covered self-expanding metal stent during hepaticogastrostomy. (*From* Nakai Y, Isayama H, Yamamoto N, et al. Safety and effectiveness of a long, partially covered metal stent for endoscopic ultrasound-guided hepaticogastrostomy in patients with malignant biliary obstruction. Endoscopy 2016;48(12):1126; with permission.)

SUMMARY

Since its introduction into clinical practice, ERCP has evolved from a diagnostic and therapeutic tool to a predominantly therapeutic tool. There is a limited role for diagnostic ERCP in current practice with the widespread availability of MRCP and EUS. However, EUS has evolved from a purely diagnostic imaging modality to one with combined diagnostic and therapeutic capabilities. The availability of specialized stents like LAMS has improved the success rates of transmural biliary drainage. The novel cautery tip delivery system available with LAMS has helped to shorten the time of complex procedures. At the present time, ERCP remains the standard of care for patients requiring biliary decompression. In the future, however, it is possible that EUS-guided transmural biliary drainage may replace ERCP for certain indications. Given the risk of adverse events related with these more invasive and innovative endoscopic procedures, a multidisciplinary (surgery, interventional radiology, and gastroenterology) team-based approach is recommended.

REFERENCES

1. McCune WS, Shorb PE, Moscovitz H. Endoscopic cannulation of the ampulla of Vater: a preliminary report. Ann Surg 1968;167:752–6.
2. Huang RJ, Thosani NC, Barakat MT, et al. Evolution in the utilization of biliary interventions in the United States: results of a nationwide longitudinal study from 1998 to 2013. Gastrointest Endosc 2017;86(2):319–26.e5.
3. Feldman DR, Kulling DP, Kay CL, et al. Magnetic resonance cholangiopancreatography: a novel approach to the evolution of suspected pancreaticobiliary neoplasms. Ann Surg Oncol 1997;4:634–8.
4. Park DH, Kim MH, Lee SK, et al. Can MRCP replace the diagnostic role of ERCP for patients with choledochal cysts. Gastrointest Endosc 2005;62:360–6.
5. Griffin N, Wastle ML, Dunn WK, et al. Magnetic resonance cholangiopancreatography versus endoscopic retrograde cholangiopancreatography in the diagnosis of choledocholithiasis. Eur J Gastroenterol Hepatol 2003;15:809–13.
6. Palazzo L, Girollet PP, Salmeron, et al. Value of endoscopic ultrasonography in the diagnosis of common bile duct stones: comparison with surgical exploration and ERCP. Gastrointest Endosc 1995;42:225–31.
7. Draganov PV, Chauhan S, Wagh MS, et al. Diagnostic accuracy of conventional and cholangioscopy-guided sampling of indeterminate biliary lesions at the time of ERCP: a prospective, long-term follow-up study. Gastrointest Endosc 2012; 75(2):347–53.
8. Baron TH. Endoscopic management of biliary disorders: diagnostic and therapeutic. Surg Clin 2014;94(2):395–411.
9. Pilot study of safety and efficacy of directed cannulation with a low profile catheter (LP) and imaging characteristics of bile duct wall using optical coherence tomography (OCT) for indeterminate biliary strictures initial report on in-vivo evaluation during ERCP. Gastrointestinal Endoscopy. 2017;85(5):AB496–7.
10. Barr Fritcher EG, Voss JS, Jenkins SM, et al. Primary sclerosing cholangitis with equivocal cytology: fluorescence in situ hybridization and serum CA 19–9 predict risk of malignancy. Cancer Cytopathol 2013;121(12):708–17. Available at: https://doi.org/10.1002/cncy.21331.
11. Cotton PB, Elta GH, Carter CR, et al. Gallbladder and sphincter of Oddi disorders. Gastroenterology 2016;150:1420–9.
12. ASGE Standards of Practice Committee. The role of ERCP in benign diseases of the biliary tract. Gastrointest Endosc 2015;81:795–803.

13. Cotton PB, Durkalski V, Romagnuolo J, et al. Effect of endoscopic sphincterotomy for suspected sphincter of Oddi dysfunction on pain-related disability following cholecystectomy: the EPISOD randomized clinical trial. JAMA 2014;311:2101–9.

14. Teoh AY, Cheung FK, Hu B, et al. Randomized trial of endoscopic sphincterotomy with balloon dilation versus endoscopic sphincterotomy alone for removal of bile duct stones. Gastroenterology 2013;144(2):341–5.e1.

15. Liu Y, Su P, Lin Y, et al. Endoscopic sphincterotomy plus balloon dilation versus endoscopic sphincterotomy for choledocholithiasis: a meta-analysis. J Gastroenterol Hepatol 2013;28(6):937–45.

16. Yang J, Peng J-Y, Chen W. Endoscopic biliary stenting for irretrievable common bile duct stones: indications, advantages, disadvantages, and follow-up results. Surgeon 2012;10(4):211–7.

17. Masci E, Bizzotto A, Arena M, et al. Removable covered self-expanding metal stent for extraction of a large biliary stone in a patient on dual antiplatelet therapy. Endoscopy 2014;46(S 01):E342.

18. Hartery K, Lee CS, Doherty GA, et al. Covered self-expanding metal stents for the management of common bile duct stones. Gastrointest Endosc 2017;85(1): 181–6.

19. Krishnamoorthi R, Jayaraj M, Kozarek R. Endoscopic stents for the biliary tree and pancreas. Curr Treat Options Gastroenterol 2017;15(3):397–415.

20. Ferreira LEdC, Baron TH. Acute biliary conditions. Best Pract Res Clin Gastroenterol 2013;27(5):745–56.

21. Sachdev A, Kohli DR. Mo1281 A Prospective Randomized Study Comparing Different Endoscopic Techniques for Treating Biliary Leaks. Gastrointest Endosc 2012;75(4):AB374–5.

22. Bridges A, Wilcox CM, Varadarajulu S. Endoscopic management of traumatic bile leaks. Gastrointest Endosc 2007;65(7):1081–5.

23. Irani S, Baron TH, Law R, et al. Endoscopic treatment of nonstricture-related benign biliary diseases using covered self-expandable metal stents. Endoscopy 2015;47(04):315–21.

24. Luigiano C, Bassi M, Ferrara F, et al. Placement of a new fully covered self-expanding metal stent for postoperative biliary strictures and leaks not responding to plastic stenting. Surg Laparosc Endosc Percutan Tech 2013;23(2):159–62.

25. Luigiano C, Iabichino G, Mangiavillano B, et al. Endoscopic management of bile duct injury after hepatobiliary tract surgery: a comprehensive review. Minerva Chir 2016;71(6):398.

26. Itoi T, Coelho-Prabhu N, Baron TH. Endoscopic gallbladder drainage for management of acute cholecystitis. Gastrointest Endosc 2010;71(6):1038–45.

27. Glessing BR, Attam R, Amateau SK, et al. Novel use of long, large-caliber, fenestrated stents for endoscopic transpapillary gallbladder stenting for therapy of symptomatic gallbladder disease. Dig Dis Sci 2015;60(12):3817–22.

28. Dumonceau J-M, Tringali A, Blero D, et al. Biliary stenting: indications, choice of stents and results: European Society of Gastrointestinal Endoscopy (ESGE) clinical guideline. Endoscopy 2012;44(03):277–98.

29. Haapamäki C, Kylänpää L, Udd M, et al. Randomized multicenter study of multiple plastic stents vs. covered self-expandable metallic stent in the treatment of biliary stricture in chronic pancreatitis. Endoscopy 2015;47(07):605–10.

30. Coté GA, Slivka A, Tarnasky P, et al. Effect of covered metallic stents compared with plastic stents on benign biliary stricture resolution: a randomized clinical trial. JAMA 2016;315(12):1250–7.

31. van der Gaag NA, Rauws EA, van Eijck CH, et al. Preoperative biliary drainage for cancer of the head of the pancreas. N Engl J Med 2010;362(2):129–37.
32. Tol J, Van Hooft J, Timmer R, et al. Metal or plastic stents for preoperative biliary drainage in resectable pancreatic cancer. Gut 2016;65(12):1981–7.
33. Song TJ, Lee JH, Lee SS, et al. Metal versus plastic stents for drainage of malignant biliary obstruction before primary surgical resection. Gastrointest Endosc 2016;84(5):814–21.
34. Adler DG, Baron TH, Davila RE, et al. ASGE guideline: the role of ERCP in diseases of the biliary tract and the pancreas. Gastrointest Endosc 2005;62(1):1–8.
35. Martinez J, Anene A, Bentley T, et al. Cost Effectiveness of Metal Stents in Relieving Obstructive Jaundice in Patients with Pancreatic Cancer. J Gastrointest Cancer 2017;48(1):58–65.
36. Almadi MA, Barkun A, Martel M. Plastic vs. self-expandable metal stents for palliation in malignant biliary obstruction: a series of meta-analyses. Am J Gastroenterol 2017;112(2):260–73.
37. Saleem A, Leggett CL, Murad MH, et al. Meta-analysis of randomized trials comparing the patency of covered and uncovered self-expandable metal stents for palliation of distal malignant bile duct obstruction. Gastrointest Endosc 2011;74(2):321–7.e1-3.
38. Lawrence C, Romagnuolo J. Double plastic stents for distal malignant biliary obstruction: preliminary evidence for a novel cost-effective alternative to metal stenting. Am J Gastroenterol 2014;109(2):295.
39. Leggett CL, Gorospe EC, Murad MH, et al. Photodynamic therapy for unresectable cholangiocarcinoma: a comparative effectiveness systematic review and meta-analyses. Photodiagnosis Photodyn Ther 2012;9(3):189–95.
40. Figueroa-Barojas P, Bakhru MR, Habib NA, et al. Safety and efficacy of radiofrequency ablation in the management of unresectable bile duct and pancreatic cancer: a novel palliation technique. J Oncol 2013;2013:910897.
41. Skinner M, Popa D, Neumann H, et al. ERCP with the overtube-assisted enteroscopy technique: a systematic review. Endoscopy 2014;46:560–72.
42. Kedia P, Tarnasky PR, Nieto J, et al. EUS-directed transgastric ERCP (EDGE) versus laparoscopy-assisted ERCP (LA-ERCP) for Roux-en-Y gastric bypass (RYGB) anatomy: a multicenter early comparative experience of clinical outcomes. J Clin Gastroenterol 2018. [Epub ahead of Print].
43. Pannala R, Brandabur JJ, Gan SI, et al. Afferent limb syndrome and delayed GI problems after pancreaticoduodenectomy for pancreatic cancer: single-center, 14-year experience. Gastrointest Endosc 2011;74(2):295–302.
44. Baron TH. Ampullary adenoma. Curr Treat Options Gastroenterol 2008;11:96–102.
45. Rustagi T, Irani S, Reddy DN, et al. Radiofrequency ablation for intraductal extension of ampullary neoplasms. Gastrointest Endosc 2017;86(1):170–6.
46. Woo SM, Ryu JK, Lee SH, et al. Feasibility of endoscopic papillectomy in early stage ampulla of Vater cancer. J Gastroenterol Hepatol 2009;24(1):120–4.
47. De Castro VL, Moura EG, Chaves DM, et al. Endoscopic ultrasound versus magnetic resonance cholangiopancreatography in suspected choledocholithiasis: a systematic review. Endosc Ultrasound 2016;5(2):118.
48. Kalva NR, Vanar V, Forcione D, et al. Efficacy and safety of lumen apposing self-expandable metal stents for EUS guided cholecystostomy: a meta-analysis and systematic review. Can J Gastroenterol Hepatol 2018;2018:7070961.
49. Bang JY, Navaneethan U, Hasan M, et al. Stent placement by EUS or ERCP for primary biliary decompression in pancreatic cancer: a randomized trial (with videos). Gastrointest Endosc 2018;88(1):9–17.

50. Paik WH, Lee TH, Park DH, et al. EUS-guided biliary drainage versus ERCP for the primary palliation of malignant biliary obstruction: a multicenter randomized clinical trial. Am J Gastroenterol 2018;113(7):987.
51. Vila JJ, Pérez-Miranda M, Vazquez-Sequeiros E, et al. Initial experience with EUS-guided cholangiopancreatography for biliary and pancreatic duct drainage: a Spanish national survey. Gastrointest Endosc 2012;76:1133–41.
52. Attasaranya S, Netinasunton N, Jongboonyanuparp T, et al. The spectrum of endoscopic ultrasound intervention in biliary diseases: a single center's experience in 31 cases. Gastroenterol Res Pract 2012;2012:680753.
53. Krishnamoorthi R, Pappu Mohan B, Law J, et al. Efficacy and safety of endoscopic ultrasound (EUS) guided choledochoduodenostomy (CDD): a systematic review and meta- analysis. Am J Gastroenterol 2018;113:S441–2.

Role of Transplant in Biliary Disease

Margaret M. Romine, MD, MS[a,b,1], Jared White, MD[a,b],*

KEYWORDS

- Liver • Transplant • Cholangiocarcinoma • Cirrhosis • Cholangitis • Biliary
- Caroli disease

KEY POINTS

- Although orthotopic liver transplantation (OLT) is a well-established curative option for hepatocellular carcinoma, transplantation for CCA has historically been unsuccessful.
- Transplantation for intrahepatic CCA remains controversial because most studies report inferior survival of OLT for intrahepatic CCA compared with hilar CCA.
- Specific challenges associated with transplantation in the setting of neoadjuvant therapy for CCA include radiation and inflammatory changes to the porta hepatis and vascular complications.

ORTHOTOPIC LIVER TRANSPLANTATION FOR CHOLANGIOCARCINOMA

Cholangiocarcinoma (CCA) is a malignant tumor of the biliary system consisting of adenocarcinoma 95% of the time, which is subtyped based on the location of the lesion as intrahepatic or extrahepatic (perihilar or distal).[1] The incidence of CCA is estimated to be 3000 to 4000 cases per year, with perihilar representing approximately 60% to 70% of cases, intrahepatic approximately 10% of cases, and distal 20% to 30% of cases.[2–4] The ductal distribution of CCA is depicted in **Fig. 1**. Surgical management remains a challenge, typically associated with a poor prognosis and median survival of 12 to 24 months without treatment. There is a 50% to 70% mortality rate at Year 1 for untreated CCA.[3,4] The 5-year survival rate after surgical resection, despite R0 resection, remains poor and rarely exceeds 40%.[5–7]

Although orthotopic liver transplantation (OLT) is a well-established curative option for hepatocellular carcinoma, transplantation for CCA has historically been unsuccessful. Recurrence rates are high and long-term survival is often quoted at less

Disclosure Statement: The authors have nothing to disclose.
[a] General Surgery, University of Alabama at Birmingham, 1808 7th Avenue South D202 Boshell Building Birmingham, Alabama 35233, USA; [b] Division of Transplantation, University of Alabama at Birmingham, 701 19th Street South 722 Lyons Harrison Birmingham, Alabama 35233
[1] Present address: 304 Kingston Circle, Birmingham, AL 35211.
* Corresponding author. 1808 7th Avenue South D202 Boshell Building Birmingham, AL 35233.
E-mail address: jaredwhite@uabmc.edu

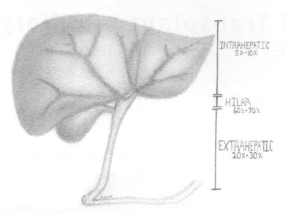

INTRAHEPATIC
5%-10%

HILAR
60%-70%

EXTRAHEPATIC
20%-30%

Fig. 1. Distribution of cholangiocarcinoma.

than 25%.[8] With the development of neoadjuvant chemoradiation protocols and well-selected patients with perihilar CCA, however, results have been encouraging for OLT in the setting of CCA.[9] Experiences published from a few centers have demonstrated improved long-term survival with neoadjuvant therapy before OLT for unresectable or potentially resectable perihilar CCA.[10–13] In 2004, the Mayo Clinic reported satisfactory results in highly selected patients transplanted for hilar CCA. They outlined a neoadjuvant chemoirradiation protocol for OLT when pretransplant staging laparotomy demonstrates no evidence of metastatic disease in regional lymph nodes. During the years 1993 to 2010, only 172 out of the original 196 patients enrolled in the Mayo protocol made it to the staging operation. A total of 38 of those (22%) were unable to proceed with transplant secondary to advanced disease. Thereafter, 126 underwent liver transplantation: 84 via deceased donor, 41 with living donor grafts, and one with a domino familial amyloid donor graft. The overall 5-year survival after the start of neoadjuvant therapy was 56%, with 65% and 44% for those with underlying primary sclerosing cholangitis (PSC) and de novo CCA, respectively. After transplantation, 5-year survival was 74% overall, and 80% and 64% for patients with underlying PSC and de novo CCA, respectively. No difference was identified between living and deceased donors. Twenty-nine (23%) patients died after transplant: 7 from complications and 17 from recurrent CCA.

Predictors of recurrence at review in 2006 were older age, prior cholecystectomy, CA19-9 greater than 100 at the time of OLT, visible mass on imaging, and extended time between neoadjuvant therapy and OLT. Pathologic findings as predictors for recurrence were residual CCA larger than 2 cm, high-grade histology, and perineural invasion.

For a patient to qualify for the protocol, the tumor must be less than 3 cm, have no evidence of intrahepatic or extrahepatic metastases, and or gallbladder involvement. The Mayo protocol specifically excludes intrahepatic CCA or gallbladder cancer. Candidates must have no active infections or medical conditions that preclude either neoadjuvant therapy or OLT. Patients with CCA extending below the cystic duct on cholangiography are also excluded because this situation makes complete extirpation difficult as these tumors are more likely to abut the portal vein. Endoscopic ultrasound is performed before neoadjuvant therapy to exclude patients with regional lymph node metastases. Other exclusion criteria include prior radiation or chemotherapy, uncontrolled infection, evidence of extrahepatic disease, in addition to patients who have had a previous attempt at resection and/or biopsy of the lesion.

Transplantation for intrahepatic CCA remains controversial because most studies report inferior survival of OLT for intrahepatic CCA compared with hilar CCA. However, a study from University of California Los Angeles demonstrated that incidentally discovered intrahepatic CCA on pathology of explant after OLT had similar survival to patients without intrahepatic CCA.[14]

Before neoadjuvant therapy for the Mayo protocol, the diagnostic criteria must be met: cytologic/histologic confirmation of CCA by transluminal brushing or tumor-associated cancer antigen (CA19-9) greater than 100 U/mL or polysomy by fluorescence in situ hybridization in the setting of a malignant-appearing stricture on cholangiography and/or visible mass on imaging. If a mass is present it must be less than 3 cm.

The University of Nebraska pioneered the use of neoadjuvant radiation therapy before OLT.[10] For the Mayo protocol, neoadjuvant therapy is administered by external beam radiation (40–45 Gy) followed by transcatheter radiation (20–30 Gy) with iridium wires. Wires are placed via endoscopic retrograde cholangiopancreatography preferentially versus percutaneous transhepatic cholangiography when this is not possible. Intravenous 5-FU is given for chemosensitization during radiation therapy. Capecitabine is given afterward and before transplantation.

All patients undergo operative staging before OLT by open or laparoscopic and/or hand-assisted strategy. Any suspicious nodules are biopsied, the liver is palpated for intrahepatic metastases, and portal lymph nodes are resected. Extrahepatic or intrahepatic metastases, lymph node involvement, or locally extensive disease preclude transplantation. The procedure is done 1 to 2 days before living donation or just before a deceased donor procurement. Before 2003, a total of 30% to 40% of patients had findings during staging operation that precluded transplantation. This was reduced with implementation of routine preoperative endoscopic ultrasound.[15] **Fig. 2** outlines the general stepwise approach of the protocol.

Specific challenges associated with transplantation in the setting of neoadjuvant therapy for CCA include radiation and inflammatory changes to the porta hepatis and vascular complications. In the Mayo series; 21% of the patients developed

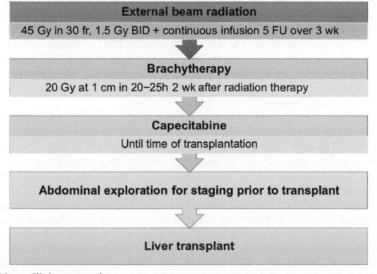

Fig. 2. Mayo Clinic protocol.

hepatic arterial complications and 20% developed complications related to the portal vein.[16] To minimize these effects, donor iliac artery is used in the setting of deceased donor grafts, whereas native hepatic artery was used in living donors. In addition to challenges faced during the procedure, patients may experience perioperative complications, such as cholangitis, intrahepatic abscess, and sepsis, which are usually related to indwelling stents, neoadjuvant radiation-induced tumor necrosis, or other treatment-related neutropenias.

For postoperative surveillance, all patients undergo Doppler ultrasound and computed tomography scan at 4 months post-transplant. Asymptomatic portal vein or hepatic artery stenosis is intervened on via percutaneous endovascular approaches.[16]

In 2006 the Model for End-Stage Liver Disease (MELD) Exception Study Group proposed granting MELD exception points to patients that meet criteria described by Gores and colleagues,[17] which are based on the Mayo protocol. A MELD score exception equivalent to 10% mortality at 3 months is granted, and the score is increased by a 10% mortality equivalent at 3-month intervals. Of note, patients with intrahepatic CCA do not receive MELD exception points under the MELD organ allocation system.

In summary, excellent results have been achieved for patients with unresectable hilar CCA. OLT offers a viable treatment option because it addresses the need for adequate resection margins in addition to underlying liver disease. With careful selection of patients with early stage disease confined to the hilum along with neoadjuvant therapy and operative staging to exclude regional lymph node involvement, successful outcomes are achieved.

ORTHOTOPIC LIVER TRANSPLANTATION FOR PRIMARY BILIARY CIRRHOSIS

Primary biliary cirrhosis (PBC) is characterized by immune-mediated inflammation of bile ducts leading to granuloma formation, chronic destructive cholangitis, and subsequent cirrhosis. Patients may progress to liver failure and ultimately death without liver transplantation. Despite the established association with antimitochondrial antibodies (AMAs) the exact cause of PBC remains unclear. There are several theories for the relationship including cross reactivity with infectious sources and environmental triggers, in addition to genetic predisposition. Screening asymptomatic family members of PBC patients using serum AMA has demonstrated a 2% to 4% rate of seropositivity, with daughters having 60 times the risk for developing PBC as compared with unrelated control subjects.[18] The overall incidence and prevalence of PBC varies based on study and ranges from 0.3 to 5.8 and 0.5 to 39 cases per 100,000 persons per year, respectively.[19] There is also evidence to suggest the incidence is increasing based on systematic review.[20]

The diagnosis of PBC requires two of the following criteria: (1) cholestatic serum profile of 6 months duration, (2) positive serum AMA, and (3) hepatic histology compatible with PBC. The only treatment approved for the treatment of PBC is ursodeoxycholic acid. It has been shown to improve survival and reduce the risk for the development of esophageal varices and cirrhosis.[21–24] Serum bilirubin has been found to be the best indicator for prognosis because the median patient survival with a bilirubin level greater than 150 mmol/L without transplant is approximately 18 months.[25]

Indications for OLT in autoimmune disease are similar to liver disease caused by hepatitis and alcohol with the exception of some disease-specific indications. These are outlined in **Box 1**. Referral for transplant should be made when the bilirubin reaches 6 mg/dL (103 mmol/L), MELD score greater than 12, and Mayo PBC risk score greater than or equal to 7.8.[26] The Mayo PBC risk score is the most validated

---

Box 1
Indications for transplantation in primary biliary cirrhosis

Symptom based
- Hepatic encephalopathy
- Intractable pruritis

End-stage liver disease
- Recurrent variceal hemorrhage
- Pulmonary hypertension
- Hepatopulmonary syndrome
- Diuretic-resistant ascites
- Progressive osteopenia
- Muscle-wasting
- Hepatocellular carcinoma (Milan criteria)

Biochemistry
- Serum bilirubin >150 mol/L
- Serum albumin <25 g/L

---

prognostic model, which is useful for predicting survival and timing for OLT in patients with PBC. PBC accounts for less than 5% of liver transplants, and this number seems to be decreasing, perhaps related to the availability of ursodeoxycholic acid.[27]

Survival with OLT is good with 1-, 3-, and 5-year patient and graft survival found to be 94%, 91%, 82%, and 89%, 83%, and 75%, respectively, in a series of 301 PBC transplant recipients in the United Kingdom.[28,29] Recurrent disease is diagnosed by characteristic histology and absence of other causes of graft damage. Elevated serum immunoglobulins and persisting AMAs do not themselves indicate recurrent disease. The histology of recurrence is comparable with pretransplant PBC. The rate of reported recurrence is variable; however, estimations range from 14% to 17% during a mean of 36-month time span and increases to as high as 35% at 1 year in one study.[30–32] Recurrence may be underdiagnosed in the absence of protocol biopsies, because many lack any biochemical abnormality.[30]

Clinical factors are not reliable in predicting which patients are at risk for recurrent disease. In addition, controversy remains regarding which type of immunosuppression should be used. In a study of 485 patients with more than 79-month follow-up, the time to recurrence with cyclosporine was found to be longer (123 months vs 62 months) compared with tacrolimus.[33] Similar results were observed in a study containing 156 patients, which demonstrated 8.4% recurrence in recipients taking cyclosporine, azathioprine, and steroids, compared with 12.2% of those receiving cyclosporin and steroids alone and 16.7% of patients taking tacrolimus and steroids.[34] These studies suggest that cyclosporin, compared with tacrolimus, is associated with a slower rate of progression of recurrent disease. Whether this means patients who undergo OLT for PBC should be offered cyclosporin-based immunosuppression rather than tacrolimus is uncertain.

Survival of patients with PBC is prolonged by ursodeoxycholic acid therapy; however, transplantation can not only prolong survival in patients not responsive to therapy but also improve quality of life. Although disease recurrence in the transplanted liver may occur, the data showing significant clinical burden from recurrent PBC are lacking to date.

ORTHOTOPIC LIVER TRANSPLANTATION FOR PRIMARY SCLEROSING CHOLANGITIS

PSC is a cholestatic disease of unknown cause characterized by recurrent multifocal strictures and dilations of the intrahepatic and extrahepatic bile ducts. An example of the classic "chain of lakes" appearance in PSC is depicted in **Fig. 3.** In 60% to 80% of cases PSC is associated with chronic inflammatory bowel disease (IBD), predominantly ulcerative colitis. Males are more commonly affected and the course is progressive in nature.[35] The diagnosis is established based on typical cholangiographic lesions of the bile ducts and exclusion of secondary causes of sclerosing cholangitis.[26] For many patients the disease runs a fluctuating course of exacerbations and remissions leading to an unpredictable natural history. There is no current effective medical treatment of PSC and patients are at increased risk for colon cancer and CCA. Liver transplantation remains the most effective treatment of PSC.

Indications for OLT in the setting of PSC is similar to those for chronic liver disease. OLT for PSC accounts for approximately 6% of all transplants. The decision to list a patient with PSC for OLT should include clinical signs and symptoms; biochemical parameters; the risk of hepatobiliary malignancy; and, in some patients, the status of concomitant IBD. The 2010 American Association for the Study of Liver Diseases guidelines warn against using previous prognostic models because there is no consensus on the optimal model to apply.[36] Other indications for OLT in PSC patients include intractable pruritus and recurrent bacterial cholangitis.

At the Mayo Clinic, 1- and 5-year survival rates for patients with PSC are 92% and 86%, respectively. In one retrospective study, risk factors for adverse outcomes after OLT for PSC were identified, which include intensive care before transplantation, age greater than 65, poor nutritional status, Child-Pugh class C, and renal failure requiring dialysis before transplantation. Risk factors specific to PSC are disease severity, previous biliary shunt surgery, concurrent bile duct cancer, and presence of IBD.[37]

A retrospective analysis of the United Network for Organ Sharing database for patients transplanted with PSC had similar 1- and 5-year survival rates of 93% and 87.5%, respectively, with deceased donor grafts. Survival was increased to 97.2% and 95.4% with living donor recipients.[38] The 1- and 5-year allograft survival rates among deceased and living donors were 87% and 79.2%, and 89.6% and 87.1%, respectively.

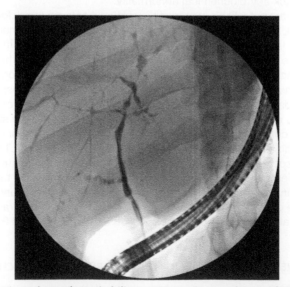

Fig. 3. Intrahepatic and extrahepatic biliary strictures in a patient with PSC before transplantation, giving the classic "chain of lakes" appearance.

Recurrent PSC may be difficult to distinguish from secondary sclerosing cholangitis, which may be associated with ischemia of the biliary tree, hepatic artery thrombosis, acute or chronic rejection, ABO mismatch, and infection.[39] The absence of other contributing factors must be ruled out before PSC recurrence is considered. Reported rates of recurrence vary and depend on the length of follow-up, increasing with time.[40] At one institution, an analysis of 150 patients who underwent transplantation for PSC demonstrated 20% recurrence.[41] Another, more recent study of 230 patients demonstrated a recurrence rate of 23.5% with median follow-up time of 82.5 months.[42] It is unclear the effect recurrent disease has on graft survival.[43,44]

Patients with severe IBD and advanced PSC requiring OLT pose a difficult challenge. Colectomy before OLT may lead to severe hepatic decompensation, rendering the patient ineligible for OLT or at least increasing the challenges of transplantation because of adhesions. There are some centers in which simultaneous OLT and colectomy is preferred.[45] Also, PSC transplant recipients with concomitant IBD are more likely to develop colon cancer, with a cumulative risk of 14% at 5 years and 17% at 10 years after OLT.[45,46]

Because of the progressive nature of the disease and lack of successful medical therapies, liver transplantation remains the only durable option for patients with PSC who have developed complications of end-stage liver disease or recurrent cholangitis secondary to biliary obstruction.

ORTHOTOPIC LIVER TRANSPLANTATION IN THE SETTING OF COMPLEX BILIARY INJURIES

Both open and laparoscopic cholecystectomy are associated with common bile duct injury. The incidence of bile duct injury with the laparoscopic approach is 0.4% to 0.6%. This is higher than the previously reported incidence (0.2%–0.3%) of bile duct injury in open cholecystectomy.[47,48] During laparoscopic cholecystectomy, in contrast to open, the biliary tree is more often injured at the proximal level and likely to have an associated vascular injury. The pattern of injury is well described and most often involves injury to the right branch of the hepatic artery or aberrantly located replaced or accessory right hepatic arteries.

When injury to the biliary tree occurs, the insult results in chronic exposure to high concentration of hepatotoxic bile acids at the canalicular membrane leading to a process of ductular proliferation and portal inflammation along with fibrogenesis and matrix deposition, known as ductular reaction. This process ultimately results in scarring.[49,50] Cholestasis results as this process progresses and bile flow develops in the intrahepatic biliary radicles, perpetuating bile and bile salt accumulation in the parenchyma. It is well accepted that the longer the duration of obstruction the more likely fibrosis is to occur, although there are no conclusive data regarding the time of progression from fibrosis to cirrhosis or factors contributing to progression. A prospective series of 64 patients with post-cholecystectomy bile duct strictures studied the amount of fibrosis at the time of repair. Thirty-four (54%) of the patients were found to have advanced fibrosis at the time of surgery with a mean duration of biliary obstruction of 16.6. months.[51] In fact, fibrotic changes occurred 1 month after biliary obstruction. Factors significantly associated with presence of advanced fibrosis were duration of biliary obstruction, basal alanine aminotransferase level, and time to normalization of alanine aminotransferase after surgical repair.[50,52] Depending on the degree of liver injury at the time of relief of obstruction, the liver may or may not recover postobstruction. Patient should be followed clinically and with repeat biopsies after obstruction has been alleviated to assess for regression.[53,54]

There are two major categories for indications for liver transplantation after bile duct injury: chronic liver disease caused by secondary biliary cirrhosis and acute liver failure caused by an associated vascular injury. The reasons for transplantation in the setting of bile duct injury are one of the following: secondary biliary cirrhosis, biliary stricture and portal hypertension, hepatic failure and complex injury, recurrent biliary sepsis, bile duct injury in a patient with underlying liver disease, pruritus, and poor quality of life. Most current data in this area are limited to case reports and small case series. These are predominantly caused by biliary injury at the time of cholecystectomy; however, there are cases of injury reported during hydatid liver disease and for nonbiliary surgery. Incidence of transplantation for biliary injury is difficult to confirm but is estimated to be 1% to 2% internationally.[54] An example of a proximal hepatic duct injury associated with portal vein thrombosis in the setting of PBC is depicted in **Fig. 4**. In this situation, liver transplantation was considered to be a more favorable approach to surgical repair given the risks associated with primary repair in decompensated liver disease.

One series describes the results following OLT for biliary injury sustained during laparoscopic cholecystectomy in a total of 27 patients over a 13-year time period. Fourteen of the patients underwent transplantation for acute liver failure and 13 for secondary biliary cirrhosis. A higher rate of vascular injuries was associated with the laparoscopic approach and the overall 5-year survival was 68%.[55] Patients transplanted for secondary biliary cirrhosis have expected long-term outcomes with a 3-year survival greater than 70%.[56,57]

A thorough preoperative evaluation should proceed as with other indications for transplantation. In the setting of bile duct injury, initial evaluation and management should ensure that the injury is appropriately treated. For example, bilomas or

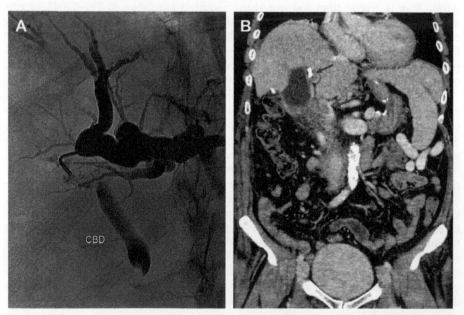

Fig. 4. Biliary injury incurred during robotic cholecystectomy in a patient with PBC. (*A*) Percutaneous cholangiogram demonstrating near transection of the common hepatic duct (*arrow*). (*B*) Computed tomography scan of abdomen demonstrating surgical clips (*short arrow*), biloma (*star*), and portal vein thrombosis (*long arrow*) in the same patient.

abscesses should be drained, adequate biliary drainage should be present, and chol-angiographic imaging should be performed to characterize the injury and current anat-omy. Many patients have percutaneous biliary drains in place at the time of evaluation. Biliary drainage should be optimized and lack of other surgical options confirmed before consideration for transplantation.

Criteria for liver transplantation in the setting of secondary biliary cirrhosis are not well established but should include at least one of the following: cirrhosis by biopsy, MELD greater than 15, fibrosis and portal hypertension in the setting of biliary stricture without percutaneous/endoscopic or surgical potential for revision, poor quality of life, and recurrent cholangitis requiring hospitalization with biliary tract stricture not amenable to surgical reconstruction.[54]

Patients transplanted in the setting of acute liver failure secondary to vasculobiliary injury have a worse prognosis and often die of infection-related complications. During evaluation in this setting one must consider the likelihood that the patient will survive the procedure based on their overall clinical stability, the presence of irreversible com-plications of liver failure, and the presence of sepsis. Given the nature of injury, contamination at the original procedure is likely; however, ongoing sepsis (with excep-tion of that confined to the native liver) is a contraindication to transplant. In addition to the standard preoperative evaluation for transplantation, contrasted imaging should clarify specific anatomic details, such as whether the vascular anatomy is suitable for transplant.

ORTHOTOPIC LIVER TRANSPLANTATION FOR BILIARY ATRESIA

Biliary atresia (BA) is the most common pediatric liver disease leading to liver trans-plantation during infancy or childhood. The exact cause of BA remains unknown; how-ever, it is an occlusive panductular cholangiopathy affecting intrahepatic and extrahepatic bile ducts.[58] It typically presents in the first few weeks of life and without early recognition and surgical intervention it progresses to biliary cirrhosis, leading to liver transplantation or death by 2 years of age.

BA is divided into three types (1–3) based on level of occlusion of the extrahepatic biliary tree. The intrahepatic bile ducts are largely preserved in types 1 and 2. Type 3 is the most common and the intrahepatic bile ducts are grossly abnormal. Clinically, the disease is divided into three groups: (1) BA splenic malformation syndrome, (2) cystic BA, and (3) isolated BA.

The incidence of BA varies by country and race, however, it is estimated to affect 1 in 12,000 to 1 in 19,500 live births in the United States.[59] A distinct female predomi-nance is seen in those with developmental BA that is not seen in the isolated BA group.[60,61] A seasonal variation has also been observed in which rates of BA are three times higher in the colder months compared with warmer.[59,62]

The macroscopic appearance of the extrahepatic biliary tree ranges from inflamed and hypertrophic yet intact to being an atrophic negligible remnant. The histologic appearance within the liver seems more consistent with early portal tract inflamma-tion, a mononuclear cell infiltrate, bile duct plugging, and proliferation with fibrosis giv-ing way to overt biliary cirrhosis from about 3 months on. One suggested cause of BA is infection with hepatotrophic viruses, either as an indirect trigger of an abnormal immune-mediated reaction or as an actual pathologic agent. Such viruses include rotavirus, reovirus, and cytomegalovirus and is based largely on studies with animal models.[63,64] However, it has been difficult to confirm these findings in humans. A more recent study demonstrated the presence of hepatotropic viral DNA and RNA in pediatric liver biopsy at the time of portoenterostomy (Kasai procedure).[65]

Infants often present with conjugated jaundice beyond 14 days of age, pale and unpigmented stools, and dark urine in an otherwise healthy, term neonate. Marked hepatosplenomegaly and ascites are rarely seen before 3 months because liver fibrosis and cirrhosis are later developments, even in infants with intrauterine BA evident at birth.[66] Fat malabsorption results in growth delay and fat-soluble vitamin deficiencies, including vitamin K. Approximately 5% of infants have an abnormal antenatal ultrasound, which appears as a "cyst," evident from at least 20 weeks' gestation.[67] This finding has no implications during pregnancy, but needs full investigation postnatally, differentiating from a choledochal cyst.

Once the diagnosis of BA is made, infants undergo portoenterostomy by the mean age of 61 days. The goal of portoenterostomy is to restore bile flow and reduce bilirubin levels to normal, which is successful in about 50% to 60% of infants.[68] When portoenterostomy is unsuccessful jaundice worsens and leads to end-stage liver disease. These patients require liver transplantation for survival by the first 2 years of life.[69] Other indications for transplantation include recalcitrant cholangitis, severe portal hypertension, hepatopulmonary syndrome, evidence of malignant change, and failure to thrive despite maximal medical therapy.

BA accounts for 40% to 50% of all pediatric liver transplants.[70] The first attempt at transplantation for BA occurred in 1963 and was rarely repeated until after the advent of effective immunosuppression.[71] Despite challenging circumstances, survival is acceptable with reported rates of 85% to 94% at 1 to 3 years post-transplant and 78% to 87% at 5 to 10 years.[72–75] Early deaths were most often caused by graft failure, whereas late deaths were more often caused by malignancy. Additionally, a history of life support at the time of OLT and decreased age were independent predictors of increased post-OLT mortality.[72]

Although transplant outcomes are among the best in pediatric liver transplantation, early recognition of BA is imperative, because portoenterostomy should be performed before 3 months of age for the best chance at cholestatic resolution. Even though most infants with BA after the Kasai procedure require transplant during their pediatric years, the surgery allows children to grow and develop for years with their native liver in place.

CAROLI DISEASE

Caroli disease is characterized by intrahepatic cystic dilation of the bile ducts that leads to intrahepatic stones, recurrent cholangitis, eventual liver failure, and potentially CCA.[76,77] It is a rare autosomal-recessive disorder of biliary cystic diseases, and is included as type V in Todani classification of choledochal cysts. When combined with hepatic fibrosis, it is known as Caroli syndrome. Remodeling of the larger intrahepatic bile ducts results in destructive inflammation and dilation with ectasia in focal, segmental, or lobar fashion. Recurrent episodes of cholangitis lead to high morbidity and mortality.

Treatment depends on the extent of intrahepatic bile duct cysts, the presence of hepatic fibrosis, secondary biliary cirrhosis, or carcinoma. Caroli can present in a localized form (isolated to one hepatic segment) or diffuse form involving the entire intrahepatic biliary tree. **Fig. 5** demonstrates numerous intrahepatic cystic dilations in a patient with Caroli. Hepatic resection, with or without Roux-en-Y cholangiojejunostomy, is the treatment of patients with Caroli disease limited to one lobe of the liver without the presence of cirrhosis or hepatic fibrosis. When cirrhosis or hepatic fibrosis is present, OLT ultimately offers the best opportunity for success **(Fig. 6)**.[78,79]

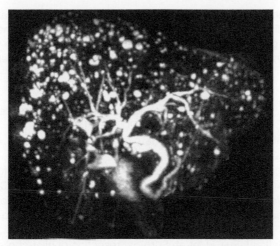

Fig. 5. Multiple cystic duct dilations in a patient with Caroli disease.

Outcomes following OLT for Caroli disease were analyzed by Millwala and colleagues[76] using the United Network for Organ Sharing Standard Transplant Analysis and Research files of liver transplant recipients between the years 1987 and 2006. The overall 1-, 3-, and 5-year graft (79.9%, 72.4%, and 72.4%) and patient (86.3%, 78.4, and 77%) survival rates were excellent following transplantation. Factors found to be associated with increased risk of graft loss include elevated bilirubin, requirement of life support or hospitalization before transplant, cold ischemia time greater than 12 hours, and Asian ethnicity.

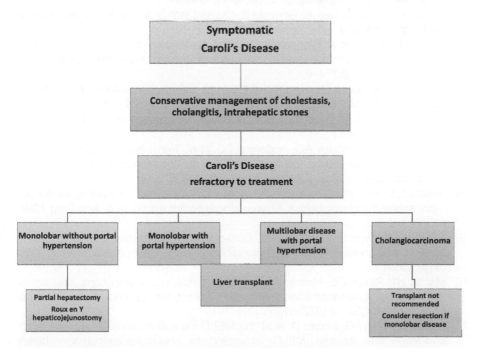

Fig. 6. Evaluation and management of patients with Caroli disease.

Liver transplantation is the treatment of choice for patients with Caroli disease and syndrome when fibrosis leads to the development of portal hypertension and esophageal varices. In patients with concomitant end-stage renal disease resulting from a polycystic kidney, combined liver-kidney transplantation is recommended.

REFERENCES

1. Razumilva N, Gores GJ. Classification, diagnosis, and management of cholangiocarcinoma. Clin Gastroenterol Hepatol 2003;11:13–21.
2. Olnes MJ, Erlich R. A review and update on cholangiocarcinoma. Oncology 2004; 66:167–79.
3. Burak K, Angulo P, Pasha TM, et al. Incidence and risk factors for cholangiocarcinoma in primary sclerosing cholangitis. Am J Gastroenterol 2004;99:523–6.
4. Farley DR, Weaver AL, Nagorney DM. "Natural history" of unresected cholangiocarcinoma: patient outcome after noncurative intervention. Mayo Clin Proc 1995; 70:425–9.
5. Hasegawa S, Ikai I, Fujii H, et al. Surgical resection of hilar cholangiocarcinoma: analysis of survival and postoperative complications. World J Surg 2007;31: 1256–63.
6. Groot Koerkamp B, Wigger JK, Gonen M, et al. Survival after resection of perihilar cholangiocarcinoma: development and external validation of a prognostic nomogram. Ann Oncol 2015;25(9):1930–5.
7. Klempnauer J, Ridder GJ, von Wasielewski R, et al. Resectional surgery of hilar cholangiocarcinoma: a multivariate analysis of prognostic factors. J Clin Oncol 1997;14:947–54.
8. Meyer CG, Penn I, James L. Liver transplantation for cholangiocarcinoma: results in 207 patients. Transplantation 2000;69(8):1633–77.
9. Goldaracena N, Gorgen A, Gonzalo S. Current status of liver transplantation for cholangiocarcinoma. Liver Transpl 2018;24:294–303.
10. Sudan D, DeRoover A, Chinnakotla S, et al. Radiochemotherapy and transplantation allow long-term survival for nonresectable hilar cholangiocarcinoma. Am J Transplant 2002;2:774–9.
11. Heimbach JK, Gores GJ, Haddock MG, et al. Liver transplantation for unresectable perihilar cholangiocarcinoma. Semin Liver Dis 2004;24:201–7.
12. Heimbach JK, et al. Transplantation for hilar cholangiocarcinoma. Liver Transpl 2004;10(10):S65–8.
13. Ethun CG, Lopez-Aguiar AG, Anderson DJ, et al. Transplant versus resection for hilar cholangiocarcinoma: an argument for shifting treatment paradigms for resectable disease. Ann Surg 2018;267(5):797–805.
14. Goss JA, Shackleton CR, Farmer DG, et al. Orthotopic liver transplantation for primary sclerosing cholangitis. A 12-year single center experience. Ann Surg 1997; 225(5):472–81.
15. Gleeson FC, Rajan E, Levy MJ, et al. EUS-guided FNA of regional lymph nodes in patients with unresectable hilar cholangiocarcinoma. Gastrointest Endosc 2008; 67(3):438–43.
16. Mantel HT, Rosen CB, Heimbach JK, et al. Vascular complications after orthotopic liver transplantation after neoadjuvant therapy for hilar cholangiocarcinoma. Liver Transpl 2007;13:1372–81.
17. Gores GJ, Gish RG, Sudan D, et al, the MELD Exception Study Group. Model for end-stage liver disease (MELD) exception for cholangiocarcinoma or biliary dysplasia. Liver Transpl 2006;12:S95–7.

18. Jones DE, Watt FE, Metcalf JV, et al. Familial primary biliary cirrhosis reassessed: a geographically-based study. J Hepatol 1999;30(3):402–7.
19. Kim WR, Lindor KR, Locke GR III, et al. Epidemiology and natural history of primary biliary cirrhosis in a US community. Gastroenterology 2000;119:1631–6.
20. Boonstra K, Beuers U, Ponsioen CY. Epidemiology of primary sclerosing cholangitis and primary biliary cirrhosis: a systematic review. J Hepatol 2012;56(5):1181–8.
21. Lindor KD, Dickson ER, Baldus WP, et al. Ursodeoxycholic acid in the treatment of primary biliary cirrhosis. Gastroenterology 1994;106:1284–90.
22. Poupon RE, Balkau B, Eschwege E, et al. A multicenter, controlled trial of ursodiol for the treatment of primary biliary cirrhosis. UDCA-PBC study Group. N Engl J Med 1991;324:1548–54.
23. Heathcote EJ, Cauch-Dudek K, Walker V, et al. The Canadian multicenter double-blind randomized controlled trial of ursodeoxycholic acid in primary biliary cirrhosis. Hepatology 1994;19:1149–56.
24. Combes B, Carithers RL Jr, Maddrey WC, et al. A randomized, double-blind placebo-controlled trial of ursodeoxycholic acid in primary biliary cirrhosis. Hepatology 1995;22:759–66.
25. Shapiro JM, Smith H, Schaffner F. Serum bilirubin: a prognostic factor for primary biliary cirrhosis. Gut 1979;20:137–40.
26. Carbone M, Neuberger J. Liver transplantation in PBC and PSC: indications and disease recurrence. Clin Res Hepatol Gastroenterol 2011;35:446–54.
27. Mendes FD, Kim WR, Pedersen R, et al. Mortality attributable to cholestatic liver disease in the United States. Hepatology 2008;47:1241–7.
28. Garcia CE, Garcia RF, Gunson B, et al. Analysis of marginal donor parameters in liver transplantation for primary biliary cirrhosis. Exp Clin Transplant 2004;2:183–8.
29. Jacob DA, Neumann UP, Bahra M, et al. Liver transplantation for primary biliary cirrhosis: influence of primary immunosuppression on survival. Transplant Proc 2005;37(4):1691–2.
30. Sylvestre PB Batts KP, Burgart LJ, Poterucha JJ, et al. Recurrence of primary biliary cirrhosis after liver transplantation: histologic estimate of incidence and natural history. Liver Transpl 2003;9:1086–93.
31. Jacob DA, Neumann UP, Bahra M, et al. Long-term Follow-up after recurrence of primary biliary cirrhosis after liver transplantation in 100 patients. Clin Transplant 2006;20:211–20.
32. Guy JE, Qian P, Lowell JA, et al. Recurrent primary biliary cirrhosis: peritransplant factors and ursodeoxycholic acid treatment post-liver transplant. Liver Transpl 2005;11:1252–7.
33. Neuberger J, Gunson B, Hubscher S, et al. Immunosuppression affects the rate of recurrent primary biliary cirrhosis after liver transplantation. Liver Transpl 2004; 10:488–91.
34. Sanchez EQ, Levy MF, Goldstein RM, et al. The changing clinical presentation of recurrent primary biliary cirrhosis after liver transplantation. Transplantation 2003; 76:1583–8.
35. Angulo P, Larson DR, Therneau TM, et al. Time course of histological progression in primary sclerosing cholangitis. Am J Gastroenterol 1999;94:3310–3.
36. Chapman R, Fevery J, Kalloo A, et al. Diagnosis and management of primary sclerosing cholangitis-AASLD practice guidelines. Hepatology 2010;51:660678.
37. Weisner RH, Porayko MK, Hay JE, et al. Liver transplantation for primary sclerosing cholangitis: impact of risk factors on outcome. Liver Transpl Surg 1996; 2:99–108.

38. Kashyap R, Safadjou S, Chen R, et al. Living donor and deceased donor liver transplantation for autoimmune and cholestatic liver disease: an analysis of the UNOS database. J Gastrointest Surg 2010;14:1362–9.
39. Jeyarajah DR, Netto GJ, Lee SP, et al. Recurrent primary sclerosing cholangitis after orthotopic liver transplantation: is chronic rejection part of the disease process? Transplantation 1998;66:1300–6.
40. Vera A, Moledina S, Gunson B, et al. Risk factors for recurrence of primary sclerosing cholangitis of liver allograft. Lancet 2002;360:1943–4.
41. Graziadei IW, Wiesner RH, Marotta PJ, et al. Long-term results of patients undergoing liver transplantation for primary sclerosing cholangitis. Hepatology 1999; 30:1121–7.
42. Alabraba E, Nightingal P, Gunson B, et al. A re-evaluation of the risk factors for the recurrence of primary sclerosing cholangitis in liver allografts. Liver Transpl 2009;15:330–40.
43. Cholongitas E, Shasang V, Papatheodoridis GV, et al. Risk factors for recurrence of primary sclerosing cholangitis after liver transplantation. Liver Transpl 2008;14: 459–65.
44. Rowe IA, Webb K, Gunson BK. The impact of disease recurrence on graft survival following liver transplantation: a single centre experience. Transpl Int 2008;21: 459–65.
45. Vera A, Gunson BK, Ussatoff V, et al. Colorectal cancer in patients with inflammatory bowel disease after liver transplantation for primary sclerosing cholangitis. Transplantation 2003;75:1983–8.
46. Fabia R, Levy MF, Testa G, et al. Colon carcinoma in patients undergoing liver transplantation. Am J Surg 1998;176:265–9.
47. Strasberg SM, Hertl M, Soper NJ. An analysis of the problem of biliary injury during laparoscopic cholecystectomy. J Am Coll Surg 1995;180(1):101–25.
48. Roslyn JJ, Binns GS, Hughes EF, et al. Open cholecystectomy: a contemporary analysis of 42,474 patients. Ann Surg 1993;218(2):129–37.
49. Barbier L, Souche R, Slim K, et al. Long-term consequences of bile duct injury after cholecystectomy. J Visc Surg 2014;151(4):269–79.
50. Sikora SS, Skrikanth G, Agarwal V, et al. Liver histology in benign biliary stricture: fibrosis to cirrhosis...and rehearsal? J Gastroenterol Hepatol 2008;23(12): 1879–84.
51. Negri SS, Sakhuja P, Malhotra V, et al. Factors predicting advanced hepatic fibrosis in patients with postcholecystectomy bile duct strictures. Arch Surg 2004;139(3):299–303.
52. Johnson SR, Koehler A, Pennington LK, et al. Long-term results of surgical repair of bile duct injuries following laparoscopic cholecystectomy. Surgery 2000; 128(4):668–77.
53. Hammel P, Couvelard A, O'Toole D, et al. Regression of liver fibrosis after biliary drainage in patients with chronic pancreatitis and stenosis of the common bile duct. N Engl J Med 2001;344(6):418–23.
54. Collins KM, Chapman WC. Liver transplantation for common bile duct injury. In: Dixon E, Vollmer C Jr, May G, editors. Management of benign biliary stenosis and injury. Cham (Switzerland): Springer; 2015. p. 366–71.
55. Parilla P, Robles R, Varo E, et al. Liver transplantation for bile duct injury after open and laparoscopic cholecystectomy. Br J Surg 2014;101(2):63–8.
56. de Santibanes E, Ardiles V, Pekolj J. Complex bile duct injuries: management. HPB (Oxford) 2008;10(1):4–12.

57. Loinaz C, Gonzalez EM, Jimenez C, et al. Long-term biliary complications after liver surgery leading to liver transplantation. World J Surg 2001;25(10):1260–3.

58. Harley JL, Davenport M, Kelly DA. Biliary atresia. Lancet 2009;374(9702): 1704–13.

59. The NS, Honein MA, Caton AR, et al, The National Birth Defects Prevention Study. Risk factors for isolated biliary atresia, National Birth Defects Prevention Study, 1997-2002. Am J Med Genet A 2007;143A:2274–84.

60. Livesey E, Borja MC, Sharif K, et al. Epidemiology of biliary atresia in England and Wales (1999-2006). Arch Dis Child Fetal Neonatal Ed 2009;94:F451–5.

61. Davenport M, Savage M, Mowat AP, et al. Biliary atresia splenic malformation syndrome: an etiologic and prognostic subgroup. Surgery 1993;113(6):662–8.

62. Yoon PW, Bresee JS, Olney RS, et al. Epidemiology of biliary atresia: a population-based study. Pediatrics 1997;99(3):376–82.

63. Riepenhoff-Talty M, Gouvea V, Evans MJ, et al. Detection of group C rotavirus in infants with extrahepatic biliary atresia. J Infect Dis 1996;174(1):8–15.

64. Petersen C, Grasshoff S, Luciano L. Diverse morphology of biliary atresia in an animal model. J Hepatol 1998;28(4):603–7.

65. Rauschenfels S, Krassman M, Al-Masri AN, et al. Incidence of hepatotropic viruses in biliary atresia. Eur J Pediatr 2009;168(4):469–76.

66. Makin E, Quaglia A, Kvist N, et al. Congenital biliary atresia: liver injury begins at birth. J Pediatr Surg 2009;44(3):630–3.

67. Caponcelli E, Knisely A, Davenport M. Cystic biliary atresia: an etiologic and prognostic subgroup. J Pediatr Surg 2008;43(9):1619–24.

68. Davenport M, De Ville de Goyet J, Stringer MD, et al. Seamless management of biliary atresia in England and Wales (1999-2002). Lancet 2004;363(9418): 1354–7.

69. Schneider BL, Brown MB, Haber B, et al. A multicenter study of the outcome of biliary atresia in the United States, 1997 to 2000. J Pediatr 2006;148(4):467–74.

70. Mack CL, Feldman AG, Sokol RJ. Clues to the etiology of bile duct injury in biliary atresia. Semin Liver Dis 2012;32:307–16.

71. Starzl TE, Marchioro TL, Vonkaulla KN, et al. Homotransplantation of the liver in humans 1963. Surg Gynecol Obstet 1963;117:659–76.

72. Barshes NR, Lee TC, Balkrishnan R, et al. Orthotopic liver transplantation for biliary atresia: the U.S. experience. Liver Transpl 2005;11(10):1193–200.

73. Cowles RA, Lobritto SJ, Ventura KA, et al. Timing of liver transplantation in biliary atresia-results in 71 children managed by a multidisciplinary team. J Pediatr Surg 2008;43(9):1605–9.

74. Diem HV, Evrard V, Vinh HT, et al. Pediatric liver transplantation for biliary atresia: results of primary grafts in 328 recipients. Transplantation 2003;75:1692–7.

75. Fouquet V, Alves A, Branchereau S, et al. Long-term outcome of pediatric liver transplantation for biliary atresia: a 10-year follow-up in a single center. Liver Transpl 2005;11(2):152–60.

76. Millwala F, Segev DL, Thaluvath PJ. Caroli's disease and outcomes after liver transplantation. Liver Transpl 2008;14:11–7.

77. Alonso-Lej F, Rever WB, Pessagno DJ. Congenital choledochal cyst, with a report of 2, and an analysis of 94, cases. Int Abstr Surg 1959;108(1):1–30.

78. De Kerckhove L, De Meyer M, Verbaandert C, et al. The place of liver transplantation in Caroli's disease and syndrome. Transpl Int 2006;19(5):381–8.

79. Habib S, Shakil O, Couto OF, et al. Caroli's disease and orthotopic liver transplantation. Liver Transpl 2006;12(3):416–21.

Moving?

Make sure your subscription moves with you!

To notify us of your new address, find your **Clinics Account Number** (located on your mailing label above your name), and contact customer service at:

Email: journalscustomerservice-usa@elsevier.com

800-654-2452 (subscribers in the U.S. & Canada)
314-447-8871 (subscribers outside of the U.S. & Canada)

Fax number: 314-447-8029

Elsevier Health Sciences Division
Subscription Customer Service
3251 Riverport Lane
Maryland Heights, MO 63043

*To ensure uninterrupted delivery of your subscription, please notify us at least 4 weeks in advance of move.

Moving?